Jürgen Drews

Immuno-pharmacology

Principles and Perspectives

With 81 Illustrations
and 22 Tables

Springer-Verlag Berlin Heidelberg New York
London Paris Tokyo Hong Kong

Professor Jürgen Drews, MD
F. Hoffmann-La Roche Ltd.

Chairman of the Research Board and
Member of the Executive Committee

Grenzacherstrasse 124
CH-4002 Basle
Switzerland

ISBN-13:978-3-642-75563-7 e-ISBN-13:978-3-642-75561-3
DOI: 10.1007/978-3-642-75561-3

2127/3130-543210

Preface to the First English Edition

The first German edition of this book was received positively by the medical and scientific press. More importantly, many medical students, students of chemistry and pharmacy but also practising physicians and pharmacology teachers have expressed their interest in this text and in its subject matter: immunopharmacology.

It is for these reasons that I decided to prepare a second edition and, in order to reach an even larger public, to write this second and expanded version in English. As in the first edition, the text is divided into seven chapters: a short history of immunopharmacology is followed by a chapter on the structure and function of the immune system. Subsequent chapters follow the operational categories of immune substitution, immune suppression, the suppression of allergic reactions and immune stimulation. The last chapter represents a modest attempt to look into the immediate future and to make a few educated guesses about forthcoming developments in immunotherapy – on the basis of clinical or experimental work that is already assessable. The second, the third and parts of the sixth chapter have been completely rewritten. Chapters four, five and seven have been revised, changed and supplemented with new information where necessary. This book is not a textbook in the usual sense; it does not make any claim to thematic completeness. It represents a selection of important examples from immunopharmacology and immunotherapy which can be used to illustrate typical problems of this discipline. It should be read as an introduction to an area which has grown out of immunology and now lies well within the scope of pharmacology and clinical therapy. The book is addressed to physicians as well as to students and to scientists interested in the applications of immunological principles to therapy.

The field of immunopharmacology is undergoing very rapid transition. Some treatment modalities which were intensively discussed a few years ago have not fulfilled the expectations once attached to them. Some of them have not yet been dropped from this edition, because they still figure in the contemporary literature though with a modest profile. It is almost impossible to pinpoint precisely those items that have the greatest topicality and at the same time are likely to be enduring. The topics discussed in this book are not always of equal importance. This is mainly due to the rate of change that is so typical of immunopharmacology and immunotherapy.

Many individuals have helped in producing this second edition. First and foremost I have to thank Dr. Werner Haas for providing much of the scientific information contained in Chapter Two, for the design of a number of figures and for his constant advice and criticism. He is certainly not responsible for any shortcomings which the book might still exhibit. I am also much indebted to Ursula Krähenbühl, to Margot Lande and to Almuth Burdeska for typing the manuscript, to Markus Hodel for the preparation of the figures and to Springer Verlag and Editiones ‹Roche› for giving the book an adequate appearance. Martin Schneider, head of Editiones ‹Roche›, deserves my special gratitude for producing the book with so much patience and efficiency. Finally, I want to thank Mitchell Bornstein and Iain MacRae for the translation of the original German text and Dr. Helga Drews for her diligent and attentive proofreading.

Basel, September 1989.

Preface

The roots of immunopharmacology can be traced as far back as the days when Julius Wagner von Jauregg treated chronic infections with artificially induced fever and, in literary terms, George Bernard Shaw elevated stimulation of the phagocytes that had recently been described by Metschnikoff to the therapeutic principle of the future ("The Doctor's Dilemma"). For a long time, stimulation of the body's "nonspecific defences" was a somewhat nebulous field of activity to which a certain notoriety was attached. The effectiveness of antibodies as mediators of specific immunity seemed to overshadow the relatively modest contribution of nonspecific resistance in defending the body against infections. Besides, too little was known about the cellular and humoral mediators of nonspecific resistance. A degree of scepticism has survived into our own times: until recently, terms such as "immunomodulation", "immunostimulation" or "immunotropic substances" tended to trigger unease among the more puristic of immunologists and pharmacologists. The tenor of this defensive approach was that "What's good about it isn't new and what's new about it isn't good".

Since then, however, the situation has changed. Nowadays, the structural and functional principles of the immune system are as well understood as those of the central nervous system or of other functional systems of the body. As a result, it is now possible to analyse and make therapeutic use of the effects of drugs on the immune system. Furthermore, components of the immune system can now be deployed first of all as experimental tools and then as therapeutic instruments. These two methodological approaches are discussed in this book. In order to lend sharper definition to the frequently, though not necessarily precisely, employed term "immunopharmacology", the subject matter has been divided up according to clinical and/or pragmatic criteria. The division into immunosubstitution, immunosuppression, antiallergic substances and immunostimulation gives the heterogeneous material a tighter structure than would any classification according to origin, chemical structure or mechanism of action.

Our knowledge of immunological functions, immunological disturbances and therapeutic interventions in the immune system is growing so rapidly that it is becoming increasingly difficult to provide a reliable approach to the basic principles and clinical uses of immunopharmacology. This book grew out of the desire to render access to a major theoretical and therapeutic field easier for medical students, practitioners, and also for pharmaceutical chemists and pharmacologists with little experience of immunology. Suggestions for the presentation of individual topics came from participants at the pharmacology lectures in Heidelberg and from many colleagues in Basel, Heidelberg and Vienna. This book is a token of my sincere gratitude to them. Particular thanks are due to my wife,

Helga Drews, MD, who devoted a great deal of her time to assuring the formal accuracy of the text and illustrations. Any mistakes that may nevertheless be present are, it goes without saying, to be laid at my door.

Basel, 16 January 1986 Jürgen Drews

Table of contents

1. Definition and History

Immunopharmacology is a still young pharmacological and therapeutic discipline that has grown out of the increasingly more closely interconnected "classical" fields of immunology and pharmacology. The term "immunopharmacology" has been in regular, though not necessarily precise use for about fifteen years only. To some people, immunopharmacology means the effect of pharmaceutical agents on the immune system and its functions, and where these agents come from is of little significance – they may be endogenous, synthetic or of microbial origin. Others tend to consider immunopharmacology as the achievement of pharmacological effects with immunological products, i.e. with antibodies, lymphokines and other factors, mostly consisting of proteins. For clinicians, on the other hand, immunopharmacology is more likely to be the basis for treatment of diseases of the immune system, particularly the autoimmune diseases and anaphylactic and atopic reactions.

Any detailed treatment of immunopharmacology must take these different viewpoints into account. This seems to be historically justified: during the last three to four decades so much has been learned about the immune system that it can now, like other major functional systems of the body such as the cardiovascular or central nervous system, be investigated pharmacologically. The cellular and biochemical mechanisms that enable the immune system to distinguish between "self" and "non-self", and the processes which occur in the immune system following the entry of a foreign substance or an antigen into the body and which lead to elimination of the substance recognized as "foreign", have been largely elucidated. Furthermore, the study of the surface structures of lymphocytes and macrophages, but also of the signal proteins, lymphokines and monokines, released by the immune cells, has resulted in a better understanding of the cybernetic interconnections existing within the immune system and between the immune system and other functional systems of the body. This knowledge can now be translated into rational approaches to the therapeutic use of antibodies and lymphokines.

The findings of clinical immunology have made it quite clear that many conditions which years ago were considered of unknown etiology should now be classified as autoimmune diseases. These include juvenile diabetes, rheumatoid arthritis, lupus erythematosus, multiple sclerosis and many other frequently observed conditions. The prospect of combating immunopathologically rooted diseases by pharmacological intervention in the immune system was a powerful motivating factor in the search for new, selective immunosuppressive agents.

The development of immunopharmacology has also profited from the fact that the limits of chemotherapy, in the fields of oncology as well as microbiology, have become more evident. Further antimicrobials with an even wider spectrum of action and even greater potency than those of the third-generation cephalosporins, the carbapenems or the monobactams, are probably less likely to bring about an improvement in the treatment of infections in immunocompromised patients than are therapeutic measures that compensate for the existing immune deficiency or even enhance the immune response beyond the "normal" level. More recent developments in experimental cancer research have shown that activated macrophages and natural killer cells (NK-cells) are able to distinguish and kill tumour cells, in contrast to normal cells, and that these functions can be enhanced by pharmacological means. The frequently expressed need of clinical oncologists for supplementation of intrinsically immunosuppressive chemotherapy by immunostimulatory measures has provided a further impulse for the development of immunopharmacology.

To summarize the main lines of development outlined above, immunopharmacology may be defined as a medical discipline, the goals of which are to elucidate the basic cellular and biochemical principles of immune regulation, to investigate the effect of endogenous, synthetic and natural substances on the immune response, and, from the insights obtained, to draw conclusions regarding the therapy of diseases that either are due to dysfunction of the immune system or can be treated by modification of the immune response. For the sake of simplicity, the immune system can be regarded as a "closed" system, and its function can be modified by a very limited number of therapeutic strategies: in the first place, components or products of the immune system of which there is a pathological quantitative or qualitative deficiency can be supplemented. This therapeutic approach applies in particular, of course, to the antibodies. Though the chapter on the therapeutic and prophylactic use of antibodies is headed "Immunosubstitution", two things must not be overlooked: firstly, immunosubstitution is possible with other components of the immune system, e.g. leucocytes, and, secondly, not every therapeutic or prophylactic use of antibodies is, strictly speaking, immunosubstitution.

Broadly speaking, the term "immunosuppression" could be applied to any pharmacological measure that brings about a reduction in immunological effector mechanisms. This broad definition would also have to include suppression of immunological reactions in cases of immediate-type hypersensitivity, i.e. treatment of allergies, and drug-induced inhibition of inflammation. Considerations of both pharmacology and therapy seemed to call for separate chapters on the different types of immunosuppression, i.e. suppression of the transplantation reaction and of delayed hypersensitivity, and on inhibition of immediate-type hypersensitivity. A separate discussion of antiinflammatory therapy in this context was ruled out for two reasons: the very indirect connections between nonsteroidal antiinflammatory agents and the immune system, and the fact that these substances are dealt with in detail in all standard pharmacology textbooks.

Measures that may enhance the immune response, regardless of the underlying mechanisms, are discussed under "Immunostimulation". It goes without saying that the attainment of a positive additive effect, i.e. one that goes beyond the baseline situation, is often only a question of dosage, and that with lower or, more frequently, higher doses, immunosuppressive effects can also be achieved. In a therapeutic context, however, the substances discussed in this chapter can be used for stimulation only and have therefore been selected for their utility value.

In the final analysis, immunopharmacology should provide a basis for clinical treatment. It therefore seemed appropriate to conclude this book with a reappraisal of the therapeutic uses of immunopharmacologically effective substances from the clinical viewpoint, and, in the light of at least some of the projects currently in progress in various laboratories, with an attempt at a preview of developments likely to occur in the field of therapy over the next few years.

2. The Immune System – A Short Introduction to its Structure and Function

The immune system consists of approximately 2×10^{12} lymphocytes, which either circulate freely in the blood or exist within organ-specific spatial structures like the lymph nodes, thymus, spleen and bone-marrow. In a wider sense it also includes the macrophages, which have important antigen-presenting functions and are, in addition, effector cells, and the granulocytes, which are mediator and also effector cells. In terms of cell mass, the lymphocytes alone are equivalent to the liver or the central nervous system and therefore occupy as much space as these organ systems.

Since the immune cells of higher organisms are almost ubiquitous, the anatomical extent of the system can be understood only if it is visualized as a single organ.

The immune system can discriminate between endogenous and exogenous structures. Structures recognized as "self" are tolerated, while "non-self" structures are eliminated from the body's cell and organ systems. Indeed, every higher form of life is engaged in a constant struggle to defend its own genetically defined identity against attack by infectious pathogens that penetrate from outside. A functioning immune system is therefore a means of maintaining the identity and integrity of the individual against a variety of threats. In terms of evolution, the development of the immune system was one of the preconditions

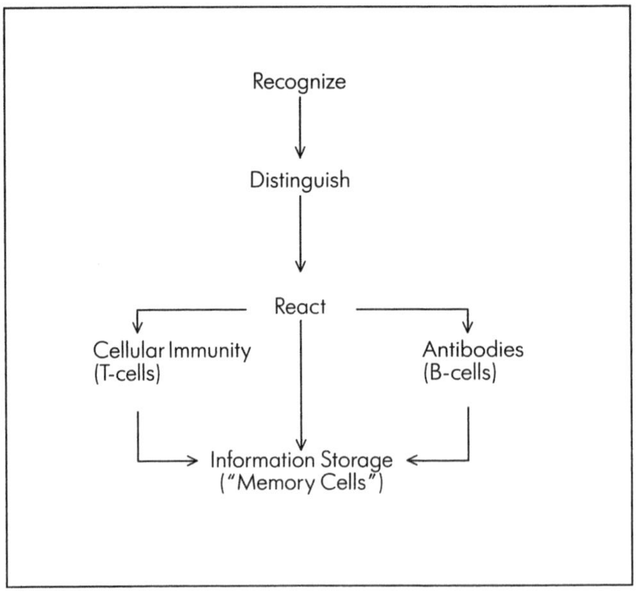

Figure 2.1. Schematic representation of the main functions of the immune system.

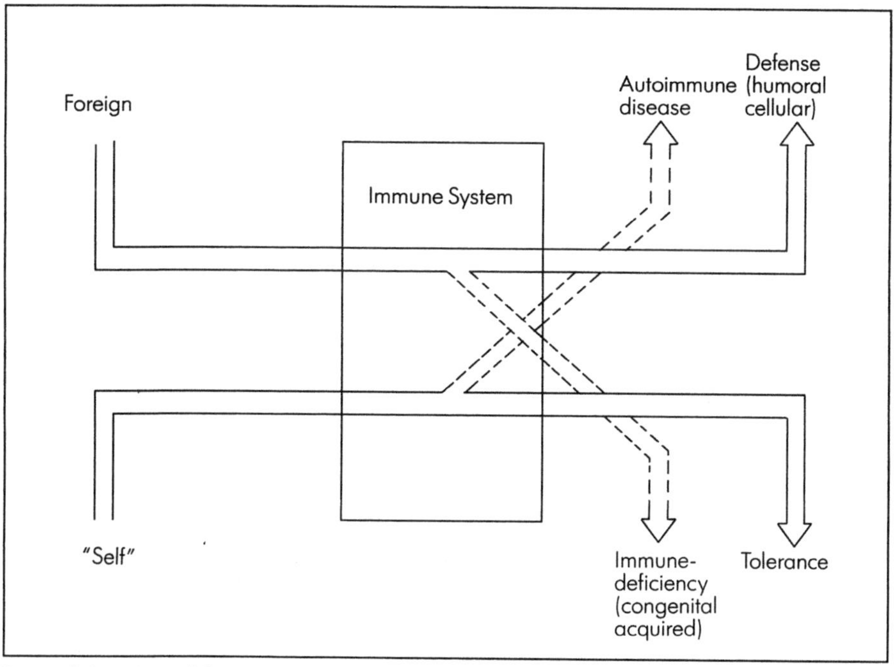

Figure 2.2. Normal functions of the immune system and possible deviations from these functions. Foreign agents are normally rejected by humoral or cellular mechanisms. If important effector functions capable of such rejection are missing, a state of immuno-deficiency ensues. On the other hand, "self" is normally tolerated. Mistakes made in the distinction between "self" and "non-self" can lead to autoimmune diseases.

that made it possible for "individualized" life in all its variety to evolve in the first place.

The immune system is able to exercise four functions *(Fig. 2.1)*. It can *recognize* a large variety of structures; it can distinguish between "self" and "non-self". It can attack, and then *eliminate*, the foreign structures by recourse to a number of humoral and cellular mechanisms; and it can *store*, and if necessary call up, information on past reactions to foreign antigens. The memory function of the immune system is confirmed by the age-old experience that individuals who have had a specific infection (e.g. measles, rubella) either do not contract the illness again or do so only in greatly attenuated form.

These functions can be disturbed. Deficiencies or disturbances of recognition can give rise to autoimmune diseases if endogenous structures are, for some reason, recognized as being foreign.

Disturbances of effector function are found in several congenital immune deficiencies. They frequently affect granulocyte or macrophage function and always increase the susceptibility of the body to a wide variety of infectious microorganisms.

Iatrogenic measures such as the use of ionizing radiation or chemotherapy with alkylating agents or antimetabolites may also impair the functions of the immune system, even to the extent of temporarily or permanently rendering the individual "defenceless" *(Fig. 2.2)*.

2.1 The cells of the immune system

2.1.1 T- and B-lymphocytes

As already mentioned, the lymphocytes are the carriers of the cognitive functions of the immune system. Lymphocytes and only lymphocytes are capable of making a distinction between "self" and "non-self". Lymphocytes guide the elimination of foreign substances or agents directly as in cytotoxic reactions or indirectly through antibodies. And finally lymphocytes can keep a record of reactions to antigens and in doing so ensure that a second encounter with a given antigen can be handled more efficiently than the first one.

There are two major populations of lymphocytes: T-cells and B-cells. T-cells develop in the thymus. On reaching maturation, they are responsible for the cell-mediated immune response, i.e. for the development of delayed-type hypersensitivity. B-cells mature outside the thymus and are responsible for the humoral immune response, i.e. for the formation of the various classes of antibodies. The designations T and B refer, respectively, to the thymus, which is essential for the maturation of T-lymphocytes, and to the Bursa of Fabricius, a lymphoid organ in the cloaca of birds, which controls the maturation of B-lymphocytes. If the Bursa of Fabricius is removed from newborn chicks, they lose forever their ability to produce antibodies.

If, on the other hand, the thymus is removed from chicks (or from newborn rodents), they are no longer able to produce a cell-mediated immune response. Interestingly enough, however, their capacity to mount a humoral immune response is also clearly inferior to that of intact animals. This finding was an early indication that T-lymphocytes also play an important role in the development of B-cell mediated immune responses. The cells which exercise this function are now identified as T-helper cells. All lymphocytes are differentiation products of pluripotent bone-marrow cells. They migrate – the B-lymphocytes directly and the T-lymphocytes via the thymus – towards the peripheral lymphatic

---

Figure 2.3. Short scheme of T-cell ontogeny. In the pre-T-cell both, the α- and β- and the δ- and γ-genes are in germ-line configuration. There are two pathways, the $\delta\gamma$ and the $\alpha\beta$ pathway. It is not understood which signals drive pre-T-cells in one or the other direction. The first receptor chain to be rearranged is the β-chain. Productive rearrangements indicated by +, non productive rearrangement by –. Cells which do not productively rearrange the receptor chains are lost. $\delta\gamma$ cells with correctly rearranged receptor chains leave the cortex of the thymus and migrate to the periphery, in particular to the skin and the submucosa of the gut. The specificity and function of these cells remain to be elucidated. $\alpha\beta$-cells interact with HLA molecules on the thymic epithelium. Cells which recognize "self" HLA molecules survive as a consequence of their encounter with epithelial cells (positive selection). The interaction of $\alpha\beta$-receptors with epithelial HLA proteins also determines the expression of CD4 and CD8 proteins. Most cortical lymphocytes express both molecules. Cortical thymocytes with class I HLA restricted $\alpha\beta$-receptors switch off CD4 expression. Cells with class II MHC restricted receptors terminate CD8 expression. A minority of cells which can recognize both classes of HLA molecules becomes double-negative. Cells which do not bind to HLA molecules on the thymic epithelium are destroyed. The positively selected "self" HLA restricted $\alpha\beta$-thymocytes move to the cortico-medullary junction where they encounter self-antigen presenting cells. Here the cells which recognize self-antigens are eliminated. This phenomenon accounts for at least a large part of self-tolerance. Not shown in the figure are various membrane proteins which also play a role in T-cell differentiation: CD2 is expressed by all cells shown. CD3 polypeptides are produced briefly before or concomitantly with $\alpha\beta$- and $\gamma\delta$-receptors.

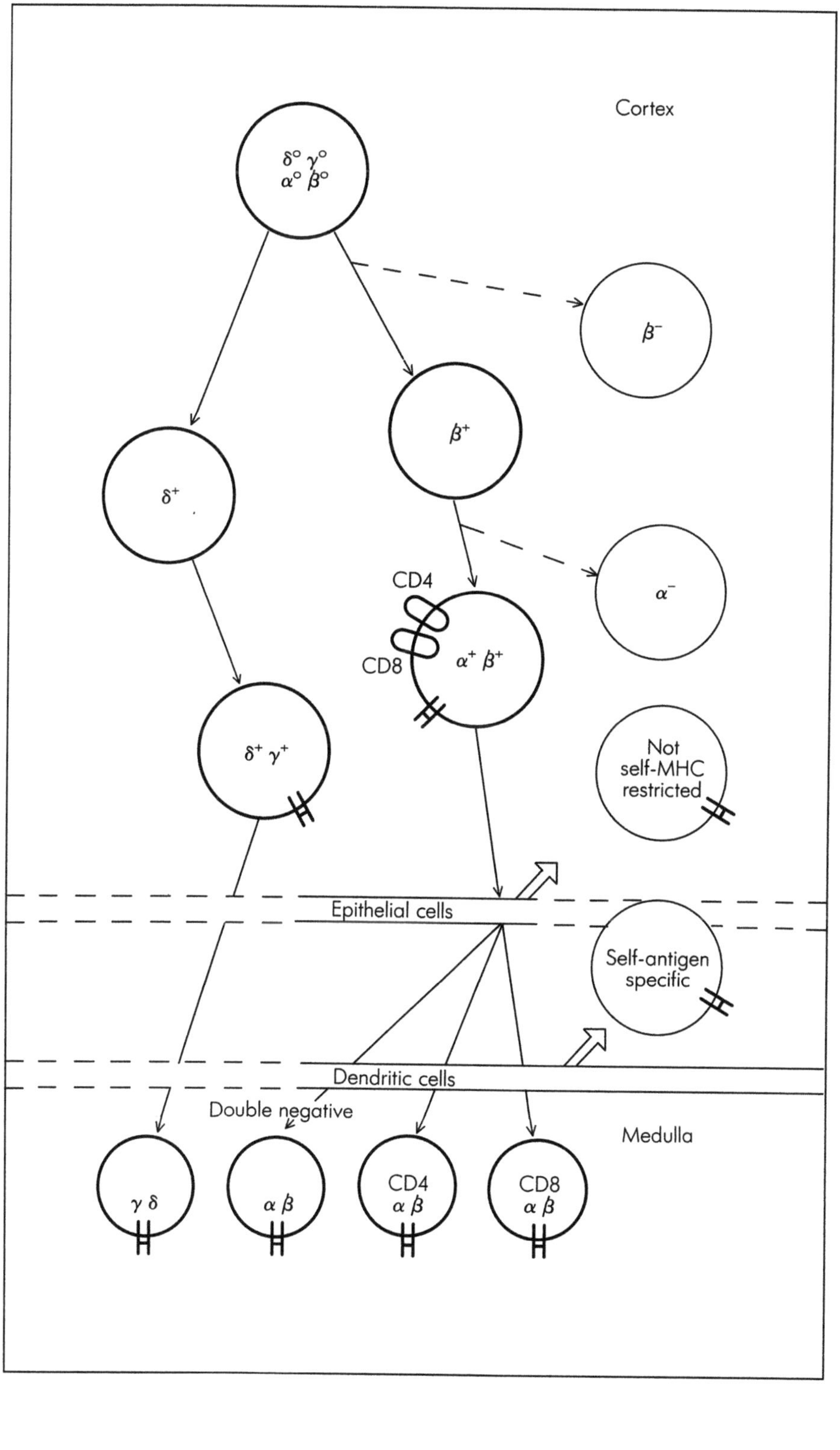
Cortex
δ° γ°
α° β°
β⁻
β⁺
δ⁺
CD4
α⁻
CD8
α⁺ β⁺
δ⁺ γ⁺
Not
self-MHC
restricted
Epithelial cells
Self-antigen
specific
Dendritic cells
Double negative
Medulla
γ δ
α β
CD4
α β
CD8
α β

tissue, i.e. the lymph nodes, tonsils and Peyer's patches, where they can react with antigens. A large proportion of the lymphocytes are in constant circulation, i.e. they leave the lymphoid organs through the efferent lymphatics, which open into the thoracic duct, and thereby pass into the bloodstream again. In this way, permanent mixing and ubiquitous interaction of all immune cells in the body are achieved.

The differentiation process of T-cells in the thymus has been largely elucidated. It can be followed by reference to the sequential appearance of surface antigens, the gradual development of function, and the changes that occur in physicochemical parameters *(Fig. 2.3)*.

In mice the fetal thymus anlage is colonized by hematopoietic cells which at day fourteen of gestation begin to generate immature thymocytes at a very high rate. In a young mouse 5×10^7 thymocytes are produced each day. Most of these cells die, only a tiny fraction ($1–2 \times 10^6$) leaves the thymus each day as mature T-cells. While the human thymus begins to involute already in the second year of life, residual T-cell generation is maintained throughout life and can be observed even in very old individuals.

The differentiation process of B-cells is less well understood. In the Bursa of Fabricius a large stem-cell which is still negative for μ-antigen (heavy chain of IgM) in the cytoplasm or on its surface develops into a mature B-cell that is μ-positive both in the cytoplasm and on the surface. This differentiation step possibly involves the participation of a secretory cell found not only in the Bursa of Fabricius but also in the white pulp, periarteriolar tissue and germinal centres of the spleen. Mammals do not possess a bursa or an equivalent organ. Mammalian B-cells differentiate at the same sites as myeloid cells, first in the fetal liver and subsequently in the extravascular space of the bone marrow parenchyma. As distinct from the situation in birds, B-cells are continuously generated in mammals throughout life. Several stages of B-cell development can be distinguished: pre-B-cells still carry the antibody genes in the germ line configuration. Pro-B-cells have already rearranged the heavy chains, while κ and λ light chains are not yet formed. Such cells are positive for cytoplasmic μ. They are also characterized as μ^+ *(Fig. 2.4)*. In addition, they can be recognized by the appearance of surface antigens such as B220. Mature B-cells have completed the rearrangement of their antibody genes and carry antibody molecules (IgM or IgD) on their surface which are anchored to the membrane. Once they carry antibodies on their surface, B-cells can be activated by the binding of antigens and by cytokines (Il-4) from T-cells. Cytokines secreted by T-cells are also

---

Figure 2.4. A short scheme of B-cell development. Pre-B-cells carry the genes for heavy and light chains in their germ-line configuration (H^oL^o). At first, the heavy chain genes are rearranged by the joining of a particular diversity (D-)gene with a corresponding J-gene. In a second step, VDJ rearrangement is completed. The complete and productive rearrangement of one heavy chain (VDJ^+) excludes the rearrangement of the corresponding allele (allelic exclusion). Cells in which neither allele can be productively rearranged are deleted. Subsequently the rearrangement of light chains takes place. Only cells which fail in rearranging their κ-genes have a "second try" with their λ-genes. Pro-B-cells are cells which have successfully rearranged and expressed their heavy chain genes. They are μ-positive in their cytoplasm. Mature B-cells carry their receptors comprising heavy and light chains on their cell surface.

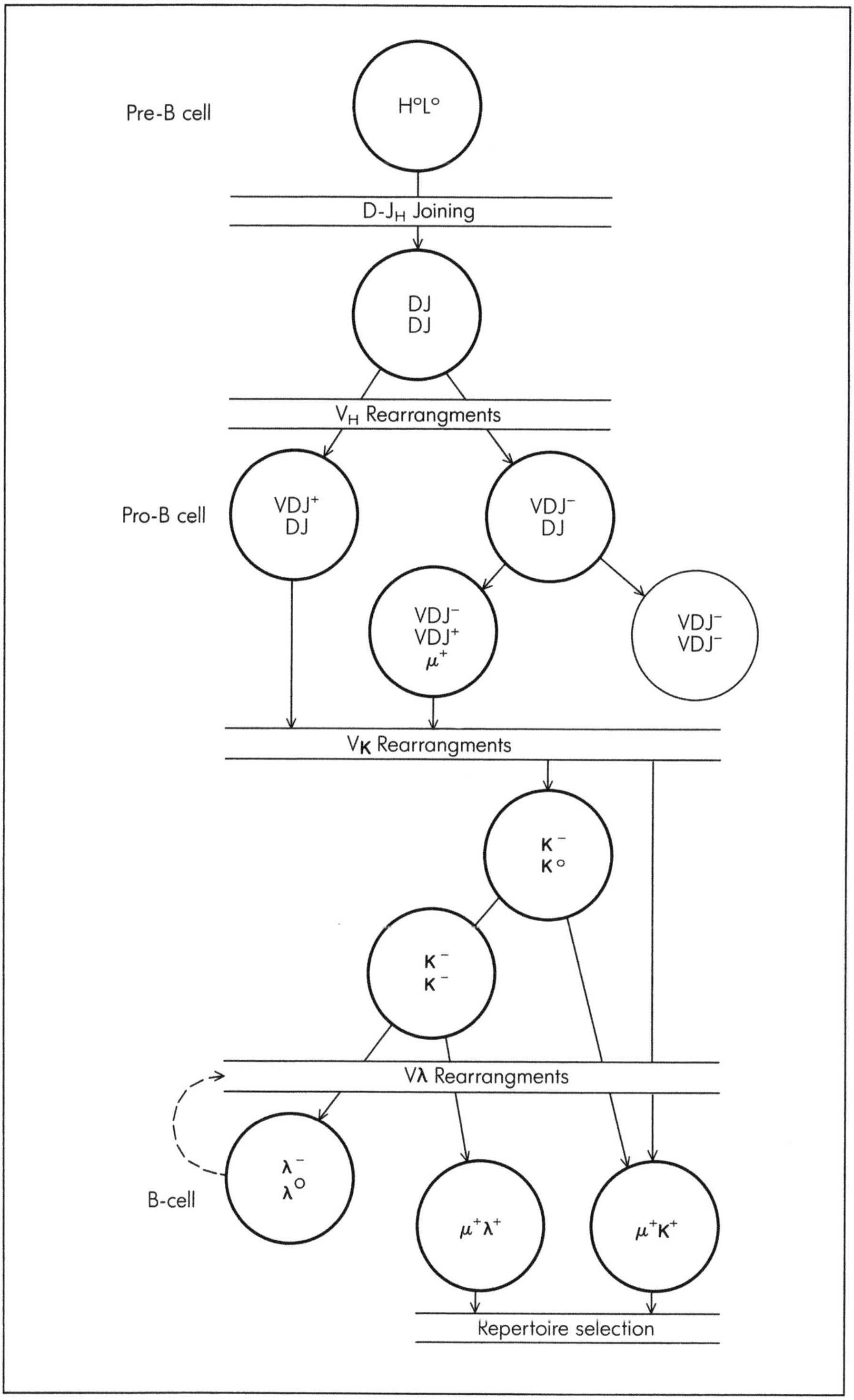
Pre-B cell
H°L°
D-J$_H$ Joining
DJ
DJ
V$_H$ Rearrangments
Pro-B cell
VDJ$^+$
DJ
VDJ$^-$
DJ
VDJ$^-$
VDJ$^+$
μ^+
VDJ$^-$
VDJ$^-$
Vκ Rearrangments
κ^-
κ°
κ^-
κ^-
Vλ Rearrangments
B-cell
λ^-
λ°
$\mu^+\lambda^+$
$\mu^+\kappa^+$
Repertoire selection

Table 2.1. Preliminary list of human leucocyte differentiation antigens clusters of differentiation (CD)

CD design	Selection of assigned monoclonal antibodies	Main cellular reactivity	Recognized membrane component
CD1a	NA1/34; T6; VIT6; Leu6	Thy, DC, B subset	gp49
CD1b	WM-25; 4A76; NUT2	Thy, DC, B subset	gp45
CD1c	L161; M241; 7C6; PHM3	Thy, DC, B subset	gp43
CD2	9.6; T11; 35.1	T	CD58(LFA-3) receptor, gp50
CD2R	T11.3*; VIT13; D66	activated T	CD2 epitopes restr. to activ. T
CD3	T3; UCHT1; 38.1; Leu4	T	CD3-complex (5 chains), gp/p 26, 20, 16
CD4	T4; Leu3a; 91.D6	T subset	Class II/HIV receptor, gp59
CD5	T1; UCHT2; T101; HH9; AMG4	T, B subset	gp67
CD6	T12; T411	T, B subset	gp100
CD7	3A1; 4A; CL1.3; G3-7	T	gp40
CD8	α chain: T8; Leu2a; M236; UCHT4; T811 β chain: T8/2T8; 5H7	T subset	Class 1 receptor, gp32, αα or αβ dimer
CD9	CLB-thromb/8; PHN200; FMC56	Pre-B, M, Plt	p24
CD10	J5, VLA1, BA-3	Lymph. Prog., cALL, Germ Ctr. B, G	Neutral endopeptidase, gp 100, CALLA
CD11a	MHM24; 2F12; CRIS-3	Leucocytes	LFA-1, gp 180/95
CD11b	Mo1; 5A4.C5; LPM19C	M, G, NK	C3bi receptor, gp 155/95
CD11c	B-LY6; L29; BL-4H4	M, G, NK, B subset	gp150/95
CDw12	M67	M, G, Plt	(p90–120)
CD13	MY7, MCS-2, TÜK1, MOU28	M, G	Aminopeptidase N, gp150
CD14	Mo2, UCHM1, VIM13, MoP15	M, (G), LHC	gp55
CD15	My1, VIM-D5	G, (M)	3-FAL, Y-Hapten
CD16	BW209/2; HUNK2; CLBFcGran1; 3G8	NK, G, Mac.	FCRIII, gp50–65
CDw17	GO35, Huly-m13	G, M, Plt	Lactosylceramide
CD18	MHM23; M232; 11H6; CLB54	Leucocytes broad	β chain to CD11a, b, c
CD19	B4; HD37	B	gp95
CD20	B1; 1F5	B	p37/32, ion channel?
CD21	B2; HB5	B subset	C3d/EBV-Rec. (CR2), p140
CD22	HD39; S-HCL1; To15	cytopl. B/surface B subset	gp135, homology to myelin assoc. gp (MAG)
CD23	Blast-2, MHM6	B subset, act. M, Eo	Fcε RII, gp45–50
CD24	VIBE3; BA-1	B, G	gp41/38?
CD25	TAC; 7G7/B6; 2A3	activated T, B, M	IL-2R β chain, gp55
CD26	124-2C2; TS145	activated T	Dipeptidylpeptidase IV, gp120
CD27	VIT14; S152; OKT18A; CLB-9F4	T subset	p55 (dimer)
CD28	9.3; KOLT2	T subset	gp44
CD29	K20; A-1A5	broad	VLA β-, integrin β1-chain, Plt GPIIa
CD30	Ki-1; Ber-H2; HSR4	activated T, B; Reed-Sternberg	gp120, Ki-1
CD31	SG134; TM3; HEC-75; ES12F11	Plt, M, G, B, (T)	gp140, Plt, GPIIa
CDw32	CIKM5; 41H16; IV.3	M, G, B	FcRII, gp40
CD33	My9; H153; L4F3	M, Prog., AML	gp67
CD34	My10; BI-3C5, ICH-3	Prog.	gp105–120
CD35	TO&; CB04, J3D3	G, M, B	CR1
CD36	5F1; CIMeg1; ESIVC7	M, PLt, (B)	gp90, Plt GPIV
CD37	HD28; HH1; G28-1	B, (T, M)	gp40–52
CD38	HB7; T16	Lymph. Prog., PC, Act. T	p45
CD39	AC2; G28-2	B subset, (M)	gp70–100

Abbreviations:

cytopl	cytoplasmic	gp	glycoprotein	LHC	epidermal Langerhans cells
DC	dendritic cells	I-CAM	intracellular cell adhesion molecule	lymph prog	lymphocyte progenitor cells
epithel	epithelial cells			M	monocytes
G	granulocytes	LFA	leucocyte function antigen	Mac	macrophages
Germ Ctr B	germinal centre B-cells				

CD design	Selection of assigned monoclonal antibodies	Main cellular reactivity	Recognized membrane component
CD40	G28-5	B, carcinomas	gp50, homology to NCF-receptor
CD41	PBM6.4; CLB-thromb/7; PL273	Plt	Plt GPIIb-IIa complex and GPIIB
CD42a	FMC25; BL-H6; GR-P	Plt	Plt GPIX, gp23
CD42b	PHN89; AN51; GN287	Plt	Plt GPIb, gp135/25
CD43	OTH71C5; G19-1; MEM-59	T, G, M, brain	Leukosialin, gp95
CD44	GRHL1; F10-44-2; 33-3B3; BRIC35	Leucocytes, brain, RBC	Pgp-1, gp80–95
CD45	T29/33; BMAC1; AB187	Leucocytes	LCA, T200
CD45RA	G1–15; F8-11-13; 73.5	T subset, B, G, M	restricted T200, gp220
CD45RB	PT17/26/16*	T subset, B, G, M	restricted T200
CD45RO	UCHL1	T subset, B, G, M	restricted T200, gp180
CD46	HULYM5; 122-2; J48	Leucocytes	Membrane cofactor protein (MCP), gp66/56
CD47	BRIC126; CIKM1; BRIC125	Broad	gp47–52, *N*-linked glycan
CD48	WM68; LO-MN25; J4–57	Leucocytes	gp41, PI-linked
CDw49b	CLB-thromb/4; Gi14	Plt, cultured T	VLa-α2 chain, Plt GPIa
CDw49d	B5G10; HP2/1; HP1/3	M, T, B, (LHC), THY	VLA-α4 chain, gp150
CDw49f	GoH3	Plt, (T)	VLA-α6 chain, Plt GPIc
CDw50	101-1D2; 140-11	Leucocytes	gp148/108
CD51	13C2; 23C6; NKI-M7; NIKI-M9	(Plt)	VNR-α chain
CDw52	097; YTH66.9; YTH34.5	Leucocytes	Campath-1, gp21–28
CD53	HI29; HI36; MEM-53; HD77	Leucocytes	gp32–40
CD54	7F7; WEHI-CAMI; PR1/1	Broad, Activ.	ICAM-1
CD55	143-30; BRIC110; BRIC128; F2B-7.2	Broad	DAF (decay accelerating factor)
CD56	Leu19; NKH1; FP2–11.14, L185	NK, activ. lymphocytes	gp220/135, NKH1, isoform of N-CAM
CD57	Leu7; L183; L186	NK, T, B sub, brain	gp110, HNK1
CD58	G26; BRIC5; TS2/9	Leucocytes, epithel.	LFA-3, gp40–65
CD59	YTH53.1; MEM-43	Broad	gp18–20
CDw60	M-T32; M-T21; M-T41; UM4D4	T subset	NeuAc-NeuAc-Gal-
CD61	Y2/51; CLB-thromb/1; VI-PL2; BL-E6	Plt	Integrin β3-, VNR-β chain, Plt GPIIIa
CD62	CLB-thromb/6; CLB-thromb/5; RUU-SP1.18.1	Plt activ.	GMP-140 (PADGEM), gp140
CD63	RUU-SP2.28; CLB-gran/12	Plt activ., M, (G, T, B)	gp53
CD64	MAb32.2; MAb22;	M	FcRI, gp75
CDw65	VIM2; HE10; CF4; VIM8	G, M	Ceramide-dodecasaccharide 4c
CD66	CLB-gran/10; YTH71.3	G	Phosphoprotein gp180–200
CD67	B13.9; G10F5; JML-H16	G	p100, PI-linked
CD68	EBM11; Y2/131; Y-1/82A; Ki-M7; Ki-M6	Macrophages	gp110
CD69	MLR3; L78; BL-Ac/p26; FN50	activated B, T	gp32/28, AIM
CDw70	Ki-24; HNE51; HNC142	activated B, -T, Reed-Sternberg cells	Ki-24
CD71	138-18; 120-2A3; MEM-75; VIP-1; Nu-TfR2	Proliferating cells, Mac.	Transferrin receptor
CD72	S-HCL2; J3-109; BU-40; BU-41	B	gp43/39
CD73	1E9.28.1; 7G2.2.11; AD2	B subset, T subset	ecto-5'-nucleotidase, p69
CD74	LN2; BU-43; BU-45	B, M	Class II assoc. invariant chain, gp41/135/33
CDw75	LN1; HH2; EBU-141	mature B, (T subset)	P53?
CD76	HD66; CRIS-4	mature B, T subset	gp85/67
CD77	38.12(BLA); 424/4A11; 424/3D9	resting B	Globotriaosycleramide (Gb3)
CDw78	Anti Ba; LO-panB-a; 1588	B, (M)	?

MCP	membrane cofactor protein	Prog	progenitor cells	VLa	very late antigen
N-CAM	neural cell adhesion molecule	RBC	red blood cells	VNR	vitroectin receptor (member of the cytoadhesion family of integrins)
NK	natural killer cells	Reed Sternberg	Reed Sternberg cells		
Plt	platelets	Thy	thymocytes		

The designation of the monoclonal antibodies does not follow a common nomenclature necessary for subsequent proliferation and final differentiation of B-cells into antibody secreting plasma cells (Il-5 and Il-6) (see below).

Under the light- or even the electron-microscope T- and B-cells can hardly be distinguished unless they have already reacted to antigenic stimulation. Then, however, the B-lymphocytes differentiate into characteristically structured plasma cells in which the abundantly developed, rough-surfaced endoplasmic reticulum is particularly striking. In a similar situation, on the other hand, T-cells only increase in size, and their cytoplasm exhibits many free ribosomes but no endoplasmic reticulum. The two cell types can be distinguished by their differing surface phenomena: only the T-cells have the glycoprotein which is known as Thy-1 antigen and which is demonstrable with the aid of antibodies.

The availability of monoclonal antibodies has made it possible to identify and characterize a great number of the surface markers of lymphocytes and to correlate their expression with the two main types of lymphocytes, with certain subsets as well as with functional states and stages of differentiation. The list of antigens detected on immune cells has become rather long: by 1989, 78 different surface structures had been distinguished on human cells by the CD (clusters of differentiation) series of monoclonal antibodies. The relationship of the CD nomenclature to other designations is shown in Table 2.1.

The most important antigens which distinguish T-cells are CD3, the T-cell receptor complex, CD4, which characterizes T-helper cells, CD8 which is found on cytotoxic cells and T-suppressor cells, and CD2, which is expressed after T-cell activation and is responsible for the formation of stable erythrocyte rosettes.

2.1.1.1. Lymphocyte receptors

Every lymphocyte, whether a T-or B-cell, has surface receptors which can bind to a specific antigenic determinant, i.e. to a chemical structure of strictly limited variability. These receptors are designated B- and T-cell receptors.The B-cell receptor is identical with the antibody which a specific B-cell can produce and secrete (see below). Every B-cell initially synthesizes membrane-bound antibodies and bears on its surface approximately 10^5 such molecules in the cytoplasmic membrane. It is only on establishing contact with the "appropriate" antigen that a B-cell divides and develops into a cell clone by further division. From the very first cell division every B-cell begins to synthesize secretory, soluble antibodies. At the same time the B-cells develop into plasma cells which devote their entire capacity for protein synthesis to the formation of antibodies, producing and secreting approximately 1,000–2,000 antibody molecules per second. Such cells are no longer able to exercise other functions and die after several days of "peak" production.

The structure of the T-cell receptor was elucidated only recently. It consists of two heavy chains, known as α- and β-chains, which are linked by a disulfide bridge, and has a basic structure very similar to that of an antibody. Binding of the T-cell receptor to an antigen is the signal for growth and division of a T-cell and for fulfilment of its function. An important "modulating" role is played by surface structures such as the CD3 complex which are narrowly adjacent to, though not identical with, the T-cell receptor.

In contrast to the B-cell receptor, the T-cell receptor does not bind native antigens. This structure has evolved in context with the major histocompatibility proteins for which it may have an inherent affinity. The α-β-heterodimer 'sees'

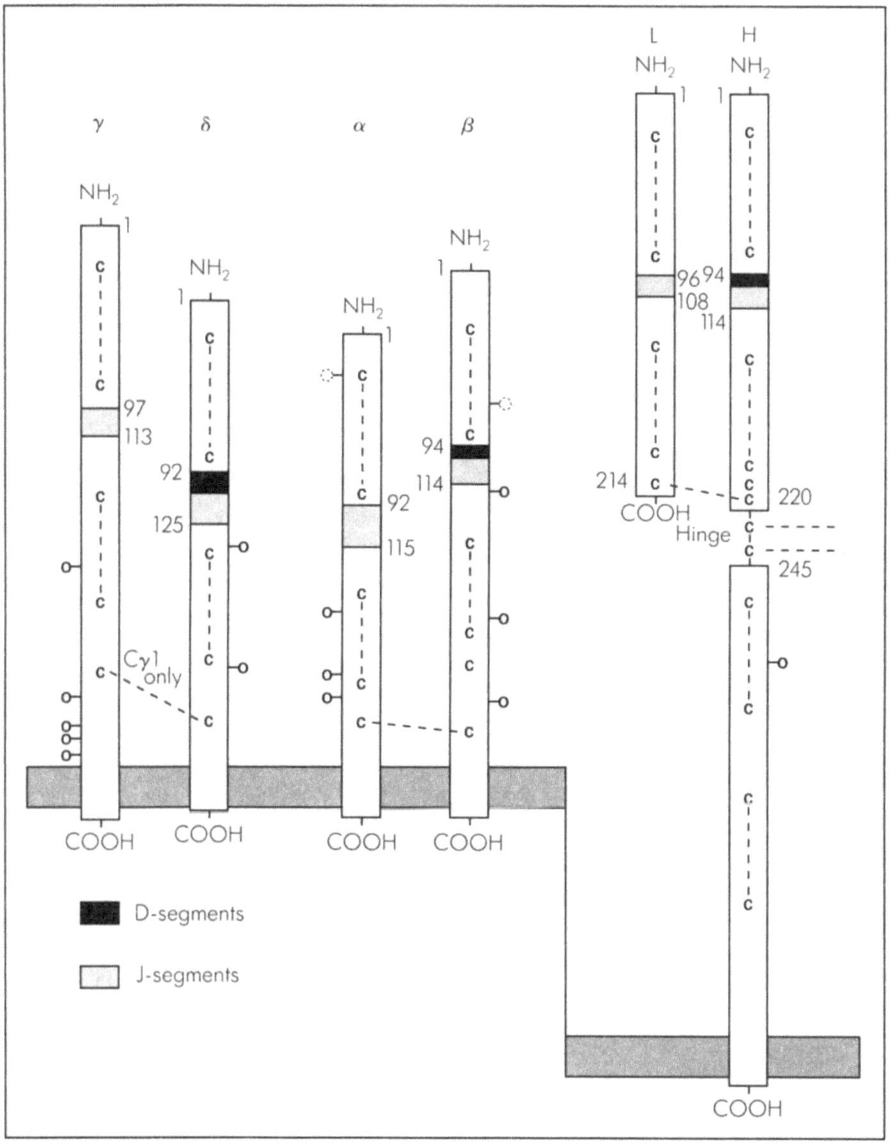

Figure 2.5. A schematic representation of the peptide chains constituting T-cell and B-cell receptors. The receptor domains are indicated by the dotted lines combining C molecules within each chain. The dotted lines between the chains represent disulfide bridges. Open circles: glycosylation sites. The figures indicate the number of amino acids at particular positions. D-segments are represented in black. The J-segments are shown as dotted areas. All chains are shown inserted into the cellular membrane.

antigen only in connection with the class I or class II histocompatibility molecule. The histocompatibility molecules play a crucial role in 'presenting' digested or 'processed' antigen to T-cells (see below). The diversity observed in the α and β chains of the T-cell receptor is produced by genetic rearrangements very much in the same way as the diversity in immunoglobulins.

Recently a second type of T-cell receptor made up of two different chains (γ

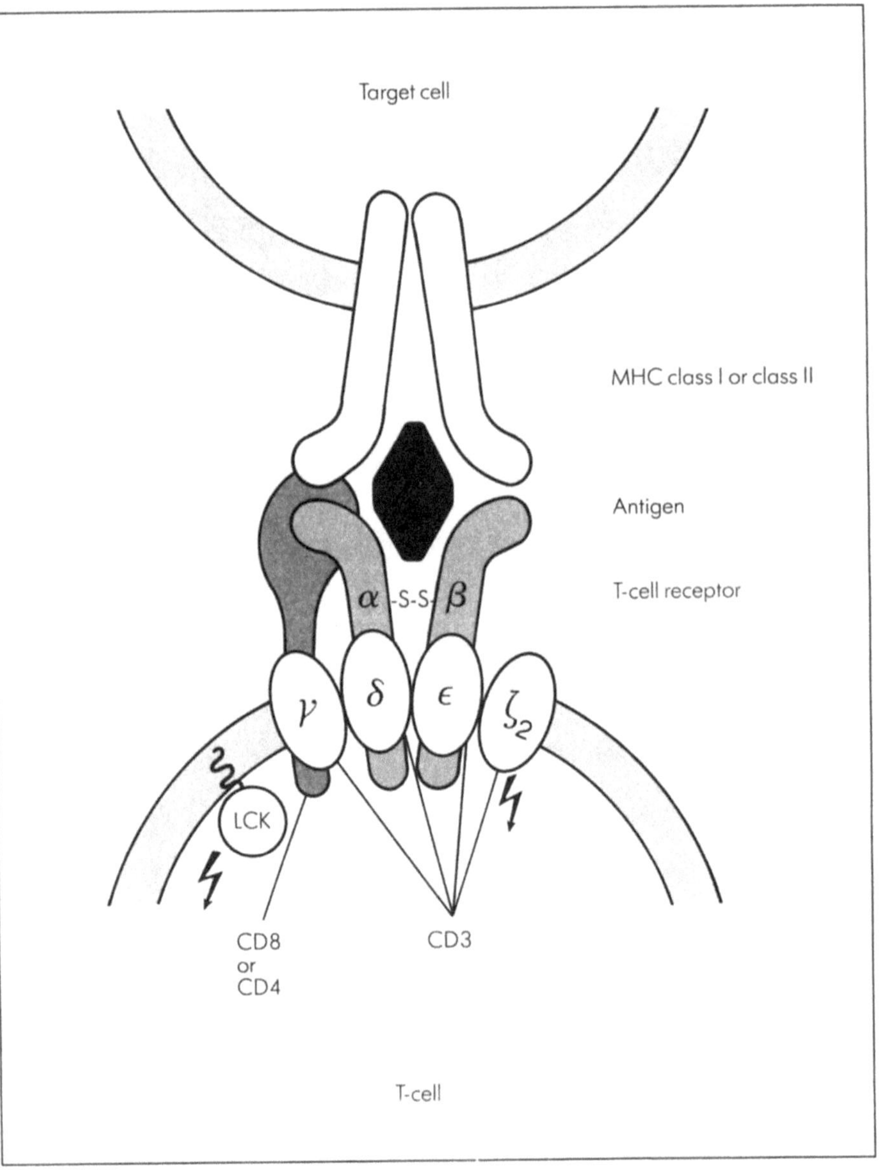

Figure 2.6. The CD3 complex associated with a T-cell receptor. The peptides γ, δ, ε and ζ have important signal transducing properties. They are, however, not covalently linked with the α- and β-chains of the T-cell receptor. LCK = lymphocyte kinase. The T-cell receptor is shown in association with a class I or class II HLA molecule presenting antigen (in black).

and δ) has been described. In mice, this receptor is expressed during fetal development two to three days prior to the appearance of the α-β-receptor in T-cells. During later fetal life cells carrying the α-β-receptor become the dominant population in the thymus. The degree of diversity expressed by γ-δ-receptors appears to be significantly smaller than that of α-β-receptors. In adult animals and in man T-cells carrying γ-δ-receptors account for 3–5% of the fetal T-cell population. The T-cell subset carrying the γ-δ-receptor does not express the CD4 and the CD8 gene. It is therefore termed: 'double negative'. The majority of peripheral T-lymphocytes which display the α-β-T-cell receptor are either $CD4^+$ or $CD8^+$. There is also a small percentage of double positive cells. The components of the B- and T-cell receptor are schematically depicted in *Fig. 2.5.*

Both T-cell receptors are closely but not covalently associated with the CD3 complex. This structure comprises three intramembranous proteins which are involved in receptor coupled signal transduction. A short scheme of T-cell ontogeny is given in *Fig. 2.6.*

2.1.1.2 Immunological memory

The way in which immunological memory functions is not understood in every detail. When virginal T- or B-lymphocytes, i.e. cells that have not come into contact with antigen, are activated by being challenged with antigen, a proportion of the cells develop into T-helper cells, cytotoxic T-cells, or – in the case of B-lymphocytes – into antibody-secreting plasma cells. Another part of these activated lymphocytes develop into "memory" cells. These cells probably participate in the antigen-mediated clonal expansion but not in the current immunological reaction. If, on a later occasion, the antigen that has triggered an immunological reaction enters the body again, it encounters the "memory cells", which, solely on account of their greater number, can mobilize a more rapid and more powerful immune response. This second – and stronger – immune reaction is designated a *secondary* immune response. It may be cell-mediated or humoral. During a secondary response, memory cells again appear to be formed: at all events, the kinetic pattern of all further confrontations with an antigen is that of a secondary immune response *(Fig. 2.7).*

2.1.1.3 Generation of receptor diversity in lymphocytes

According to current estimates, a mouse can produce from 10^6 to 10^7 different antibody molecules. We may assume that the corresponding figure for humans is at least one, probably two, orders of magnitude higher. How is this diversity of antibodies generated? For some time scientists considered the possibility that the formation of each of the antibodies which a mouse or human could make was directed by a special gene. However, the production of only one million antibodies would require the coding capacity of 2×10^9 base pairs if one takes into account only the structural information and disregards regulatory

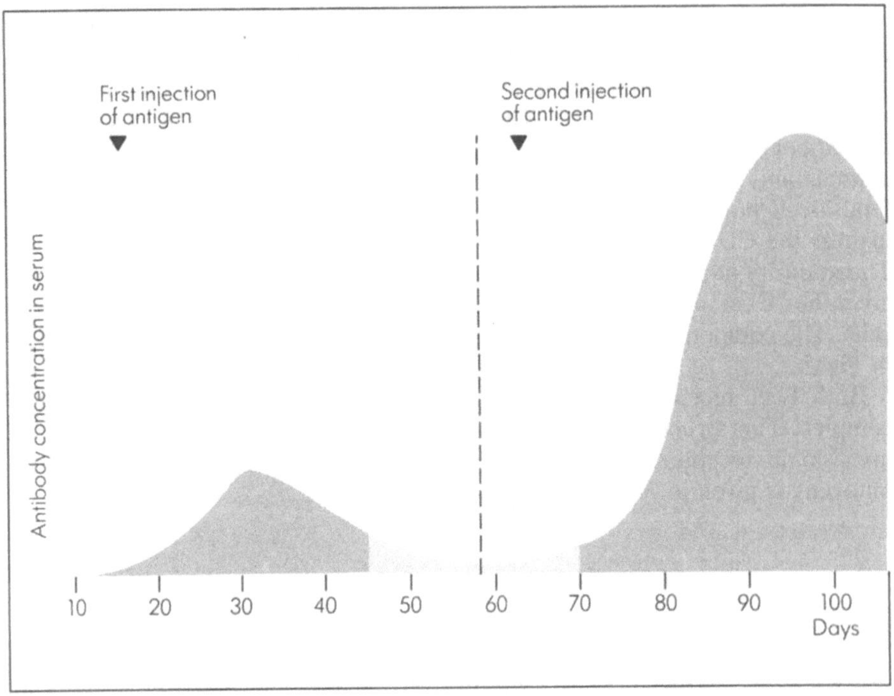

Figure 2.7. Diagram of a humoral immune response. The first injection of antigen is followed 15–20 days later by a relatively weak immune response which regresses after several weeks. A second injection of the same antigen brings about a relatively rapid rise in the antibody titre to a much higher level. This phenomenon is due to the existence of memory cells. During day 45 and 70 antibody titres may be too low to be detectable.

signals which would be necessary for the selective expression of each of these genes. Since the nucleus of an animal cell contains on average 3×10^9 nucleotide pairs, almost the whole genome would be occupied in this case with programming antibody synthesis and there would be no spare capacity for other proteins. The path taken in evolution to produce a large number of different antibodies and of course T-cell receptors must therefore have been different.

T-cell receptors consist either of an α- and β- or of an γ- and δ-chain. B-cell receptors, membrane-bound antibody molecules, are formed by the combination of two heavy chains and two light chains, each of the same type. All of these receptor chains belong to a superfamily of proteins which are characterized by a common structural feature: they all contain a number of homologous units, each of which comprises approximately 100 amino acids. These units fold into domains of similar structure. The antigen receptor polypeptides have one unique property: they consist of one highly variable NH_2-terminal domain linked to one or several constant domains. The genetic basis for the immense diversity of antibodies and T-cell receptors is generated by a large number of separate genes which code for the variable parts of the lymphocyte receptors. There are three types of genes which contribute to the variable parts of antibodies: V (variable) genes, D (diversity) genes and J (joining) genes. The V genes in particular are always present in a great number of different copies, but D and J genes also contribute to diversity. During the development of lymphocytes the V, J and D genes can be recombined among each other and with the genes of the constant parts of the receptor chains to yield a large variety of different structures. Since in B-cells there are always a heavy and a light chain for which this somatic recombination occurs independently and since either of two types of light chains can be used, the number of possible combinations becomes extremely high. In T-cells, α- and β-receptor chains are also formed by recombination events from a pool of genes for the variable gene segments and for a single gene for each of the constant parts. These genes are inherited in the germ line configuration. Their appropriate recombination is the essential molecular equivalent of functional maturation in the thymus for T-cells and in the bone-marrow for B-cells. The degree of diversity which is generated by the random recombination of different germ line genes is further enhanced by the fact that the joining process between V, J and D is imprecise. Up to 10 nucleotides can be deleted (junctional diversity) and up to 20 nucleotides can be added by terminal deoxynucleotide transferase (N-region diversity) at the junctions between the joined segments. Because of these variations and because most variable gene segments have only one reading frame not all recombinations are productive. After somatic recombination the variable segments are transcribed with the constant parts of the receptor genes and the coding sequences are then brought into contiguity by transcriptional processing, called splicing.

The rearrangement of variable region gene segments is mediated by a putative multienzyme complex, the Ig recombinase. The same recombinase is expressed in both B- and T-lymphocytes. However, in B-cells it only assembles the variable regions of Ig heavy and light chains and in T-cells it only assembles the variable regions of T-cell receptor polypeptide chains. This means that the action of the recombinase must be regulated by cell type specific nuclear factors. These factors generate "open" chromatin structures that are accessible for the recombinase as well as for the proteins which mediate transcription. The regulated generation of distinct sites in the various receptor gene loci which are accessible for the recombinase accounts not only for the cell type specific action of the recombinase but also for the programmed order in which the receptor gene segments are rearranged in each cell type. A productive rearrangement within one chromosome can then prevent rearrangement on the homologous chromosome and induce rearrangements at another receptor gene locus. The result is that each lymphocyte expresses only one type of antigen binding site that is formed by the pairing of the variable domains of two types of receptor chain. The diversity of the antigen repertoire is considerably increased by the fact that each receptor chain of one type can associate in different cells with many if not all chains of the other type. The various steps of differentiation which lead to mature lymphocytes expressing complete antigen receptors are shown schematically for B-cells in *Fig. 2.4* and for T-cells in *Fig. 2.3*.

Mutations of variable region sequences do not seem to make a significant contribution to the diversity of pre-immune receptor repertoires. However, a hypermutation mechanism is operating in antigen stimulated B-cells and makes an important additional contribution to B-cell receptor diversity.

Newly generated antigen receptor expressing cells are still immature lymphocytes. The interactions of these cells with endogenous ligands result in the deletion or the positive selection of cells with particular specificities.

For most if not all T-cells the recognition of polymorphic structures of major histocompatibility antigens at the surface of thymic epithelial cells is a prerequisite for a late differentiation step. Immature T-cells which fail to recognize these structures or which recognize other self antigens are deleted (see below). In B-cell development it seems that a complex network of interactions between the variable domains of receptors (idiotype-anti-idiotype interactions) result in the selection of cells which produce useful antibodies against common bacterial antigens. Self antigen specific cells which escape the premature deletion are usually not harmful. Some are even thought to perform useful functions while others fail to be destructive because they do not encounter the self antigens in immunogenic forms.

The details of the recombination events leading to the synthesis of functional antibodies will be described in connection with the discussion of antibodies.

2.1.1.4 Effector functions of T-cells

Different groups or "subsets" of T-cells may exercise different functions after contact with an antigen. Cytotoxic T-cells kill cells on whose surface they have "recognized" foreign antigens together with their own histocompatibility antigens.

The vast majority of cytolytic T-lymphocytes (CTL) belong to the CD8 subset which is class I MHC restricted (see below). CTL precursors (CTL-P) that are activated by an antigen presenting cell differentiate into CTLs in the presence of Il-2, IFN-γ and a poorly defined CTL differentiation factor (CDF). CTLs normally kill only target cells which express the same MHC-antigen complex that was presented to their precursors by an antigen presenting cell, although the actual killing of the target cells is mediated by nonspecific factors. Many CTL and NK cell lines maintained in tissue culture have granules which contain a protein called perforin. This 70 kd protein resembles the ninth component of the complement system in its primary structure as well as in its ability to form membrane pores by polymerization. The pores are channels of up to 16 nm in diameter which disrupt the plasma membrane barrier. Recognition of antigen on the target cell surface by CTLs results in degranulation. Together with perforin several other granule components are released including a family of highly homologous serine esterases (referred to as granzymes A-H) as well as other enzymes and proteoglycans which are found in many secretory cells.

Figure 2.8. The function of cytotoxic T-lymphocytes. Antigens (in this case viruses) are taken up by an antigen presenting cell. The processed antigen is subsequently presented to CD4 helper cells and to CD8 cells. A resting CD8 cell becomes activated by antigen recognition in the context of an HLA class I molecule and by secretory stimuli (IL-1, IL-6). It receives additional stimulation from the activated CD4 helper cell (IL-2, TCDF). The activated T-cell now develops into a T-cell clone, which can specifically lyse cells which carry viral antigens in association with HLA class I antigens. a = activated.

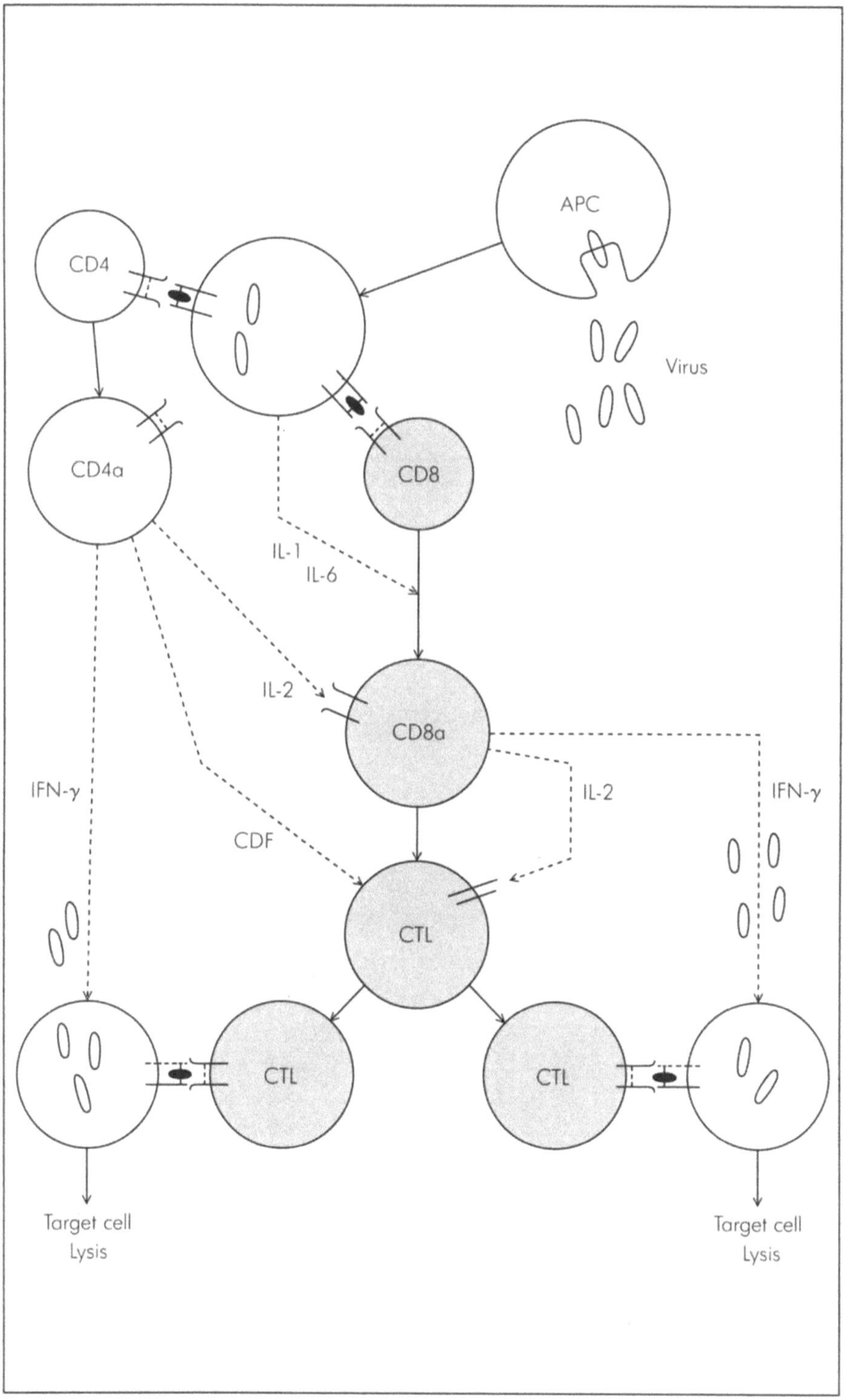

APC
CD4
Virus
CD4a
CD8
IL-1
IL-6
IL-2
CD8a
IFN-γ
IL-2
IFN-γ
CDF
CTL
CTL
CTL
Target cell
Lysis
Target cell
Lysis

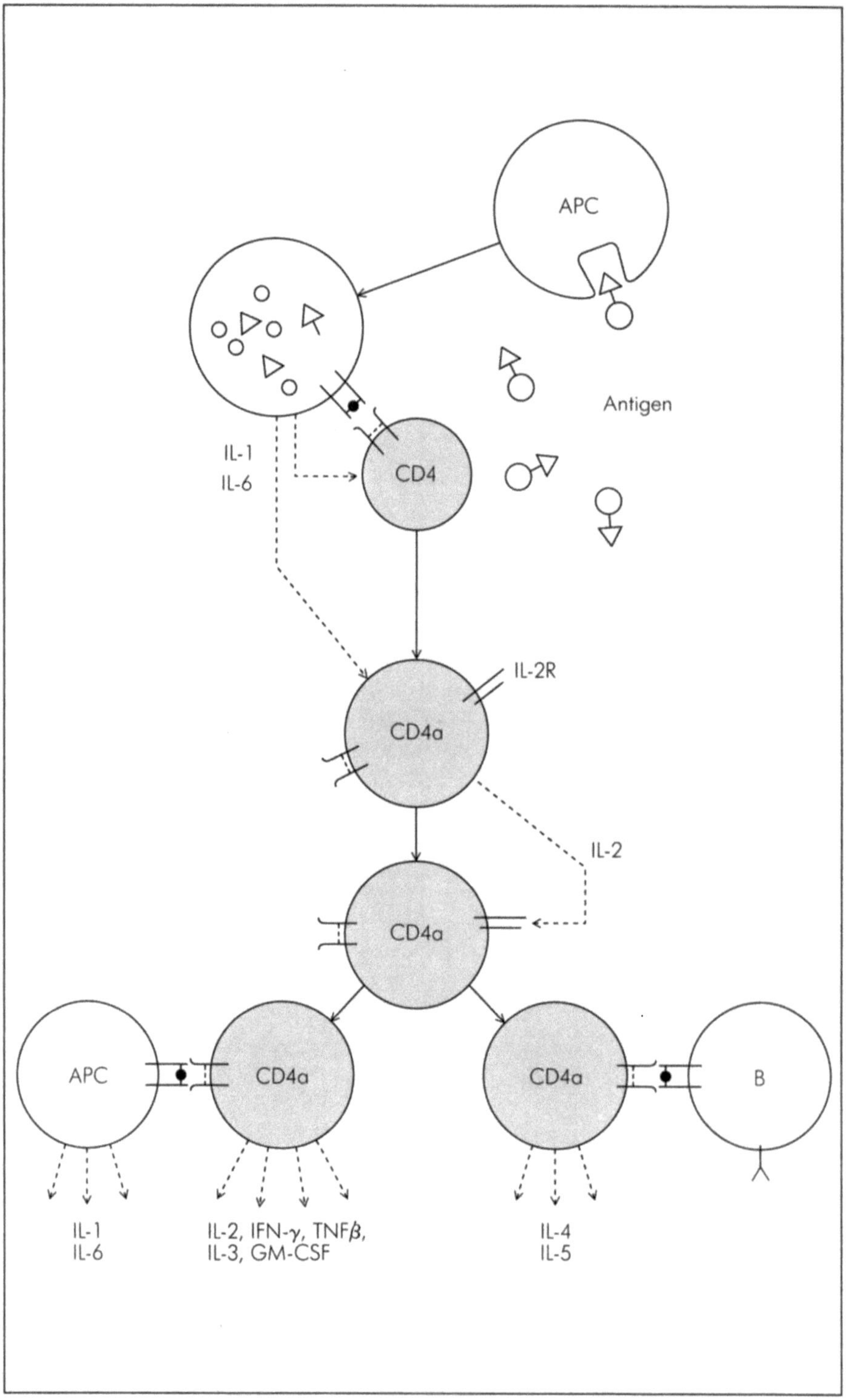
APC
Antigen
IL-1
IL-6
CD4
CD4a
IL-2R
IL-2
CD4a
APC
CD4a
CD4a
B
IL-1
IL-6
IL-2, IFN-γ, TNFβ,
IL-3, GM-CSF
IL-4
IL-5

The proteoglycans which are highly charged molecules have the purpose of binding and inactivating perforin at the low pH within the granules. In this way self-damage to the CTLs is prevented. At the neutral pH of the extracellular space, however, perforin dissociates from the proteoglycans and attacks the membrane of the target cell. The reason why perforin acts only on the target cell membranes rather than on the CTL membrane is not known.

Several observations indicate that there are alternative mechanisms by which CTLs and probably also NK-cells can kill their target cells. However, none of these mechanisms have been sufficiently characterized to be discussed here.

Under physiological conditions virus infected cells which carry class-I molecules in association with viral antigens *(Fig. 2.6)* are the most likely targets for the CTLs.

T-helper cells reinforce both the humoral immune response elicited by B-cells and the cytotoxic T-cell-mediated immune response. They do so by secreting certain proteins or glycoproteins that are essential for proliferation of the lymphocytes involved in the immunological reaction. One such signal protein that plays an important role in the T-helper function of cytotoxic T-cells and, according to recent research, also of B-cells is interleukin 2 or T-cell growth factor (TCGF). This protein is discussed in more detail elsewhere. T-suppressor cells suppress immune reactions of B- or T-cells. They, in turn, have to be stimulated by T-helper cells, but they then inhibit helper cell function. T-helper and T-suppressor cells are thus functionally connected in a kind of feedback circuit, in which a T-helper cell that has activated a T-suppressor cell is itself then inhibited by the same suppressor cell.

The interaction of the "regulatory T-cells" (T-helper and T-suppressor cells) maintains the functional balance of the immune system. Opinion differs on the way in which the regulatory T-cells interact with cytotoxic T-cells. The possibility that such interactions are humorally mediated by lymphokines is illustrated in *Figs 2.8* and *2.9*. The importance of these substances will be discussed in detail in a later section.

How do B-cells and T-helper cells interact? Like macrophages or dendritic cells, B-cells can present antigen in conjunction with class II molecules. But since B-cells carry surface immunoglobulins they can 'catch' antigen much more efficiently than other antigen presenting cells. This specific mechanism of binding enables B-cells to bind, incorporate and present antigen at antigen concentrations which are about a thousandfold lower than those needed for antigen uptake and presentation by macrophages. B-cells carrying Ig receptors with an affinity for tetanus toxin of 10^{-8} l/mol^{-1} are capable of presenting this antigen at concentrations of 10^{-11} M! At this concentration, only 10–50 molecules

Figure 2.9. Scheme of CD4 T-cell responses. Antigen (bacterial) is taken up by an antigen presenting cell, processed and presented to a T-helper cell. Recognition of the antigen in conjunction with HLA class II plus secretory stimuli emanating from the antigen presenting cell (IL-1 and IL-6) lead to an activation of the T-helper cell (expression of IL-2 receptors and activation of IL-2 secretion). Through this autocrine mechanism, the activated T-cell develops into a clone. Upon renewed contact with antigen presented by accessory cells (macrophages, dendritic cells) or B-cells this clone secretes a large array of cytokines, most of which have the ability to stimulate the proliferation (recruitment) and activation of immunological effector cells.

will be bound per cell. This becomes possible through the intracellular enrichment of the antigen. Ig receptors which have bound antigen are internalized quite rapidly so that every hour five to ten times the amount of antigen which is bound to the cell at any given time is delivered to the interior of the B-cell. Secondly, the long half-life of antigen within the B-cell (24 hours) leads to a considerable accumulation of antigen in T-cells. A. Lanzavecchia has called this phenomenon the 'vacuum cleaner effect'. B-cells which have 'seen' their antigen through their Ig receptor become partially activated. A state of full activation, however, is only reached after the same cells present this antigen which is now processed and associated with a class II molecule to a T-helper cell. The T-helper cell will respond to this presentation with a battery of humoral and membrane associated signals which send the B-cell irreversibly towards its final differentiation into a secretory plasma cell. *Fig. 2.10* gives an illustration of the possible chain of events.

A particular possibility for the interaction between B-cells and T-helper cells was described many years ago: small molecules such as dinitrophenol are immunogenic only when they are bound to a larger molecule, e.g. a protein. Studies in whole-body irradiated mice have now shown that B-lymphocytes produce antibodies to dinitrophenol (DNP) only if they are "supported" by T-lymphocytes that react to the carrier protein coupled with DNP. T-lymphocytes from mice that have been immunized against another protein are ineffective as helper cells in the formation of DNP antibodies. The interaction of B-cells and T-helper cells that is needed for "helping" and for antibody formation is possibly mediated by an antigen bridge consisting of hapten and carrier protein. Even then, however, the helper cells would be expected to release a humoral signal such as interleukin 2. Interaction between regulatory cells and cytotoxic T-cells could also be made possible by reciprocal anti-idiotypic activity.

2.1.1.5 Transplantation reactions and MHC antigens

Tissue (e.g. skin) transferred from one individual to another of the same species (allografts) will in most cases be rejected. The same applies to grafts from different species (xenografts). When lymphocytes from donor A are transferred to recipient B, the graft-versus-host reaction is observed, i.e. a reaction of the graft against the host's tissue. Both reactions – rejection and the graft-versus-host reaction – are due to the fact that T-lymphocytes from the donor and the recipient recognize each other as "foreign" and react against each other. This

---

Figure 2.10. Antigens are taken up by an antigen presenting cell and by a B-cell via its receptor molecule exposed on the surface. Within the antigen presenting cell, the antigen is processed and then exhibited in conjunction with an HLA class II molecule on the surface of the cell. A T-cell which recognizes the antigen becomes activated. The antigen is also processed within the B-cell and exposed on class II molecules of the B-cell. T-helper cells which recognize the antigen in connection with HLA class II molecules will now secrete cytokines like IL-2, IL-4 and interferon-γ. These secretory stimuli will drive the B-cell along its developmental pathway to become an antibody-forming cell and eventually a plasma cell, which is highly specialized to secrete antibodies. APL = antigen presenting cell; TH = T-helper cell (CD4); AFC = antibody forming cell; PC = plasma cell; a = activated.

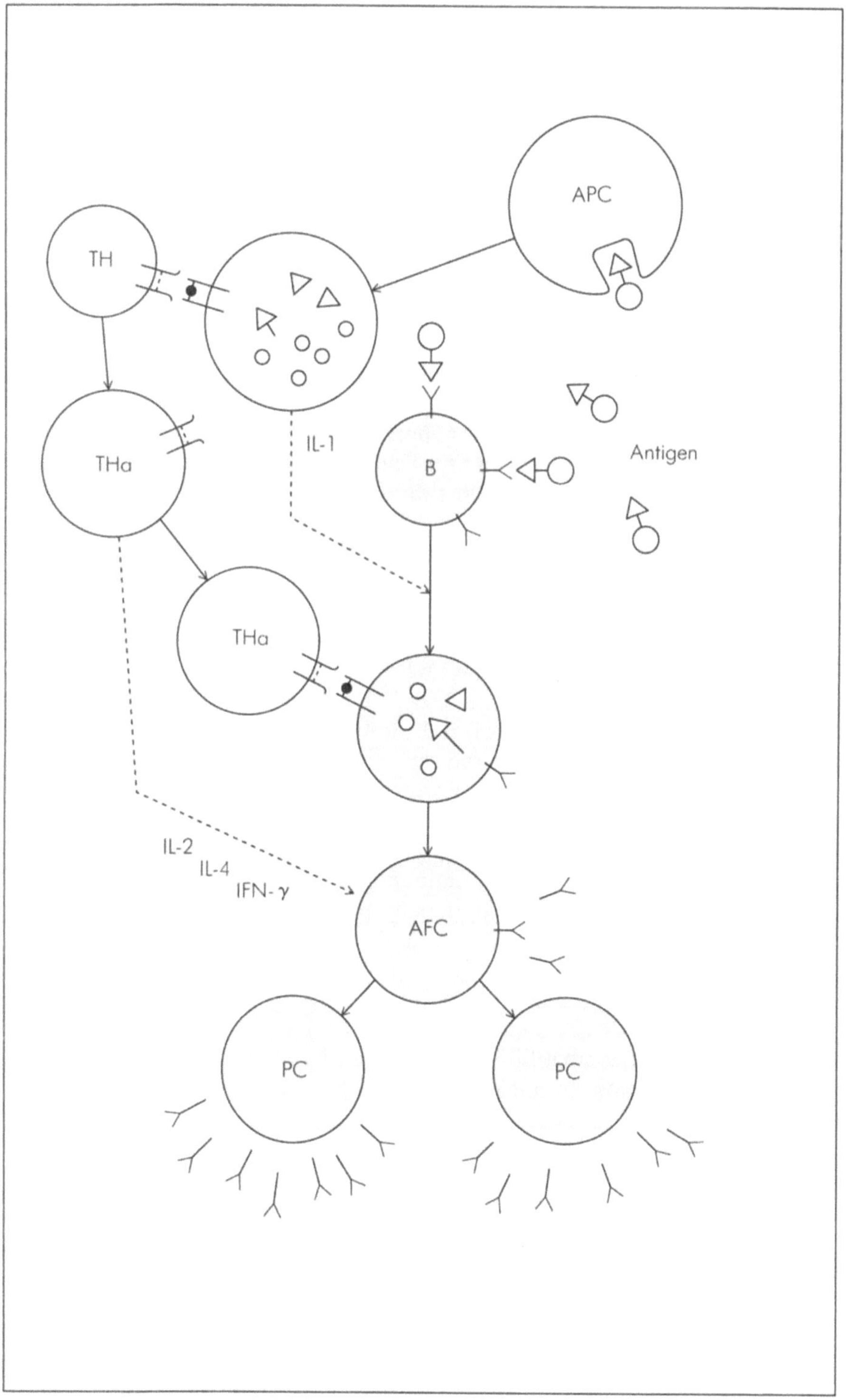
APC
TH
IL-1
B
Antigen
THa
THa
IL-2
IL-4
IFN-γ
AFC
PC
PC

reaction can be simulated in vitro by incubating lymphocytes from two different individuals (mixed lymphocyte reaction). In the course of the reaction the two T-cell populations generate cytotoxic T-cells which initiate lysis of the foreign cells. Better quantification of the reaction is obtained by lethally irradiating the lymphocytes of one individual or treating them with cytostatics before the reaction. Though these cells then still act as an antigenic stimulus for the undamaged lymphocytes of the other individual, they themselves are no longer able to divide. In this situation the formation of lymphoblasts is clearly attributable to the cells of the non-irradiated partner.

These in-vivo and in-vitro graft reactions do not, however, occur in grafts or lymphocyte cultures with tissue or cells from identical twins. There must be genetically programmed differences in the surface antigens which are virtually always present – even in grafts between relatives – and which are responsible for the reactions described. These antigens are called transplantation or histocompatibility antigens. Of particular importance are the major histocompatibility complex (MHC) and, in man, the human leukocyte-associated antigen (HLA) complex. Nowadays a distinction is drawn between two "classes" of HLA and MHC antigens: class I antigens, which are found on virtually all nucleated cells, and class II antigens, which are found only on immune cells, i.e. B- and T-lymphocytes, and antigen-presenting cells such as macrophages, dendritic cells or Langerhans' cells.

Class I antigens consist of a single polypeptide chain of 345 amino acids (Mr 45 kd). Their structure is determined by three genetic loci (HLA-A, HLA-B and HLA-C in man). The molecule bridges the cytoplasmic membrane with a short hydrophobic group. The carboxyl terminal end protrudes into the cytoplasm. 80% of the molecule is on the cell surface. In this external segment are three successive, largely homologous segments, the so-called domains $\alpha1$, $\alpha2$, $\alpha3$, which have probably developed as a result of gene duplications. Associated non-covalently with $\alpha1$ is a $\beta2$-microglobulin (Mr 11,500 dalton) which shows a high degree of homology with an immunoglobulin segment. The loci coding for HLA class I antigens are exceptionally polymorphic, i.e they occur in 23 alleles for the A locus, in 49 for B and in 8 for C. Since in any individual two alleles may be expressed from each locus there can be six class I antigens expressed altogether. The same number of antigens can be generated from each of the class II loci DR (20 alleles), DQ (3) and DP (6), so that up to twelve different major histocompatibility antigens can be present in each individual. Considering the number of alleles in each of the six loci and the fact that two

Figure 2.11 A genetic map of the human HLA complex. The HLA genes are located on the short arm of chromosome-6 (A). The area in which the class I, class II and class III genes are located is shown in detail. The DP locus contains 5 loci, two of which (α- and β) represent functional genes. The DR region, approximately 150 kb telomeric from DP contains four loci, two of which (α and β) are functional. DQ contains the genes for two β-chains ($\beta1$ and $\beta2$) and one α-chain. The black boxes represent functional genes, open boxes are pseudogenes (B). The principal structure of the β light chain and of the α heavy chain of class II molecules includes a leader sequence, $\beta1$, $\beta2$ or $\alpha1$ and $\alpha2$ domains, a transmembrane region and a cytoplasmic tail. In black the 3'-untranslated part of the gene. The α heavy chain of class II molecules is depicted in a similar fashion (C). Analogously the genes for class I heavy chains and for β-microglobulins are shown. The basic structure of the class I and class II molecules is depicted in panel D in a strongly simplified fashion. Class I heavy chains have 3 domains, $\alpha1$, $\alpha2$ and $\alpha3$. $\beta2 = \beta2$ microglobulin.

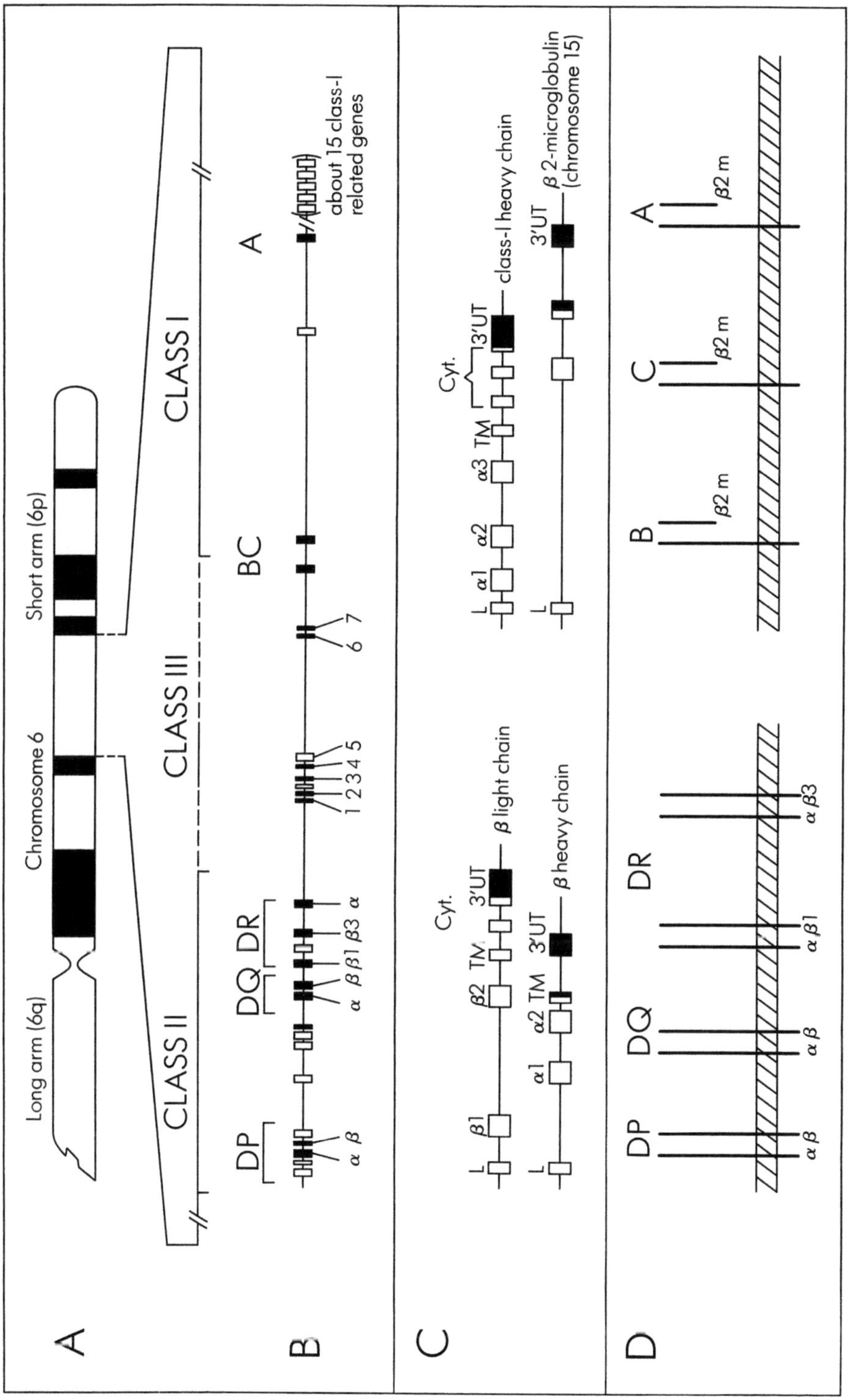
A
B
C
D
Long arm (6q)
Chromosome 6
Short arm (6p)
CLASS II
CLASS III
CLASS I
DP
DQ
DR
BC
A
α β
α β β1 β3 α
1 2 3 4 5
6 7
about 15 class-I related genes
L
β1
β2
TM
Cyt.
3'UT
β light chain
α1
α2
β heavy chain
α3
class-I heavy chain
β 2-microglobulin (chromosome 15)
β2 m
α β
α β1
α β3

alleles can be simultaneously expressed from each locus, the number of possible combinations and thus of individual histocompatibility 'profiles' becomes enormous – in the order of several billions! Because of the close genetic linkage of some of these alleles, however, the number of combinations which actually occur is considerably smaller. MHC antigens are intraindividually very homogenous and interindividually highly variable.

The class II genes of the HLA complex were initially thought to be Ir genes, i.e. genes that modulate the intensity of the immune response to a certain antigen. Unlike class I antigens, they are – as already mentioned – expressed only on lymphocytes, macrophages or other antigen presenting cells. They consist of two peptide chains – an α- and a β-chain (Mr 33,000 and 28,000 daltons, respectively). Both of them bridge the plasma membrane with hydrophobic groups, short COOH-terminal ends protrude into the cytoplasm and their longer NH_2-terminal ends are outwardly directed. Both chains are glycosylated. Each of the two chains has two major domains outside the cell, $\alpha1$ and $\alpha2$ and $\beta1$ and $\beta2$ respectively. In man the synthesis of these class II antigens is also coded by the D region comprising the loci DP, DQ and DR *(Fig. 2.11)*. The product of the DR locus (within the D region) is responsible for the restriction of antigen presentation. There is a correlation between the structure of this region and susceptibility to certain diseases (see Chapter 7). *Fig. 2.12* shows a schematic depiction of MHC class I and class II molecules.

The function of MHC antigens in the body's antiinfectious defences was elucidated 1974 by Zinkernagel and Doherty. In their experiment, a mouse

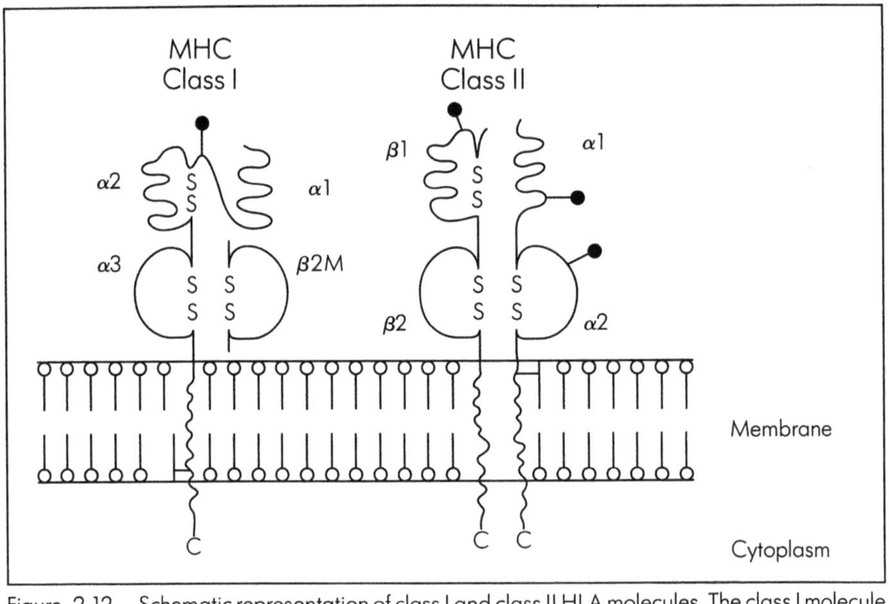

Figure 2.12. Schematic representation of class I and class II HLA molecules. The class I molecule contains 3 domains $\alpha1$, $\alpha2$ and $\alpha3$ outside of the cell membrane. A transmembrane region spans the cell membrane and ends in a short cytoplasmic tail. The $\beta2$ microglobulin chain is non-covalently linked to the α heavy chain. HLA class II molecules: each chain comprises two extra-cellular domains: $\alpha1$, $\alpha2$ and $\beta1$, $\beta2$, respectively. Carbohydrate side chains are indicated by filled circles.

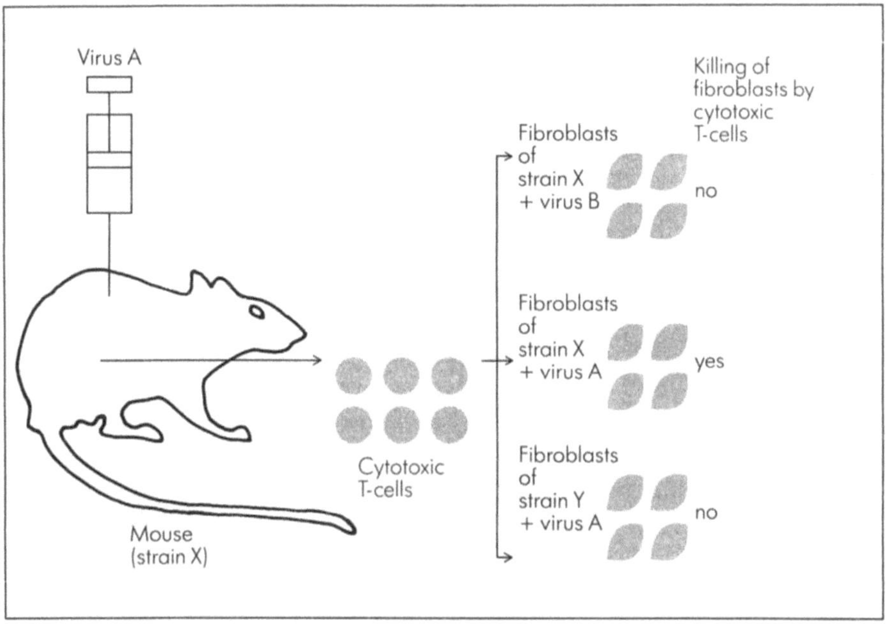

Figure 2.13. Cytotoxic T-cells recognize foreign antigens only in association with certain cell-surface structures. The T-lymphocytes of a mouse infected with virus A kill cells infected with virus A only if the cells have the same class I histocompatibility antigens on their surface as the immunized animal. This is designated restriction of the cell-mediated immune response.

strain, X, was infected with a virus, A. The cytotoxic T-cells of the immunized mice were then incubated in vitro with fibroblasts from the same mouse strain which had previously been infected with the same virus, A, or with another virus, B. As expected, the cytotoxic T-cells reacted only against fibroblasts that had been infected with virus A. Surprisingly, however, cytotoxic T-cells from mouse strain X did *not* attack fibroblasts from a genetically different mouse strain which had been infected with the "right" virus A. Thus, virally infected cells were lysed only when they exhibited not only the viral antigen but also the surface structures that were recognized by the cytotoxic lymphocytes as "self". Further experiments showed that the antigens which, besides the viral antigens, had to be recognized by the cytotoxic T-cells were class I glycoproteins. In other experiments it was demonstrated that T-helper cells recognize foreign antigens in association with MHC class II antigens *(Fig. 2.13)*. These findings made it easier to answer a number of outstanding questions concerning the MHC antigens. It had been observed that in the mixed lymphocyte reaction not 0.1%, or less, of all cells were converted to blast cells but rather 3–5%, i.e. a much higher proportion of cells than that part of a population that should react against any antigen. The fact that, during the evolution of the immune system, the T-lymphocytes were "trained" to recognize foreign antigens, usually in association with the antigens of the MHC or HLA complexes, makes this high percentage plausible: it is possible that many T-cells react to foreign MHC glycoproteins because these molecules resemble their own MHC glycoproteins of the T-cells, in association with foreign antigens. An explanation can also be found for the extreme polymorphism of the MHC molecule: many viral antigens are recognized by cytotoxic T-cells only in association with MHC class I molecules. By the same token, T-helper cells will see many bacterial antigens only in association with MHC class II antigens. This signal enables T-helper cells to promote the formation of antibodies to a particular bacterial antigen by B-cells. Opsonization with antibodies renders the bacterial cell identifiable for lysis by macrophages or neutrophils. From the viewpoint of the microorganism, new antigens whose physicochemical properties enable them to avoid association with the glycoproteins of the MHC complex should therefore be constantly developed. The immune system would have to counter this evolution by developing a large number of different MHC molecules which associate chemically with all, or almost all, microbial antigens. This reduces the likelihood that the existence of a particular species is endangered by failure to recognize a specific viral or bacterial antigen within the range of recognition mechanisms which the animal species (population) concerned has at its disposal.

MHC or HLA antigens play a crucial role in the evolution of T-cells which tolerate 'self' and react against 'non-self'. Stem cells or pro-T-cells enter the fetal thymus where they proliferate vigorously. In the mouse, a large part of the resulting immature T-cells are $CD4^+/CD8^+$ and carry a $\gamma\delta$ or $\alpha\beta$ T-cell receptor. These immature cells then react with class I or class II antigens which are expressed on thymus epithelium. At this stage, the ability of young T-cells to recognize 'self' in the form of class I or II molecules is a prerequisite for their survival. Only cells which bind to thymic epithelium escape destruction. How cells which do not bind are eliminated is not clear. The surviving T-cells are 'MHC-specific'. They may also at this point differentiate into $CD4^+$ (helper) cells or into $CD8^+$ (killer) cells depending on their contact with either class II or class I antigen.

In a subsequent selection step these T-cells are confronted with accessory cells, macrophages or dendritic cells, which also express class I and class II antigens on their surface, probably in association with processed 'self' proteins. This time, all the cells which react strongly with 'self' in connection with class I or class II antigens are killed by an unknown mechanism. The cells which survive will therefore recognize and tolerate their own MHC antigens and they will also not react against MHC antigens in association with self-determinants. Of all the T-cells which are generated in the thymus only a small fraction survives the double selection step. The thymus of a young adult mouse contains 2×10^8 thymocytes, largely of the $CD4^+/CD8^+$ type. 5×10^7 cells of this phenotype

---

Figure 2.14. Role of the thymus epithelium for the acquisition of MHC restriction. Young mice which carry a mixed DR genotype (k × b) are thymectomized. Half of the animals are then transplanted with thymus epithelium expressing the k-haplotype and the other half receive cells with a b-haplotype. After 2 weeks all animals are irradiated in order to destroy any accessory k or b-cells.
Subsequently, the animals received k × b stem-cells. After reconstitution all mice are immunized with KHL in complete Freund's adjuvant. After 9 days, the T-lymphocytes are obtained from the draining lymph nodes and incubated with KLH and either k or b-antigen presenting cells. The results show that T-cells which were selected on thymic epithelium carrying the b-haplotype are only activated by KLH presenting macrophages of the same genotype. The same is true for T-cells "educated" in a k environment. KLH = keyhole limpet hemocyanin.

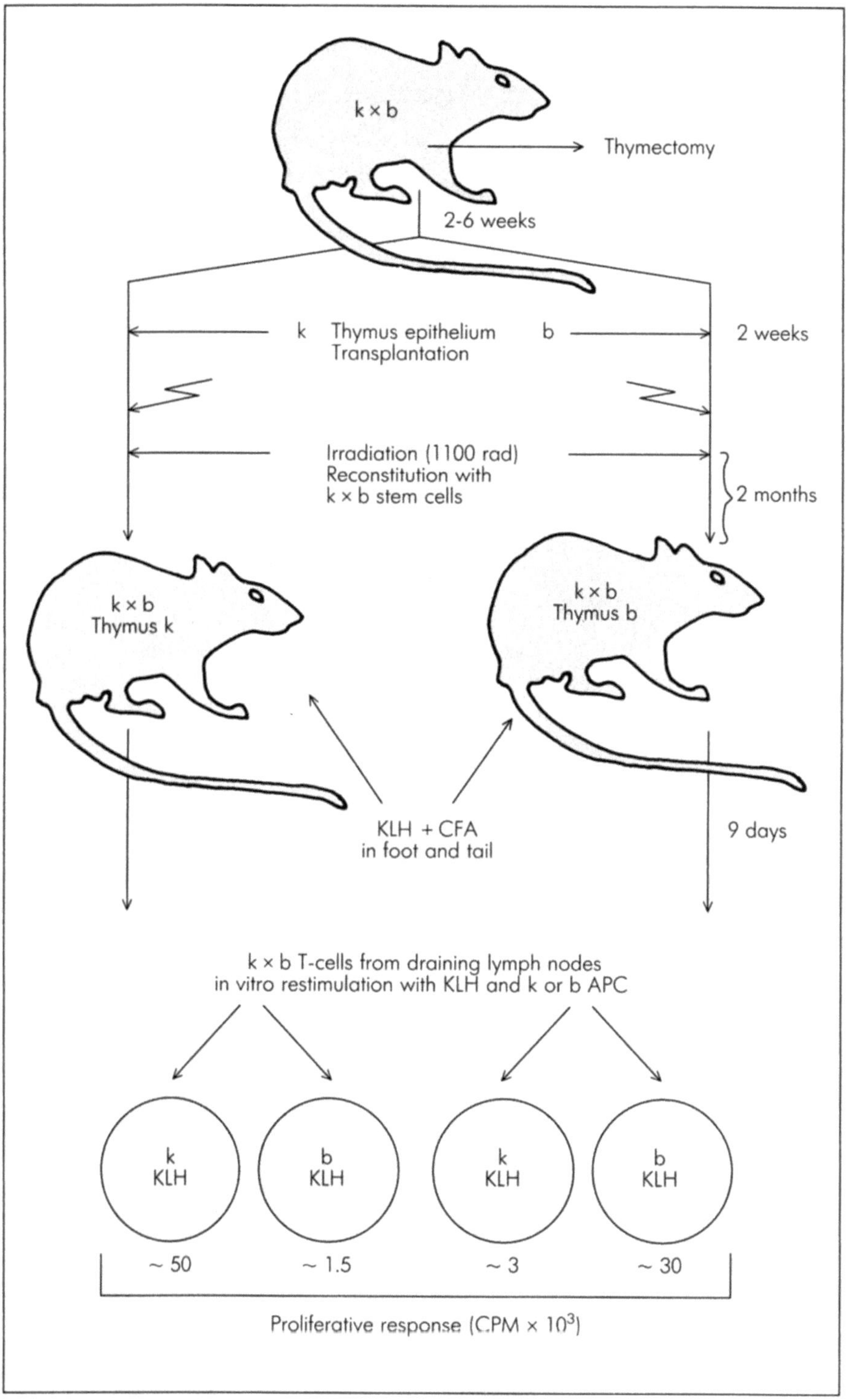
k × b
Thymectomy
2-6 weeks
k Thymus epithelium b
Transplantation
2 weeks
Irradiation (1100 rad)
Reconstitution with
k × b stem cells
2 months
k × b
Thymus k
k × b
Thymus b
KLH + CFA
in foot and tail
9 days
k × b T-cells from draining lymph nodes
in vitro restimulation with KLH and k or b APC
k
KLH
b
KLH
k
KLH
b
KLH
~ 50
~ 1.5
~ 3
~ 30
Proliferative response (CPM × 10³)

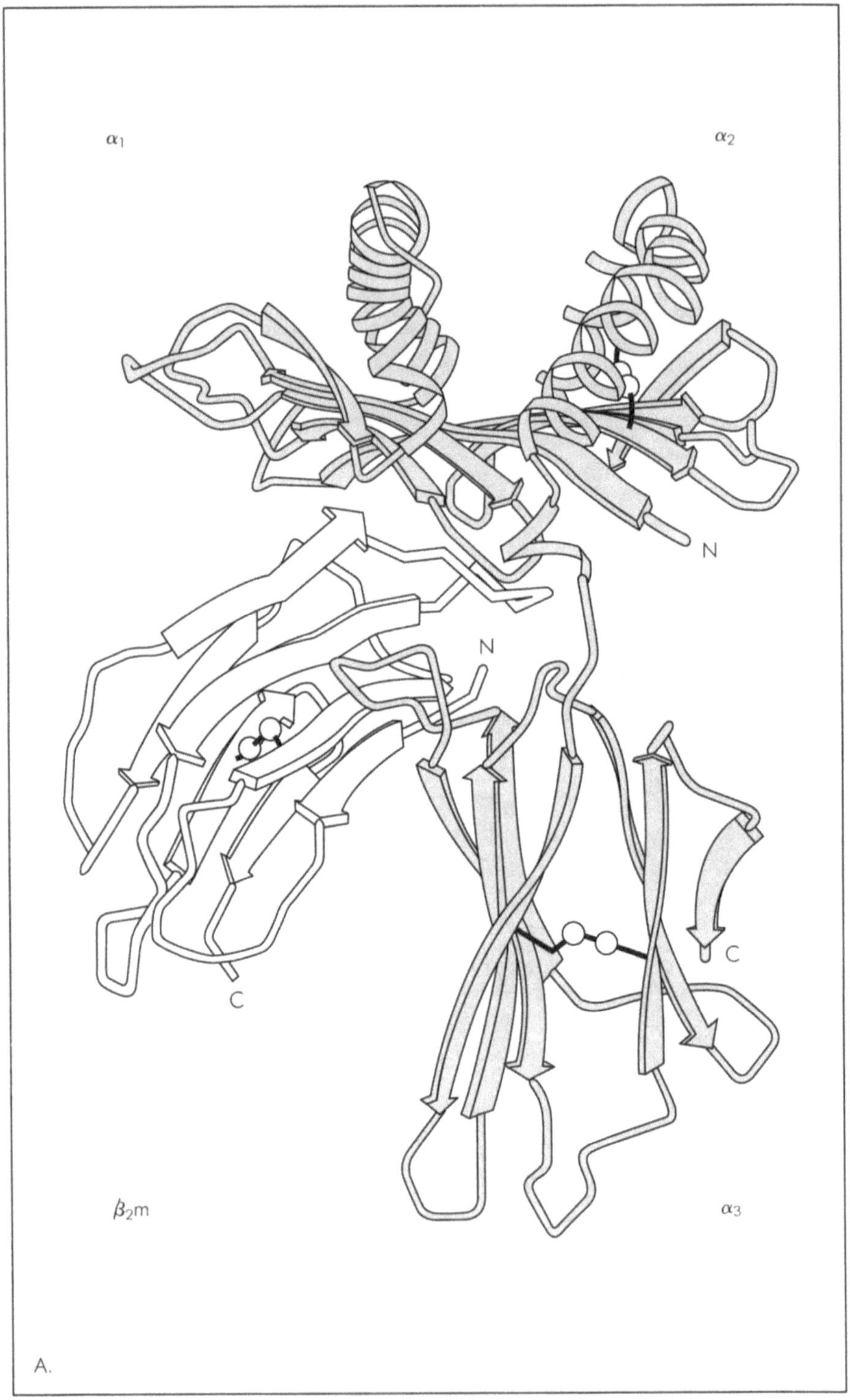

α1
α2
N
N
C
C
β2m
α3
A.

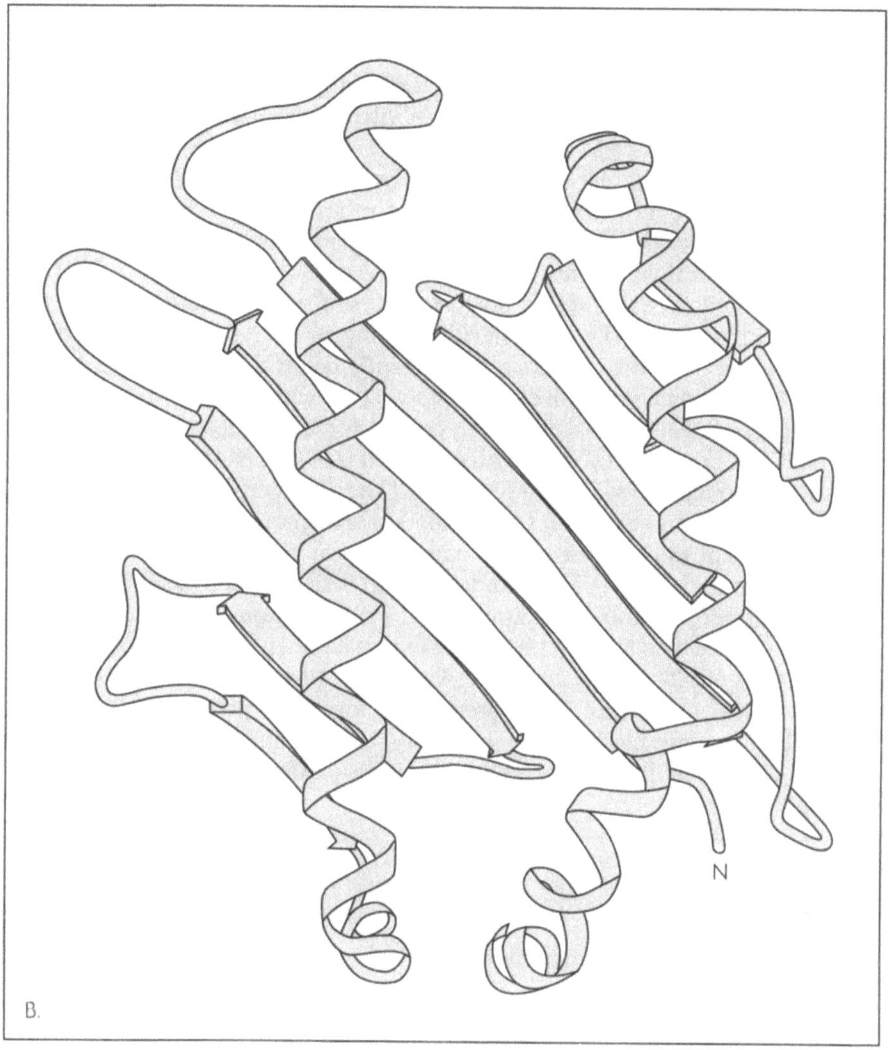

Figure 2.15. Three-dimensional representation of a class I MHC molecule. The α1-, α2- and α3-domains of the class-I heavy chain are shown in association with β2 microglobulin in a three-dimensional configuration. (A) The groove between the α1- and α2-domains is formed by β-pleated sheets (bottom) and two α helical structures on either side. Seen from above (2.15 B) one can see the bottom of the groove which is the attachment site for antigenic peptides presented to T-cells.

are produced per day but only $1-3 \times 10^6$ mature functional $CD4^+/CD8^-$ or $CD4^-/CD8^+$ cells leave the thymus during the same time (see also Chapter 4).

The importance of the thymus epithelium for the acquisition of MHC restriction is nicely demonstrated by the experiment illustrated in *Fig. 2.14*. Young mice which carry a mixed DR genotype (k × b) are thymectomized. One half of the animals are then transplanted with thymus epithelium expressing the k haplotype and the other half receives transplants of the b haplotype. The animals are then irradiated in order to destroy any accessory k or b cells and are subsequently reconstituted with k × b stem cells. After reconstitution all animals are immunized with keyhole limpet hemocyanin (KLH) in complete Freund's adjuvant (CFA). After nine days, the T-lymphocytes are obtained from draining the lymph nodes and incubated in vitro with KLH and and either k or b antigen presenting cells. T-cells which were selected on thymic epithelium carrying the b haplotype are only activated by KLH presenting macrophages of the same MHC genotype. The same is true for T-cells 'educated' in a 'k environment'. This experiment shows clearly that young T-cells 'learn' restriction by interacting with thymic epithelium.

For a long time it was unclear how exactly 'self' or 'non-self' proteins are associated with class I or class II molecules. Using x-ray crystallography, a team of researchers at Harvard University has recently determined the three-dimensional structure of a class I molecule. The structure which they obtained shows that the class I molecule has a binding pocket for the antigen which is to be presented. The pocket is formed by the $\alpha1$ and $\alpha2$ regions of the heavy chain while the $\alpha3$ domain of the same chain and the $\beta2$ microglobulin sit next to the cellular membrane to which the $\alpha3$ domain is anchored by a short peptide. Eight segments of the two $\alpha1$ and $\alpha2$ domains form a β-sheet which serves as the flat floor of the pocket. It is bounded by two helical protein segments. Most of the polymorphic amino acids are located in the bottom of the groove and in the helical sides. The antigen binding pocket is large enough to accommodate a peptide of about 20 amino acids. We know that this is about the size of the pieces to which an antigen is fragmented before it is presented. So far, a polymorphic antigen binding site has only been demonstrated for class I molecules. However, it appears likely that it also exists in class II structures *(Fig. 2.15)*.

2.1.2 Macrophages

Macrophages are extremely flexible cells. Their most obvious property is their ability to phagocytose, i.e. ingest, live or inert particles. This ability, to which the cells owe their name, is revealed in three individual steps. Firstly, the cell establishes contact with the particle to be ingested – this depends solely on its surface components and is non-energy-dependent. Then it generates and transmits a biological signal that ultimately results in phagocytosis. Finally, it absorbs the particle by sending out cellular pseudopodia which engulf the particle and cause it to be ingested into a phagocytic vacuole after the respective plasma membranes have approached and fused with each other. These phagocytosis-induced vacuoles are known as phagosomes. This last step, and presumably the second one as well, require energy. The presence of membrane-surface *receptors* which can react with ligands of the particle to be digested is crucial for the interaction, the development of the signal, and the actual mechanism of phagocytosis. The most important of these receptors are special binding sites for Fc fragments, IgG antibodies and for the complement protein C3b. It is by way of these receptors that, for instance, bacteria opsonized by IgG are bound to the cell surface, killed and ingested. Bacteria can be classified according to their ability to survive in macrophages. "Extracellular" microorganisms such as gram-positive cocci, corynebacteria, *Haemophilus influenzae* and others are killed either by a complement-dependent mechanism on the surface of the macrophage, or by the myeloperoxidase system within minutes or even seconds of being engulfed. Pathogens such as *Brucella, Toxoplasma* and *Salmonella* are designated "intracellular" microorganisms which can resist aggressive oxidation and can even survive for some considerable time in macrophages. Intracellular organisms stimulate macrophages to maximum cytotoxicity: thus activated, they are then able not only to digest and intracellularly break down bacteria and other opsonized cells or cell debris but also to attack and kill tumour cells. This, however, requires a ratio of approximately 10 to 20 macrophages for each tumour cell. The underlying mechanism of this effect has not yet been fully elucidated.

It can, however, be assumed that the oxygen compounds synthesized by the peroxidase system of the macrophages, H_2O_2 and a number of oxygen radicals play an essential role in the destruction of bacteria and, perhaps even more so, of tumour cells.

Among the most important functions of "activated" macrophages is the secretion of proteases, e.g. elastase, of thrombolytic substances such as plasminogen activators and of monokines such as interleukin-1, colony stimulating factors (CSF) and tumour necrosis factor (TNF). On the one hand all of these functions are manifestations of a still primitive system – on the other hand they are already part of a complex regulatory network which directly or indirectly controls the actual immune cells, i.e. the lymphocytes. *Table 2.2* contains a list of the most important products secreted by activated macrophages.

The ability of the macrophage to present antigens in association with histocompatibility antigens on its surface clearly belongs to the second category. This function is a pivotal one for the development of a cell-mediated immune response. Antigens are phagocytosed, broken down into smaller units and then "presented" on the cell surface in close association with the genes of the histocompatibility complex. Antigenic structures that are presented in association with class II HLA antigens are "seen" by T-helper cells. Cytotoxic T-cells and T-suppressor cells recognize foreign structures in association with class-I antigens.

As already described, our understanding of the structural environment in which an antigen is presented by class-I histocompatibility molecules has recently been significantly enriched. We are still awaiting the details of antigen presentation by class II molecules. Significant progress has been made in following the intricacies of protein processing by macrophages and – probably – other antigen presenting cells. Most – if not all – proteins must be taken up and processed by macrophages before they can be presented in conjunction with class-II molecules. In any case, proteins which, after intracellular degradation, are presented by macrophages, are a thousand times more immunogenic to T-cells than undegraded native proteins. Our present view of the events leading to presentation of an antigen is the following: a globular protein is taken up by a macrophage and becomes internalized through an acid vesicular compartment called an endosome. Here it is denatured and partially fragmented. The endo-

Table 2.2. Products secreted by activated macrophages

A. Enzymes

Product	*Function*
Plasminogen activators, elastase	Inflammatory, tissue repair
Collagenase I, II, III, IV, V	Inflammatory
Cytolytic proteinase	Tumoricidal
Components of complement pathways: C_1, C_2, Factor B, Factor D, Factor I	Antimicrobial, inflammatory, opsonic
Coagulation factors: Factor VII, Factor IX, Factor X, tissue factor	Coagulation, tissue repair
Angiotensin-converting enzyme	Activation of angiotensin
Acid hydrolases	
Arginase, lysozyme	Antimicrobial, tumoricidal, immuno-regulatory
Lipoprotein lipase	Metabolism of lipoproteins

B. Plasma proteins

Product	*Function*
Components of complement pathways: C_1, C_2, C_3, C_4, C_5, Factor B, Factor D, Factor I, Factor H, properdin	Antimicrobial, inflammatory, opsonic
Fibronectin	Opsonic, adhesive
Apoliprotein E	Cholesterol transport to liver
Transcobalamin II	Transport of Vitamin B_{12} to tissues
Coagulation factors: Factor VII, Factor IX, Factor X, Factor V	Coagulation, tissue repair
α_2-Macroglobulin	Regulation of plasma-enzyme activities

C. Cytokines

Product	*Function*
Interferons	Antiviral, immunoregulatory
Interleukin I	Acute phase response, tissue repair, inflammatory
Angiogenesis factor	Tissue repair
Granulocyte-monocyte colony-stimulating activity	Production of granulocytes and monocytes
Tumor necrosis factor/cachectin	Inflammatory, tumoricidal

D. Low-molecular-weight products

Product	*Function*
Superoxide: hydrogen peroxide:	Microbicidal, tumoricidal
Hydroxyl radical: singlet oxygen	Microbicidal, tumoricidal
Prostaglandins E_1, E_2	Inflammatory, immunoregulatory
Thromboxane B_2: leukotriene C_4	Inflammatory, immunoregulatory
Platelet-activating factor	Inflammatory, activates platelets
cAMP	Cellular regulation
Thymidine	Tumoricidal
Uracil: uric acid	Not known

Modified from the comprehensive review by Takemura and Werb (1984) Am. 9. Physiol. 246, (1–69)

[1] Guyre and Munck (1989) In "Anti-inflammatory steroid actions. Basic and clinical aspects", Academic Press pp 199–225

somes contain or are closely associated with freshly synthesized class-II molecules. Those fragments of the digested antigen which show an affinity for the class-II molecule bind to it and are subsequently transported to the cell surface where the complex is displayed for interaction with a T-cell. Fragments which, due to a lack of affinity, do not interact with class II molecules are taken up by lysosomes and degraded completely. Chloroquine and NH_4Cl inhibit antigen presentation. The reason for this phenomenon is twofold: both compounds are enriched in the acid vesicles of macrophages and both are also weak bases. Their accumulation in endosomes will therefore lead to a rise in pH within these vesicles which would critically disturb controlled degradation of proteins. In the case of chloroquine, this mechanism may well be the reason why this compound can be of therapeutic benefit in certain autoimmune diseases, particularly in rheumatoid arthritis. Whether there is any general structural 'pattern' according to which certain fragments bind to MHC class-II molecules and are presented while others do not bind and are degraded is at present not clear. One could envisage a model in which MHC class-II molecules are constantly recycling from the cell interior (acid vesicles) to the cell surface carrying 'self' determinants. Since the binding of young T-cells to class-I and II-antigens in association with 'self' components is a negative selection parameter during T-cell development in the thymus, such class-II 'self' complexes would not elicit an immune response. Any 'foreign' fragment with a stronger affinity to the class-II molecules, however, would disrupt this 'cycle' and displace an endogenous peptide from the class-II molecule. In doing so it would also – on account of its high affinity to MHC class II – alter the tertiary structure of the binding site and its environment and be subsequently recognized as 'foreign'.

The expression of class-II molecules on macrophages is transitory. It appears to be a feature of young cells. Eventually all macrophages become class II negative and, therefore, loose their antigen-presenting capacity. Prostaglandins in nanomolar concentration inhibit class II expression while γ-interferon clearly enhances the transcription of the MHC gene, which is needed for antigen presentation.

Macrophages are derived from blood monocytes. These in turn derive from bone marrow promonocytes, the precursor of which is a "colony-forming unit" (CFU-GM) from which both myeloblasts and promyelocytes can develop *(Fig. 2.16)*. Differentiation of a mature monocyte from this earliest monocyte precursor requires about three cell generations. In man, each cell cycle lasts two days. The mature monocytes leave the bone marrow 24 hours after the last division. Unlike the granulocytes, there is no reserve pool of mature monocytes in the marrow. After about 70 hours in the bloodstream, the mature monocytes migrate into the various organs and tissues. Their biological half-life in blood is 71 hours. The total number of monocytes circulating in the blood is about 1.7×10^9. Every hour, about 1.6×10^7 cells leave the bloodstream and start evolving into macrophages. Macrophages are found as Kupffer cells lining the sinusoids of the liver, and as splenic macrophages in the sinuses of the spleen. They are found in the bone marrow and play an important defensive role in the alveoli of the lung and in the peritoneal cavity. The extent to which the morphology of macrophages adapts to their location and its specific functional

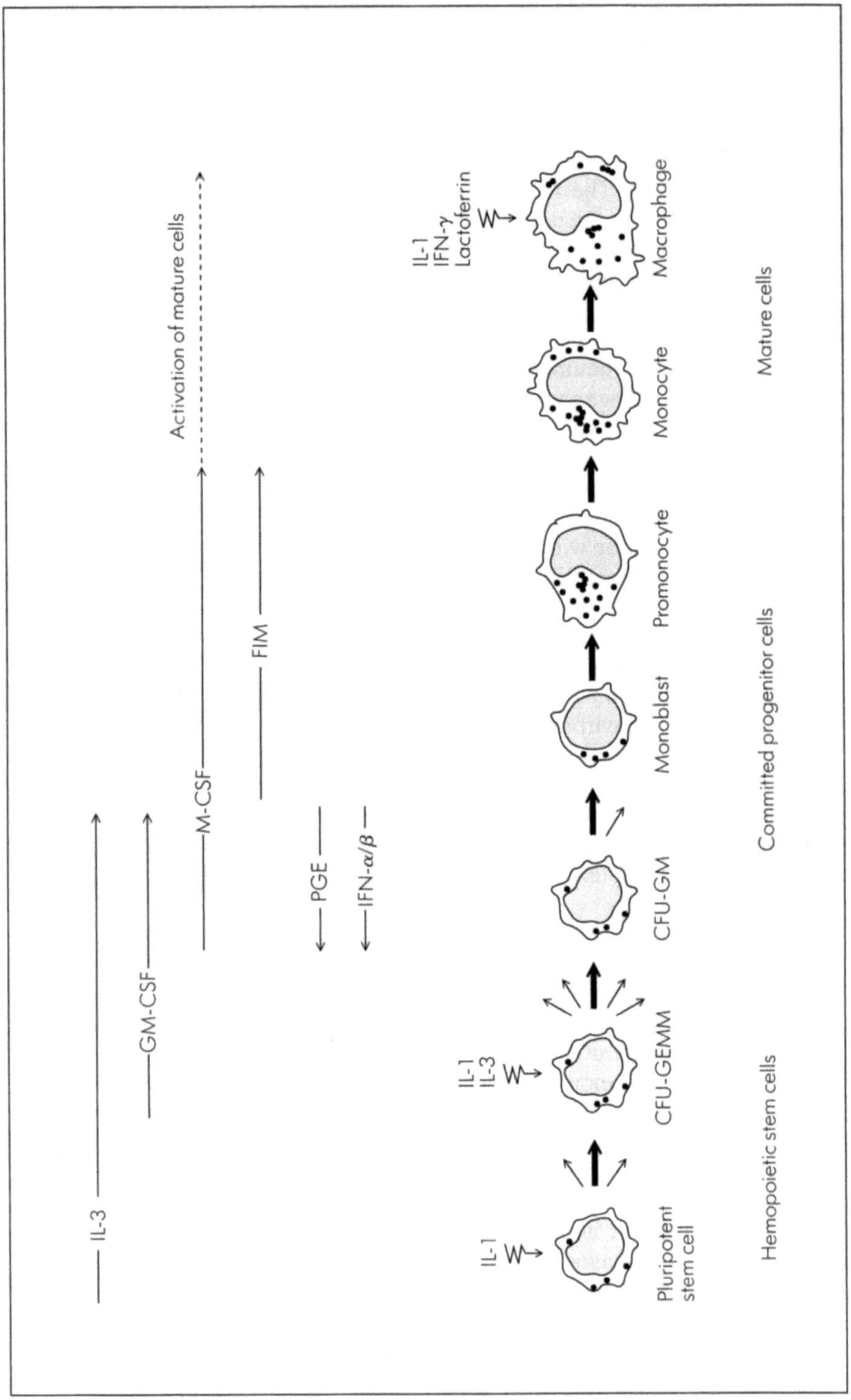
IL-3
GM-CSF
M-CSF
Activation of mature cells
FIM
PGE
IFN-α/β
IL-1
IL-1
IL-3
IL-1
IFN-γ
Lactoferrin
Pluripotent stem cell
CFU-GEMM
CFU-GM
Monoblast
Promonocyte
Monocyte
Macrophage
Hemopoietic stem cells
Committed progenitor cells
Mature cells

requirements is demonstrated by osteoclasts and giant cells from granulomas, both types being of monocytic origin and therefore varieties of macrophages. Dendritic cells and Langerhans' cells from subcutaneous tissue seem to be of particular importance for the presentation of antigen referred to earlier.

Macrophages are mobile cells, and their mobility is influenced by various endogenous substances (lymphokines, prostaglandins). Immature cells show a positive peroxidase reaction, but become peroxidase-negative with increasing age. Macrophages are long-lived, i.e. irrespective of location and function they can live for up to 40 days. What is more, alveolar macrophages are known to be able to renew themselves by division. Thus, once a population of alveolar macrophages has become established, it is no longer dependent on "reinforcements" from the bloodstream. The extent to which this "independence" also applies to the other types of macrophage is not known. Compared with granulocytes, lymphoblasts and plasma cells, macrophages are relatively resistant to ionizing radiation and cytostatics. In association with the functions of phagocytosis, secretion of lymphokines and cytotoxicity already mentioned, these properties make them an interesting target for stimulation by pharmaceutical agents, particularly in individuals who, as a result of partial failure of granulocyte- and lymphocyte-dependent functions, are susceptible to infection. This will be discussed in greater detail in a later chapter.

2.1.3 Neutrophils

Neutrophils (neutrophilic leucocytes) are the most important instruments used in the acute defence of the body against bacterial and fungal attack. This defence is based on three mechanisms: adherence, phagocytosis and secretory functions. Neutrophils are derived from a myeloid bone marrow stem cell by a clearly defined process of differentiation *(Fig. 2.17)*. A healthy adult produces between 10 and 15×10^{10} of these short-lived blood corpuscles daily; their half-life in blood is 6–20 hours and they are functionally competent in the tissue for a further 1–2 days. Neutrophils have the important ability to adhere to surfaces and to other cells. The molecules which mediate this adherence are a group of related cell-surface glycoproteins which comprise CR3, the receptor of a component of complement (C3b, see below) and two other receptors called LFA-1 and P 150,95. These molecules show common architectural features. Each of them has a distinct α-subunit in the 150000–180000 dalton range but they share a common β-subunit with a molecular weight of 150000 daltons. The

Figure 2.16. A schematic representation of factors controlling monocyte production in the bone marrow and maturation of monocytes to macrophages. Solid lines connect the relevant hematopoietic stages and thin arrows indicate the descendence of other hematopoietic cell lines, e.g. lymphocytes from pluripotent stem-cells. The arrows in the upper part of the figure indicate the influence of hematopoietic factors and its duration on cell differentiation. Arrows pointing to the right indicate stimulation, those pointing to the left inhibition of development. IL = interleukin; GM-CSF = granulocyte macrophage colony-stimulating factor, M-CSF = macrophage CSF; FIM = factor increasing monocytopoiesis. PGE = prostaglandin of the E series; IFN = interferon; CFU-GEMM = colony-forming units, capable of forming granulocyte-erythrocyte-monocyte-megakaryocyte progeny; CFU-GM = CFU, able to form granulocytes and macrophages.

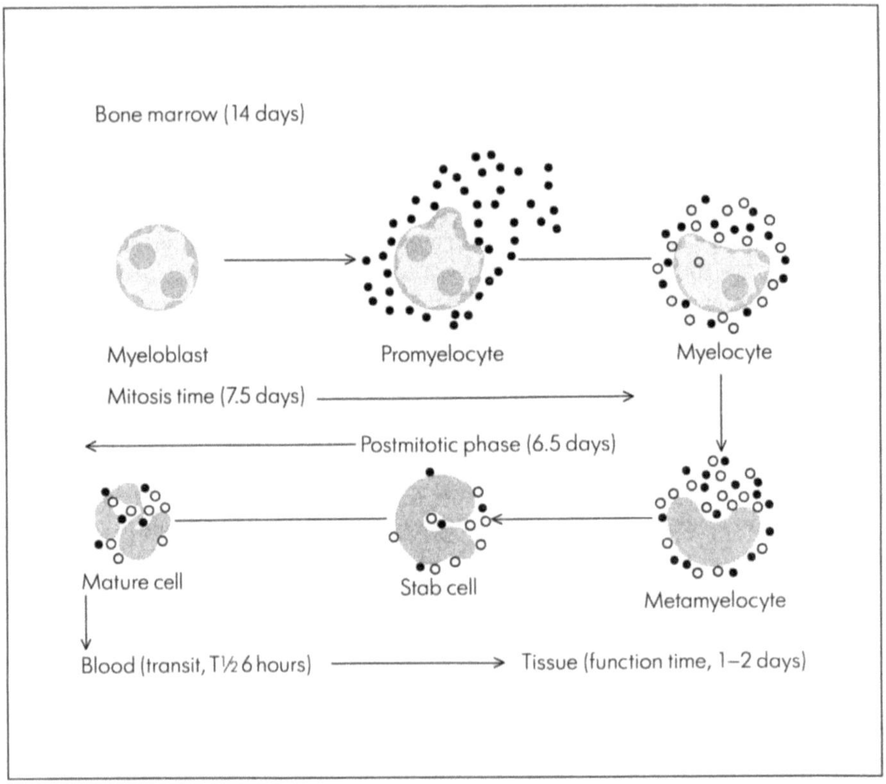

Figure 2.17. Maturation of human neutrophilic leukocytes. The black cytoplasmic granules represent the peroxidase-positive, primary or azurophilic granules. The open forms represent the peroxidase-negative, secondary or specific granules.

most important of these molecules appears to be CR3. This receptor has been shown to enhance the adherence and the phagocytosis of opsonized microorganisms. LFA-1 also improves adherence while the function of P 150,95 is not yet known. The physiological importance of adherence as a distinct function of neutrophils (and macrophages which also carry LFA-1) is illustrated by the fact that there is a rare autosomal recessive disorder which stems from the inability of the affected individuals to synthesize normal β subunits. These patients suffer from frequent skin infections, mucositis and otitis throughout childhood. Gingivitis and paradontosis often lead to a loss of teeth. Severe, even life-threatening bacterial or fungal infections like pneumonia may also occur intermittently.

Phagocytosis, the second major function of neutrophil is greatly facilitated by Fc receptors as well as by the complement receptor mentioned above. Other receptors like the one binding C5a, the soluble fragment of complement component 5 and N-formyl methionyl peptides convey chemoattractant stimuli which are exerted by these ligands. It has recently been shown that mammalian mitochondria produce N-formyl-methionyl peptides just like bacteria. This finding raises the strong possibility that mitochondrial leakage in damaged or hypoxic tissues may provide strong chemotactic signals even in the absence of bacterial infection.

The neutrophil precursors contain azurophilic granules initially stainable with acid dyes. Later, at the differentiation level of myelocytes, neutrophilic granules appear which are ultimately twice as numerous as the azurophilic cells and which confer upon the cell their staining reactions to acid and basic dyes but also their name. The two types of granules – primary azurophilic and secondary neutrophilic – can be readily separated by centrifugation in continuous saccharose gradients and then analysed. They contain different enzymes: the primary azurophilic granules are related to the lysosomes of other cells and therefore contain mainly acid hydrolases, while the secondary granules contain lactoferrin and vitamin B_{12}-binding protein in addition to lysozyme *(Table 2.3)*.

Myeloperoxidase is an important constituent of the primary granules. It is an iron-heme containing protein. In the presence of hydrogen peroxide and halide, myeloperoxidase produces hypochlorous acid and chlorine. Both of these products can be instrumental in destroying target cells. Hereditary myeloperoxidase deficiency, an autosomal recessive disorder is, surprisingly, not characterized by an increased proneness to bacterial infections. This is probably due to the compensatory functions of other microbicidal mechanisms. However, the respiratory burst in leucocytes from such patients is prolonged upon neutrophil activation. This finding offers an explanation for the absence of overt clinical symptoms in this disorder. At the same time, it points towards a modulating function of myeloperoxidase in the response of the neutrophil. Neutrophils lacking myeloperoxidase are, however, deficient in killing fungi.

A prominent constituent of the secondary (neutrophil) granule is lactoferrin, an important chelating agent for iron. Since iron is a prerequisite for bacterial growth the removal of this metal ion from a particular environment constitutes

Table 2.3. Constituents of granules from human neutrophils

Primary (azurophilic) granules	Secondary granules
Acid hydrolases	Lysozyme
– beta-glucuronidase	Lactoferrin
– acid beta-glycerophosphatase	Vitamin-B_{12}-binding protein
– N-acetyl-beta-glucosaminidase	Collagenase
– alpha-mannosidase	Acid proteins
– arylsulfatase	
– beta-galactosidase	
– 5'-nucleotidase	
– cathepsin D	
Neural proteases	
Chymotrypsin	
– elastase	
– collagenase	
Cationic proteins	
Myeloperoxidase	
Lysozyme	
Acid mucopolysaccharides	

an important antimicrobial defence mechanism. Lactoferrin also enhances the formation of hydroxyl radicals. Furthermore, it may help in the regulation of myelopoiesis by inhibiting the release of colony-stimulating factors from macrophages and monocytes.

All the granules are enveloped in a typical trilaminar membrane. The membranes of the secondary granules contain more phosphatidylethanolamine than the "primary" granules. The structural differences in the granules are matched by corresponding functional differences. While the phagocytosis of bacteria, the presence of bacterial toxins, or adsorption to opsonized surfaces ("frustrated phagocytosis") lead to exocytosis of primary and secondary particles, there are a number of chemical stimuli that effect almost exclusively the release of secondary granules to the outside *(Table 2.4)*. The substances that cause specific degranulation of this kind include, in particular, hydroxy-eicosatetraenoic acids (5-HETE and 12-HETE), i.e. products of the effect of lipoxygenase on arachidonic acid. Endogenous pyrogen, which is identical with interleukin 1, has the same effect. These in-vitro phenomena are confirmed by *in vivo* findings: sterile exudates contain collagenase, vitamin B_{12}-binding protein and lactoferrin in proportion to the number of neutrophils present at the site of inflammation. The release of secondary granules seems to occur at all functional stages of the neutrophils, i.e from diapedesis and adhesion to opsonized surfaces up to phagocytosis, while exocytosis of primary granules occurs only during phagocytosis and under the influence of toxic stimuli (lipopolysaccharides, crystals, O_2-metabolites).

Exocytosis of secondary granules may be considered a secretory function with which the cell can react to environmental changes within 30 minutes. Once emptied, the granules cannot be refilled. Nevertheless, neutrophils are, to a limited extent, able to synthesize RNA and protein. Secretion of mediators not found in the granules, e.g. leukocyte pyrogen, chemotactic factor or plasminogen activator, can be suppressed by inhibitory substances of protein synthesis. Radioactive amino acids are incorporated in vitro into these molecules by neutrophils.

The phagocytic and humoral stimuli that lead to exocytosis of secondary granules and to synthesis and secretion of non-granule-bound proteins also trigger the release of oxygen metabolites, i.e. H_2O_2, superoxide anion, OH- and singlet oxygen. This respiratory burst is generated by a number of electron transfers in which NADPH serves as the electron donor and a flavoprotein containing flavin-adenine dinucleotide. A quinone and a unique cytochrome b558 are the other partners. Cytochrome b558 has a molecular weight of 22,000. It is normally attached to a 91,000 dalton protein which is membrane associated. There are forms of chronic granulomatous disease, an x-chromosome linked hereditary disorder in which the gene coding for the transmembrane protein is defective. In these cases the cytochrome b558 does not function properly. These findings indicate that the enzymatic tools required for production of oxygen radicals are closely associated with the plasma membrane of the neutrophils. This in turn means that, during neutrophil activation, oxygen radicals are also released towards the outside of the cell. In this way neutrophils can kill certain bacteria such as gram-positive cocci extracellularly. Activation of phospholipase

Table 2.4. Stimuli causing exocytosis of granules

Stimulus	Primary granules	Secondary granules
Phagocytosis	++	+++
Adsorption to opsonized, non-phagocytosable surfaces	+++	+++
Bacterial toxins	+++	+++
Nonspecific adsorption	±	++
Hydroxy-eicosatetranoic acids	–	++
Calcium ionophores	+	+++
Calcium-dependent spontaneous exocytosis	–	+
Lectin	–	+++

and biotransformation of the arachidonic acid liberated by this enzyme result in the synthesis by neutrophils of hydroxy-eicosatetraenoic acids, of type E and F prostaglandins, and of thromboxane. The HETE derivatives in particular give rise to the specific degranulation already described and are therefore part of the "reinforcement" effect.

What is the physiological significance of the neutral proteases that enter the tissues on exocytosis of secondary granules? Considering the destructive role played by these enzymes in certain chronic inflammatory diseases such as rheumatoid arthritis, their evolutionary function might well be questioned. We must, however, assume that neutrophils are primarily cells of acute inflammation and that the enzymes they secrete are also functionally active primarily in this context. The neutral proteases have an "insulating" effect which can prevent the spread of an inflammatory process. Generally speaking, the functions listed in *Table 2.5* can be equated with the secretory functions of neutrophils.

So far we have been discussing the secretory signals that are sent out by the actual neutrophil involved in defensive acute inflammatory reactions. We must, however, bear in mind that this cell is itself the target of regulatory mechanisms emanating from other cells, including those of the immune system. Cells of monocytic origin secrete a factor that activates neutrophils and at the same time restricts their mobility (NAF, see chapter 6). By means of such signals, neutrophils are also functionally involved in chronic inflammatory processes.

In summary, neutrophils can be characterized as cells that specialize in keeping the tissues free from intruding bacteria by means of phagocytosis, secretion of antimicrobially active oxygen metabolites, and by the rapid release of large numbers of tissue-degrading enzymes.

The enzymes secreted by neutrophils are regionally active, though some proteins not contained in the granules, e.g. leucocyte pyrogen, also have sys-

Table 2.5. Effects of the secretory function of neutrophils on defence reactions

Extracellular antimicrobial activity
Elimination of infected cells
Modulation and amplification of inflammatory reactions
Release of mediators for stimulation of myelopoiesis
Recruitment of monocytes to the site of inflammation

temic effects. Neutrophils react to a variety of stimuli emanating from microorganisms or from damaged tissue. Afferent and efferent humoral signals link them with other cells of the immune system.

2.1.4 Eosinophilic granulocytes

The neutrophilic granulocyte may be regarded as an indicator of acute inflammatory processes, which serve to eliminate bacteria rapidly from the body. It might even be said that the specific functions of the neutrophils are the provisional outcome of an evolutionary adaptation made by higher organisms to the constant threat posed by bacteria. In contrast, the existence and the special functions of the eosinophilic granulocytes can be seen as the result of defence mechanisms against *parasitic invasion.* These mechanisms developed during evolution and have since been steadily improved. The reactions triggered by parasites such as helminths, schistosomes, trichinae and cercariae comprise, on the one hand, immediate-type hypersensitivity, elicited by the interaction of IgE antibodies with Fc_{ε} receptors of mast cells and basophils and the consequent release of mediators, and, on the other, chronic granulomatous inflammation, mediated by antigen-specific T-cell activation followed by the release of lymphokines and the recruitment to the inflammatory site of macrophages, histiocytes and eosinophils.

The eosinophilic granulocyte exhibits granules which stain with eosin by virtue of their cationic properties. This staining is due to the presence of several cationic proteins. *Table 2.6* gives a short overview. The most prominent cationic protein is the major basic protein which forms the core of the eosinophilic granules. In direct in-vitro comparisons this protein appears to have the strongest toxic effect on newborn larvae of trichinella spiralis and on other worms. At concentrations of 5×10^{-5} M, major basic protein killed close to

Table 2.6. Properties of principal eosinophil, granule proteins

Name	Molecular weight ($\times 10^{-3}$)	pl	Activities	Site
MBP	10 (man) 11 (guinea pig)	>11	Toxic to parasiters, murine tumor cells, many mammalian cells; causes histamine release from basophils and rat mast cells, neutralizes heparin	Core
ECP	21	>11	Shortens coagulation time, alters fibrinolysis; toxic to parasites; potent neurotoxin; inhibits cultures of peripheral blood lymphocytes; causes histamine release from rat mast cells	Matrix
EDN	17.9	Basic	Potent neurotoxin	Matrix
EPX	18	Basic	Neurotoxin; inhibits cultures of peripheral blood lymphocytes; toxic to parasites	
EPO	71–77 (man) 75 (horse)	>11	In the presence of H_2O_2 + halide kills microorganisms and tumor cells, initiates mast cell secretion, inactivates leukotrienes, causes histamine release from rat mast cells	Matrix

100% of the larvae within one hour. At the same concentration eosinophilic cationic protein had a lethal effect on these organisms only after three hours of incubation while eosinophil-derived neurotoxin (EDN) was distinctly less toxic in this situation. All of the cationic granule proteins can be secreted by exocytosis and have been found deposited on the surface of parasites after exposure of these organisms to eosinophilic cells.

Eosinophils develop from stem cells, which differ from the neutrophilic precursor cell (the promyelocyte). From maturation to release, mature eosinophils spend about 63 hours in the human bone marrow; the subsequent sojourn in blood is 3–8 hours. In normal circumstances, the concentration of eosinophilic granulocytes in blood is 450–700 per μl. The cells then migrate into tissue, primarily subepithelial connective tissue of the skin, bronchi, gastrointestinal tract and vagina.

During acute inflammatory episodes, eosinopenia occurs as a result of rapid margination of circulating eosinophils, chemotactically induced migration to the focus of inflammation and inhibition of the release of mature eosinophils from the marrow. High-molecular-weight glycoproteins which cause eosinopenia can be isolated from inflammatory exudate. Such substances might be involved in the pathogenesis of eosinopenia. Rising eosinophil concentrations in blood and their overrepresentation at the site of inflammations of metazoal etiology are caused by a number of factors, some of them with acute, others with protracted effects. Recent studies have shown that GM-CSF, the colony-stimulating factor which acts on the progenitor of granulocytes and monocytes also influences eosinophils in culture. It maintains their viability in a concentration-dependent fashion, increases their ability to generate a leukotriene (LTC-4) and stimulates the antibody-dependent killing of *S. mansoni* larvae by a factor of seven when compared with freshly isolated unstimulated cells. It is generally assumed that GM-CSF acts on early committed precursors of eosinophils.

Il-5, the so called T-cell replacement factor or B-cell differentiation factor II (Mr 20,000 daltons), is at present the best candidate for a specific eosinophilic colony-stimulating or differentiation factor. The relationship of this factor to other proteins which have been described as stimulators of eosinophil proliferation and activity is not yet clear.

Both factors are produced only if an intact population of T-lymphocytes is present. The production of these factors may be directly influenced by T-helper cells. The in-vivo increase of eosinophils in the blood correlates with the in-vitro kinetics. Mice which have been sensitized to antigens from trichinae develop eosinophilia two days after renewed exposure to the antigen.

If lymphocytes from the thoracic duct of sensitized mice are transferred to normal animals, the latter also develop eosinophilia within two days. The present interpretation of these findings is that certain T-lymphocytes are activated by metazoal antigens to release specific cytokines, among them Il-5 and GM-CSF. Within a short space of time, these substances enforce maturation of highly differentiated precursor cells and, at the same time, stimulate proliferation of early precursor cells. These effects result in enhanced release of newly formed eosinophils after one to two weeks.

As mentioned above, eosinophils are instrumental in two types of tissue reaction: immediate-type hypersensitivity and chronic granulomatous inflammation. In the first reaction basophilic granulocytes and mast cells play the main role, in the second one lymphocytes dominate. Immediate-type hypersensitivity is caused by IgE antibodies which occupy Fc_{ε} receptors on mast cells and basophils. When cytophilic antigens bind to these cell-located antibodies, the ensuing conformational change of the antibody molecules is translated into a biochemical signal which causes the release of mediator substances contained in the cell granules. These mediators include three types of substance which act on eosinophils: chemotactic substances such as eosinophil chemotactic factor of anaphylaxis, (ECF-A) whose activity can also be generated by two acidic tetrapeptides with the sequences Ala-Gly-Ser-Glu or Val-Gly-Ser-Glu. These substances act chemotactically on eosinophils, i.e. they cause eosinophils to accumulate at the site at which an antigen has penetrated the body and reacted with cell-bound IgE antibodies. A second set of chemotactic molecules is derived from arachidonic acid. Cyclooxygenase in mast cells gives rise primarily to the synthesis of prostaglandin PGD_2, a potent chemokinetic factor for eosinophils. It is known that this prostaglandin possesses very marked bronchoconstrictor properties. Finally, histamine, which is released from the granules of basophils, stimulates the migration of eosinophilic granulocytes at concentrations of 3×10^{-7} to 10^{-6} M. At higher concentrations, however, this mediator has an inhibitory effect on eosinophil migration. This is also true of chemokinetic activities, which are mediated by the complement fraction C5a or by other chemotactic factors.

The relationship between mast cell degranulation and accumulation of eosinophils is also apparent morphologically. The skin of monkeys immunized with parasitic antigens exhibits, after another injection of cercariae of the liver fluke *Schistosoma japonicum,* small vessels surrounded by degranulated mast cells; the vessel wall is penetrated by eosinophilic granulocytes. With respect to chronic inflammation, there is apparently a connection between the secretion of lymphokines by lymphocytes which are stimulated by specific parasitic antigens, and glycoprotein recruitment of eosinophils, which are found in particular at the margins of granulomas. If lymphocytes are cultivated in vitro from patients with parasitic infestation and the cell supernatants injected into healthy volunteers, eosinophil infiltrates are created. The substances responsible for this reaction are possibly identical with ESP (eosinophil stimulation promoter), a glycoprotein produced by T-cells with a molecular weight of 25 kd.

Eosinophils are less markedly bactericidal than neutrophils. It is not quite clear which factor is responsible for this difference. Discussion has centred on differences in the peroxidase systems which produce oxygen metabolites. Eosinophilic granulocytes, however, have an efficient battery of defence mechanisms against parasites such as schistosomes, helminths, trichinae, etc. These mechanisms act through the peroxidase systems mentioned above and through major basic protein (MBP), which is perhaps more important but at any rate *typical of eosinophils.* This protein, which has a molecular weight of 16,000 daltons under reducing conditions in SDS gels, is a component of the granules of eosinophils. The basicity of this molecule is based on the presence of 13 mol of arginine. The molecule contains two SH groups, which lead to the formation of polymers through the formation of -S-S bridges under oxidative conditions. This property makes it difficult to investigate the molecule in vitro, but it could also be the key to understanding the biological action of MBP: a rapid and irreversible reaction with membrane proteins might explain why eosinophils which have deposited MBP on the surface of a parasite become irreversibly bound to the parasite. MBP is a toxic protein not only for parasites but also for the cells of the host. Since infiltration of the bronchial submucosa with eosinophils is one of the histological features of bronchial asthma, mucosal damage, in particular damage to the ciliary function, has been attributed to the secretion and action of MBP. Both in-vitro experiments, in which the action of the basic protein on the mucosal structure and function of tracheal rings was investigated, and clinical findings point to a pathophysiological role of MBP in bronchial asthma. Further investigations are necessary, however, to confirm this. The morphological findings in mammalian cells, particularly in ciliated epithelia of the bronchial mucosa, suggest that this protein impairs the function of contractile proteins belonging to the cellular skeleton.

2.1.5 Mast cells and basophils

Mast cells which are in many ways similar to the basophilic granulocytes of the bloodstream are ubiquitous cells which are mainly found at the interface of the environment and the organism. These cells are located in particularly high numbers just beneath mucosal surfaces and in the subepithelial layers of the skin. One finds them also in the meninges and in the connective tissue sheaths surrounding blood vessels and nerves.

Under the microscope, mast cells exhibit large numbers of granules which stain with basic dyes. The granules contain heparin or an oversulfated proteoglycan known as chondroitin sulfate di-B. They also contain histamine or, in rodents, serotonin (5-hydroxytryptamine), chemotactic factors and a large number of enzymes, among which three groups can be differentiated: acid hydrolases, enzymes which generate and detoxify oxygen like peroxidase and superoxide dismutase and neutral proteases. The acid hydrolases like β-hexoseaminidase, arylsulfatases A and B and proteases like trypsin and chymotrypsin do not selectively occur in mast cells. However, there are two major enzymes located in the secretory granules of mast cells which can be regarded as specific markers of these cells and their subsets. These enzymes are chymase and tryptase – not to be confused with chymotrypsin and trypsin. Both are serine esterases. Chymase seems to exist as a monomer with a molecular weight of 30,000; tryptase contains two subunits α and β with molecular weights of 34,000 and 33,000 respectively. The intact enzyme ($\alpha 2\beta 2$) has a molecular weight of 134,000 daltons. The function of these two mast-cell specific enzymes is not clear. They can, however, be used to divide human mast cells into subsets. One subset (T) contains only tryptase, the other one (TC) contains both enzymes. T and TC mast cells appear to be roughly comparable to those subsets defined in rats as mucosal and connective tissue type mast cells. The names indicate the location where these cell types are found. The human T-subset like the rat mucosal mast cell is mainly found in mucosal membranes as well as in bronchi and in alveoli, whereas the TC-type corresponding to the connective tissue subset in rats, is predominant in the submucosa and skin. Both enzymes have a strong affinity for heparin and other proteoglycans.

The biological functions of tryptase and chymase have not been elucidated. The fact, however, that tryptase generates the anaphylatoxin C3a from complement component 3 indicates a possible role of this enzyme in mediating anaphylactic responses. Chymase has the activity of an angiotensin converting enzyme; it splits angiotensin 2 from angiotensin 1. The vasoconstricting activity of chymase-generated angiotensin 2 may well attenuate mucosal edema generated by histamine, by leukotrienes, PGD_2 or platelet activating factor. The presence of chymase may thus lead to an attenuation of acute inflammatory responses and bring an element of chronicity to such reactions. Within minutes after a signal which triggers degranulation the contents of the granules can be delivered to the environment.

Mast cells and basophils have high affinity Fc receptors for IgE antibodies on their surface. These "homocytotropic" antibodies bind to Fc receptors with extraordinary tenacity. IgG molecules are also capable of binding; but after subcutaneous injection they are demonstrable on the mast cell surface for about a day only. When cell-bound antibodies are cross-linked by an antigen, the Fc region undergoes a change in conformation which induces a membrane signal. This not precisely defined signal causes an influx of calcium ions into the cell. Factors that promote or inhibit mast cell degranulation are relatively well understood. A common denominator of some of them is changes in the concentration of cyclic nucleotides: an increase in the concentration of cGMP and a decrease in that of intracellular cAMP cause degranulation. High cAMP concentrations, however, have a stabilizing effect on the granules. The biochemical details of mast cell degranulation are dealt with in the section on antiallergic substances (Chapter 5). Alpha-adrenergic and cholinergic stimuli cause degranulation while β-adrenergic agonists and prostaglandins inhibit degranulation. *Fig. 5.4* provides an overview of the most important pharmacological factors influencing degranulation.

It has recently been shown that the exocytosis which leads to degranulation is absolutely dependent on two parameters only: a rise in intracellular calcium over the resting level of about 10^{-7} M and on GTP or a stable analogue of this nucleotide. ATP shifts the concentration curves for both 'activators' to the left: it 'sensitizes' the mast cell but does not serve as a trigger for degranulation.

Substances originating in the granules almost all cause an acute (histamine, serotonin) or chronic increase in cell contractility. Since this contraction also affects capillary endothelial cells, extravasation of fluid and cells, i.e edema formation and migration of cells, occurs in the regions of the mast cell degranulation.

The proliferation and differentiation pathways of mast cells are not too well understood. Apparently T-cell-dependent lymphokines like Il-3 are needed for both proliferation and differentiation but some of the factors necessary for the maturation and activation of mast cells are not well characterized. Mast cells are morphologically and functionally influenced by their environment. It was already mentioned that there seem to be several subsets. It has been shown in mast cells from dogs and rats that these subsets reacted to different triggers with varying patterns of response. Dog mastocytoma cells will excrete only histamine when challenged with substance 48/80 but will respond with generation of arachidonic metabolites when exposed to 15-hydroxy-eicosatetraenoic acid (15-HETE). An antigenic stimulus or the calcium binding agent 23187 will, in contrast, lead to the excretion of both groups of mediators. The physiological differences between mast cells in various anatomical locations may offer a chance for the selective treatment of allergic conditions which occur at different sites.

Recent investigations have supported the hypothesis that mast cells are involved not only in anaphylactic reactions but also in the development of allergic reactions of the delayed type (DTH, delayed-type hypersensitivity). In the supernatants of purified T-cells isolated from immunized mice, a factor was identified which effects antigen-specific sensitization of mast cells. This sensitization is not IgE-dependent, and is also of shorter duration than that effected by IgE. The two types of sensitization have, however, some points in common: peak antigen-specific cutaneous hypersensitivity is reached after two hours in both cases. Neither of the two forms can be triggered in mast-cell-deficient mice (W/W^v and SI/SI^d), and both reactions can be inhibited by serotonin antagonists such as methysergide.

In trying to assign a physiological key role to mast cells one could perhaps say the following: *mast cells have the main task of removing allergens of primary toxic potential which may enter the body via the skin or the mucous membranes. They also seem to be closely connected with tissue repair: mast cells are frequently found in association with scars, callus formation in bone and rheumatoid synovitis.*

2.1.6. NK- and K-cells

About 2–6% of circulating human leucocytes belong to the morphological category of large granular lymphocytes (LGL). They have kidney-shaped nuclei, a relatively (for lymphocytes) high ratio of cytoplasmic to nuclear volume, and prominent cytoplasmic granulation, though the granules are not so densely packed as in mast cells or eosinophilic granulocytes. These cells can be isolated through discontinuous Percoll gradients with a high degree of purity. Together with erythrocytes they form rosettes of low affinity. This means that the greater part of these cells form rosettes with erythrocytes at 4 °C, whereas T_G-cells, i.e. T-lymphocytes that carry Fc receptors, can still form rosettes at 29 °C. In vitro, the cells associated with the LGL-fraction exert a lytic effect on a number of different tumour cells. This activity is independent of any form of sensitization by tumour cell antigens and is not restricted by histocompatibility antigens or species barriers. Cells possessing these properties are called "natural killer" cells (NK-cells). A second form of activity is, however, associated with the LGL-group: antibody-dependent, cell-mediated cytotoxicity (ADCC). This activity is observed only in the presence of IgG antibodies to certain target cells. Cells exerting this form of activity were originally called "killer" cells (K-cells). Today, however, most authors are of the opinion that NK-and K-cells are identical, i.e. that one and the same population of large granular lymphocytes exhibits both forms of cytotoxicity. The main arguments for this theory come from experimental results. In all cases of separation by density gradient centrifugation, the two activities were absolutely parallel and were found in the same cell fractions. It may therefore be assumed either that the same cells mediate both K- and NK-activity or that cells which are identical in morphology and density mediate either one or the other function.

The origin of NK-and K-cells is still not entirely clear. The surface receptors expressed on these cells could point in the direction of monocytic cells (Qa-3, Qa-4, Qa-5) or towards an association of NK-cells with the T-cell lineage. One surface structure NK-1 (Leu 7) seems to be fairly but not absolutely NK-cell specific.

Biochemical features, e.g. the occurrence of NaF-resistant α-naphthyl acetate esterase, an enzyme typical of T-cells, also suggest that NK-cells are close to T-lymphocytes. Another tentative piece of evidence for the association of NK-cells with the T-cell lineage was recently produced by the finding that the β chain of the Il-2 receptor (Il-2 Rβ) which is also called the p70 subunit of this receptor is expressed on the large granular lymphocyte fraction in quantities, proportional to the sensitivity of these cells to Il-2. It has been shown that p70 can bind Il-2 alone and can subsequently associate with the smaller Il-2 receptor (p55) to form the high affinity structure. In NK-cells, Il-2 is first bound by p70 which is expressed in 'resting' cells. The complex between p70 and Il-2 may be sufficient to induce the first phase of the induction of lymphokine activated killer cells (LAK-cells) from NK-cells. At a later stage, the Il-2 Rα-chain is also expressed so that fully induced LAK-cells now carry the complete high affinity receptor.

Some rat LGL-lines which possess NK-activity were shown to express aberrant transcripts of the β chain of the T-cell receptor comprising only 1000 base-pairs. This finding – also arguing in favor of a T-cell relationship for NK-cells – has prompted the suggestion that NK-cells may be pre-T-cells that acquired all the functional effector mechanisms but which never developed the proper recognition instruments typical of mature T-cells.

Our understanding of the mechanism by which NK-cells recognize and lyse their targets is far from complete. At present, the single steps belonging to this sequence of events can be described at a phenomenological rather than at a mechanistic level. The NK-cell first has to bind to its target cell via an NK receptor which recognizes particular structures on a target cell. What exactly these structures are is not known. Transferrin receptors which are present on all rapidly dividing cells have been implicated as features to which NK-cells react. On YAC-cells, three species of glycosylated proteins with molecular weights in the range of 130, 160 and 240 kd seem to be recognized by the NK receptor, the structure of which is also not known. After the contact between the NK-cell and its target cell has been established, granules within the NK-cells are oriented towards the site of binding. Subsequently, granules from the effector cells are released at or close to the attachment site. The final step is the actual lysis of the target cell. Lysis is probably caused by a highly lipophilic protein from NK-cell granules which 'punches' holes or circular channels into the plasma membrane of the target cell through which water and electrolytes can pass unhindered. These membrane defects may in themselves suffice to kill the target cell. Alternatively they may provide easy access for a 'cytotoxic factor' (NKCF) which is also produced by activated NK-cells (see above).

Besides their cytotoxic properties, NK- or LGL-cells have secretory functions. They secrete a number of lymphokines, including interleukin-1 and interleukin-2, α- and γ-interferons, colony stimulating factor (CSF) and a B-cell growth factor (BCGF). The significance of these secretory properties has not yet been elucidated. NK function is known to be enhanced by interleukin-2 and γ-interferon. Possibly, then, the lymphokines secreted by NK-cells are "self-activating". According to C. Brooks, interleukin-2 acts via the activation of γ-interferon secretion by NK-cells (see below). But the secretory signals emanating from NK-cells possibly have other immunoregulatory functions: there have been a number of reports that NK-cells inhibit growth of myeloid cells and, conversely, promote proliferation of erythrocytic precursor cells.

NK-cells are also subject to regulatory impulses emanating from other cells. For instance, the cytotoxicity of NK-cells is inhibited by the prostaglandins, particularly PGE_2 and PGD_2 released by activated macrophages and monocytes. Granulocytes have a similar effect on NK-cells. It is not quite clear whether NK-cells play a role in vivo, for instance in the destruction of tumour cells or virally infected cells. Two findings from animal experiments suggest that NK-cells do play a genuine role: firstly, mice with a genetic defect that impairs the cytotoxic potential of their NK-cells are particularly susceptible to tumour growth. Secondly, NK-cell clones which were allowed to proliferate in vitro in the presence of interleukin-2 inhibit the growth and metastasis of tumour cells in vivo. Diminished NK-cell activity has been found in patients with various types of leukemia or other lymphoproliferative diseases. Whether this is a result or a cause of the malignant disease is open to debate. But it is noteworthy that this diminished NK-cell activity is found even in patients with preleukemic syndromes.

It has recently been postulated that NK-cells play a role in 'immunological surveillance'. If – as Lewis Thomas has claimed – a surveillance mechanism which ensures the universal requirements of multicellular organisms to preserve uniformity of cell type and to prevent mutant cells from "colonising and flourishing" represents an evolutionary advantage for higher organisms, then NK-cells might indeed be logical candidates for playing a role in such system. This point must, however, still be regarded as speculative. In view of the fact that the majority of tumours occur after the reproductive phase of a given individual, one might even doubt whether natural defenses against tumours could be selected in evolution. Defences against bacteria and parasites, on the other hand, are definitely effective for the survival of many mammalian species and should therefore have been selected.

2.2 Humoral components of the immune system

2.2.1 The structure and function of antibodies

Antibodies are products of B-cells. They are initially synthesized as membrane-proteins, the two antigen-binding arms of which are "outwardly" directed. After interaction between these membrane-bound antibodies, which function as receptors, and antigen, soluble antibodies are produced which leave the cell. Thus, there are two types of antibody molecules, membrane-bound and secreted, which differ in the structure of their heavy chains. All membrane-bound antibodies have a connecting peptide, a hydrophobic transmembrane sequence and a cytoplasmic tail at the carboxyl-terminal end of their heavy chain. In contrast, the heavy chains of secreted antibodies terminate with that domain of their constant region which is closest to their C-terminal end. The additional information which is necessary to achieve anchoring of a heavy chain in the membrane is contained in two exons which are located down-stream of the last exon of the constant region *(Fig. 2.18)*. In mature plasma cells transcription terminates at a point just down-stream of exon C_4. The exons specifying the synthesis of the membrane-spanning domain remain untranscribed. In developing B-cells, however, transcription terminates down-stream of the two additional exons M1 and M2. An RNA region spanning part of C_4, the sequences between C_4 and M1 as well as the nucleotide sequence between M1 and M2 is then removed by RNA splicing. Thus the synthesis of membrane-bound versus secreted antibodies is regulated by a balance of two different mechanisms: termination of transcription at alternative sites and the alternative use of different RNA cleavage sites during the splicing process. The latter mechanism seems to play the main role in the regulation of membrane versus secreted γ-globulins. In other words: γ-genes seem to be transcribed including the M1 and M2 exons. Whether a secreted or membrane-bound antibody is synthesized is then largely dependent on the use of alternative splicing pathways.

Antibodies consist of two "heavy" chains (440 amino acids) and two "light" chains (220 amino acids) which are linked by a "hinge" region and several disulphide bridges to form a Y-shaped molecule. Both the light and the heavy chains consist of constant (at the COOH-terminal) and variable regions (at the NH_2-terminal) *(Fig. 2.19)*. The heavy chains are linked by two -S-S bonds at the "hinge region". The light and the heavy chains are each linked by an -S-S bond: an antibody molecule thus consists of four disulphide bonds which ensure interbonding of the peptide chains. In addition to these disulphide bonds *between* the chains, however, there are also intrachain -S-S bonds, which form

---

Figure 2.18 Expression of membrane-bound versus secreted IgM antibody. The example refers to results obtained with the gene for the murine μ chain. Dashed lines indicate splicing events, e.g. the removal of RNA from the primary transcripts. The vertical dashed lines S within C4 describe the RNA splicing site for M1 (membrane-bound form). The solid vertical arrows indicate potential points for the termination of transcription for both forms of primary transcript. L = leader sequence; TATA and OCT, regulatory signals; V = variable, D = diversity, J = joining region; M1 and M2 = membrane exons. The dots indicate polyadenylation signals.

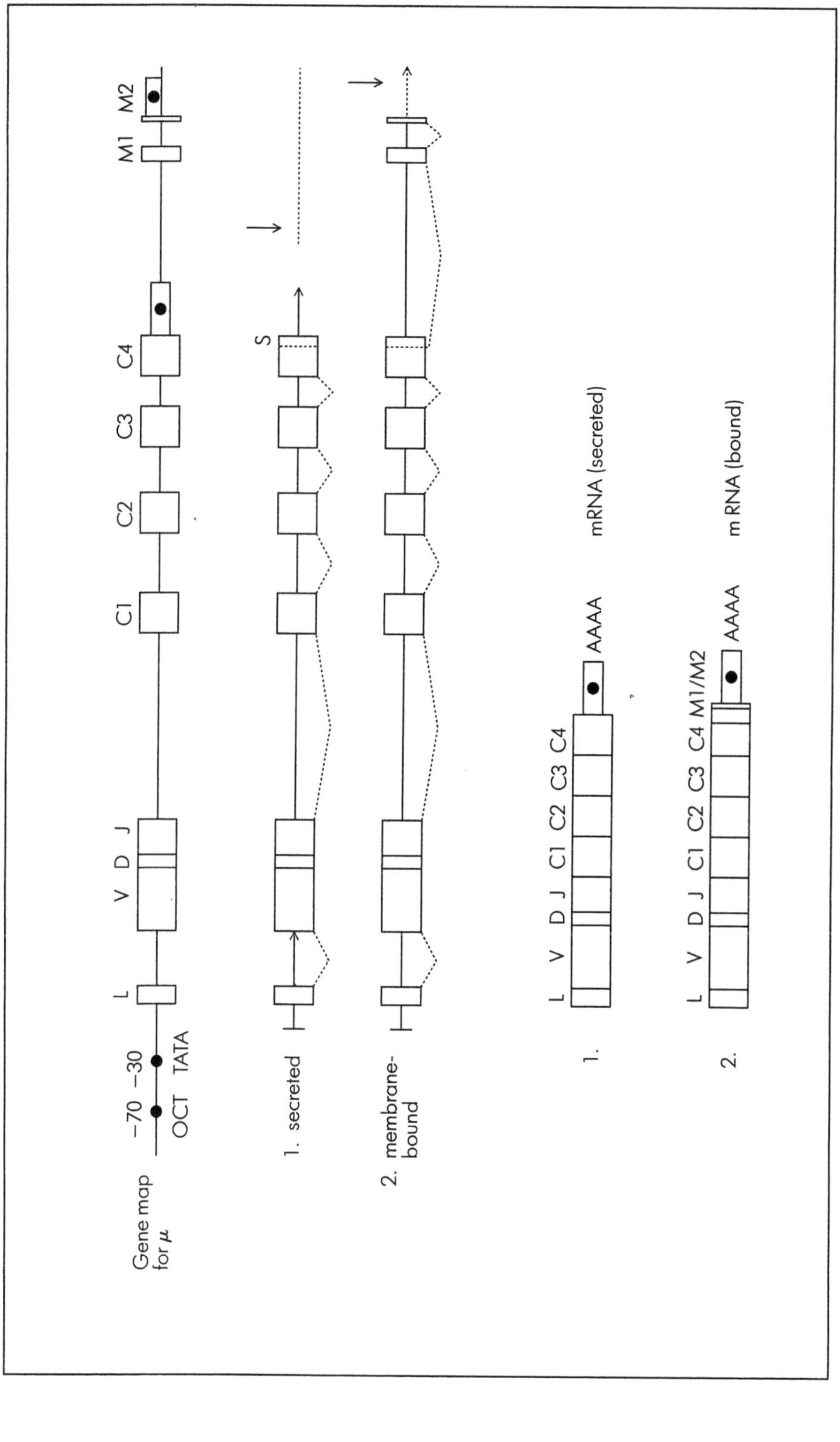
Gene map for μ
−70 −30
OCT TATA
L
V D J
C1
C2
C3
C4
M1 M2
1. secreted
S
2. membrane-bound
1.
L V D J C1 C2 C3 C4
AAAA
mRNA (secreted)
2.
L V D J C1 C2 C3 C4 M1/M2
AAAA
m RNA (bound)

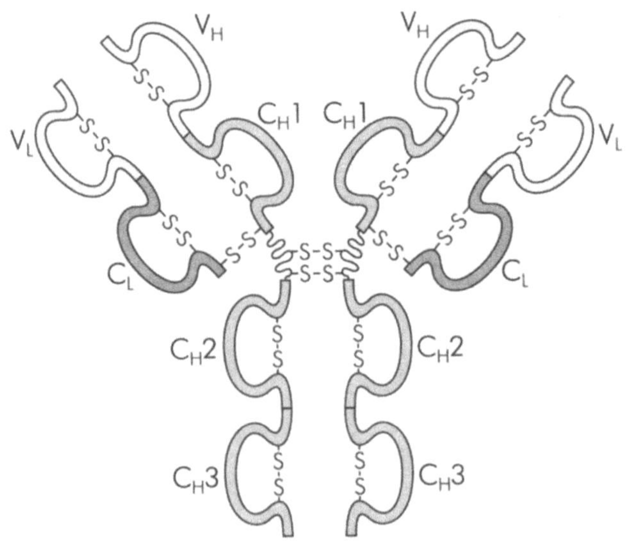

Figure 2.19. Schematic diagram of an antibody molecule. The heavy and the light chains are folded into domains. The variable domains of the light and heavy chains V_L and V_H are the sites at which antigen is bound. The constant domains of the heavy chains (mainly C_H2 and C_H3) are responsible for further biological properties of the molecule (see Chapter 3). The heavy chains of IgM and IgE have an additional constant domain (C_H4).

four loops in the heavy chains and two in the light chains. These loops are also known as domains. The amino acids are densely packed within these domains by hydrophobic interactions. Each domain has its particular function: because of the variability of their amino acid sequences, the V_H and V_L domains form the antigen-binding portion.

Inspection of many variable region sequences shows that the diversity of each type of receptor chain is concentrated in three hypervariable regions. These regions are also called complementarity determining regions (CDR) because, at least in antibodies, they have been shown to contain the amino acids which form the noncovalent contacts with the antigen. CDR 1 and CDR 2 are encoded by sequences within the V-segments, while CDR 3 segments are encoded by the VJ or VDJ joining regions.

The CH_2 domain in the IgG molecule is the binding site for C1q, the complement component with which the complement cascade starts, while the CH_3 domain is responsible for binding of an antibody to its Fc receptor. As homology in the amino acid sequences of the domains suggests, these domains originated from gene duplications. The proteolytic enzymes papain and pepsin split antibody molecules into several characteristic fragments (see Chapter 3, *Fig. 3.2*).

Papain splits the heavy chains at the N-terminal of the -S-S bonds that unite them, giving rise to two individual Fab ("fragment antigen binding") fragments and one Fc ("fragment crystallizable") fragment, so called because of its tendency to form crystals. Pepsin also cleaves in the "hinge" region, though "below" the -S-S bond, i.e. nearer the carboxyl-terminal, thus leaving a $F(ab')_2$ fragment of which the two antigen-binding arms are still linked by the disulphide bonds between the heavy chains. This $F(ab')_2$ fragment can still combine with antigen and therefore precipitate with antigen. It does not, however, have the Fc fragment, which is broken down into small units. This, of course, eliminates the biological functions of this antibody part: binding to macrophages or granulocytes by way of their Fc receptors, and the ability to activate complement (see also chapter 3).

It has already been stated that all antibodies consist of two identical heavy and two identical light chains. There are five classes of heavy chain: γ, α, μ, δ and ε. Since the physicochemical and the functional properties of an antibody molecule are determined by the heavy chains, there are also five classes of antibody. Only two classes of light chain exist, κ and λ; they are found in all classes of antibody.

In functional terms, κ and λ are equivalent. However, an antibody molecule has either 2 κ- or 2 λ-chains, and never one chain of each of the two types. The various classes of antibody together make up about 20% of plasma proteins and have different functions (see *Table 2.7* for an overview).

IgG antibodies (with γ-chains) are the most common immunoglobulins. They bind via their Fc fragments to the Fc receptors on macrophages and on white blood cells and thus induce phagocytosis of the microorganisms to which they are bound. After binding to antigens (microorganisms), they are also able to activate complement and to kill bacteria already outside phagocytosing cells. IgG antibodies also bind to the Fc receptors of placental cells, eventually entering the fetal circulation by an endocytotic process. Other antibodies are not capable of binding to these Fc receptors and are therefore unable to pass from the maternal to the fetal bloodstream.

Table 2.7. The biological features of human immunoglobulins (IgG, IgA, IgM, IgD and IgE)

Class	IgG				IgA		IgM	IgD	IgE
	G_1	G_2	G_3	G_4	A_1	A_2			
Serum concentration (mg/ml)	7.2	3.5	0.8	0.3	1.9	0.2	1.9	0.03	0.0001
Number of antigen-binding sites in molecule (valence)	2	2	2	2	2	2	5(10)	2	2
Half-life (days)	21	21	7	21	6	6	5	3	2,5
Complement binding	++	+	++	0	0	0	++	?	0
Binding to homologous mast cells	0	0	0	±	0	0	0	0	+
Binding to phagocytosing cells	++	+	++	±			0		
Placental transfer	+	+	+	+	0	0	0	0	0

IgM antibodies are synthesized during a primary immune response. An IgM-producing cell typically switches over later on – during a secondary immune response – to the production of a different kind of antibody, e.g. IgG (this is known as "class switching"). IgM antibodies contain μ-chains and are linked by -S-S bridges to form pentameric aggregates. A particular polypeptide, the J chain (J=joining chain) (Mr 20,000 daltons), plays an important role in the formation of this pentamer. It allows the generation of covalent bonds between the Fc parts of two individual IgM molecules. IgM molecules play a special role in B-cell development. They are the first antibodies to be synthesized in a young B-cell, even though they later "switch over" to the production of other classes of antibody. "Pro-B-cells" synthesize only μ-chains. During maturation to B-cells, they acquire the ability to synthesize κ- or λ-chains which then combine with the μ-chains to form IgM molecules. These molecules are inserted into the membrane by way of the hydrophobic amino acid sequence in the heavy chains that was discussed earlier. Such a cell is then ready to function as a B-cell, i.e. to produce soluble antibodies after contact with a suitable antigen. Like IgG antibodies, the IgM antibodies are able to opsonize microorganisms and – even more effectively than IgG – to activate complement.

IgA molecules contain α-chains. They are found primarily in secretions, i.e. the lacrimal fluid, saliva, breast milk, gastrointestinal juices and bronchial secretion. IgA molecules may occur as monomers. More commonly they are united by a J chain which spans their Fc fragments to form dimers. When these dimers appear in secretions, they additionally contain a secretory component, a peptide with a molecular weight of 71,000 daltons. Unlike the α-chain and the κ- or λ-chain, it is not a product of a B-lymphocyte but of the secretory epithelium. The secretory component is located (similar to a receptor) on the cell side facing the bloodstream and binds IgA dimers. By means of endocytosis and subsequent exocytosis the newly formed IgA complex then arrives on the side of the epithelium facing the glandular lumen and finally enters the lumen itself. IgA protects the surface of the mucosa against penetration by microorganisms. These antibodies are important components in the immunological "defence" of body surfaces.

The protective role of IgE is not quite clear. These antibodies, which contain one epsilon-chain, bind by way of their Fc fragments to specific receptors which are found only on mast cells or basophilic leucocytes in the blood. Whenever two or more adjacent antibody molecules are bound by an antigen, the binding of an antigen to these cell-bound antibodies always results in a change in the conformation of the Fc fragment and in a number of biochemical events (described below) culminating in the secretion of serotonin or histamine. These mediators bring about an increase in capillary permeability for macromolecules and white blood cells. IgE antibodies are the key molecules of the immediate-type hypersensitivity reaction, and their interaction with antigen gives rise to allergic disorders such as hay fever or bronchial asthma. Their physiological importance may reside in the linking of their function with the release of mediators and the subsequent migration of leucocytes, antibodies and complement components into the pericapillary space. The significance of IgD antibodies is still unclear. They are found almost exclusively as membrane-bound receptors. B-cells with IgD molecules on their surface seldom appear to be stimulated by contact with antigen into synthesizing soluble IgD molecules. It remains to be seen whether IgD-bearing B-cells are of any specific (regulatory) significance.

2.2.1.1 Antibody diversity

In 1976, Hozumi and Tonegawa showed that the gene segments which code for the constant and variable parts of antibody molecules are present in embryonic cells on different DNA fragments and that the segments of an antibody gene which in the final analysis control the synthesis of a given antibody are combined only by somatic recombination. Today we know that for the synthesis of each antibody chain – whether heavy or light – one "gene pool" is available from which only a single polypeptide is synthesized per cell.

In humans, gene segments coding for κ-light-chains are located on the short arm of chromosome 2. Approximately 20–30 variable gene segments (V_K) are located upstream of 5 joining segments (J_K) and a single gene coding for the constant region of κ-chains (C_K). The distance between the J_K segments and the constant region amounts to 3 kilobases (kb) *(Fig. 2.20)*. Each V_K segment carries a number of transcription signals in its 5' flanking region: a TATA box 30 bp upstream of the starting point of transcription, an octamer at −70 base pairs and a pentadecamer at −90 base pairs. In order to give rise to the synthesis of a light-chain mRNA a Vκ segment must first be brought into contiguity with one of the Jκ segments. This is accomplished by recombination. Each V_K segment carries in its 3'-flanking region two signals, a heptamer nucleotide (CACAGTG) and a nonamer (ACATAAACC). These two signals are separated from each other by a sequence of twelve base pairs. These signals are recombination sites which correspond to two complementary signals on the 5' side of the J_K segments. These complementary signals are separated by 23 base pairs. The pairing of a 12 base pair spacer with a 23 base pair segment, both carrying the heptamer and nonamer signals in opposing directions, seems to be a prerequisite for recombination to occur. It is referred to as the 12/23 bp rule. The mRNA transcribed from the recombined DNA is then spliced so that the recombined VJ segment is brought into contiguity with the C_K transcript. The completed κ-chain is then generated by the translation of the VJC_K mRNA.

The κ-light-chain gene cluster is usually rearranged before λ. If the recombination is productive the cell will continue to synthesize κ-chains. If, however, the κ rearrangement did not result in a functional gene, λ rearrangement will ensue. In such cells the κ-locus is often lost or deleted. This loss occurs via another recombination step of $V5_K$ with a DNA segment located 24 kilobases down-stream of C_K.

The rearrangement of the heavy chain genes follows the same rules as those just described for the κ-genes. As already mentioned, rearrangement of the heavy chain genes precedes that of the light chains. The heavy chain gene cluster is located at the tip of the long arm of chromosome 14. It is by far the most complex of the three Ig loci (κ, λ and H). There are at least 100 V_H regions, probably more, which are located at the 5' end of several groups of

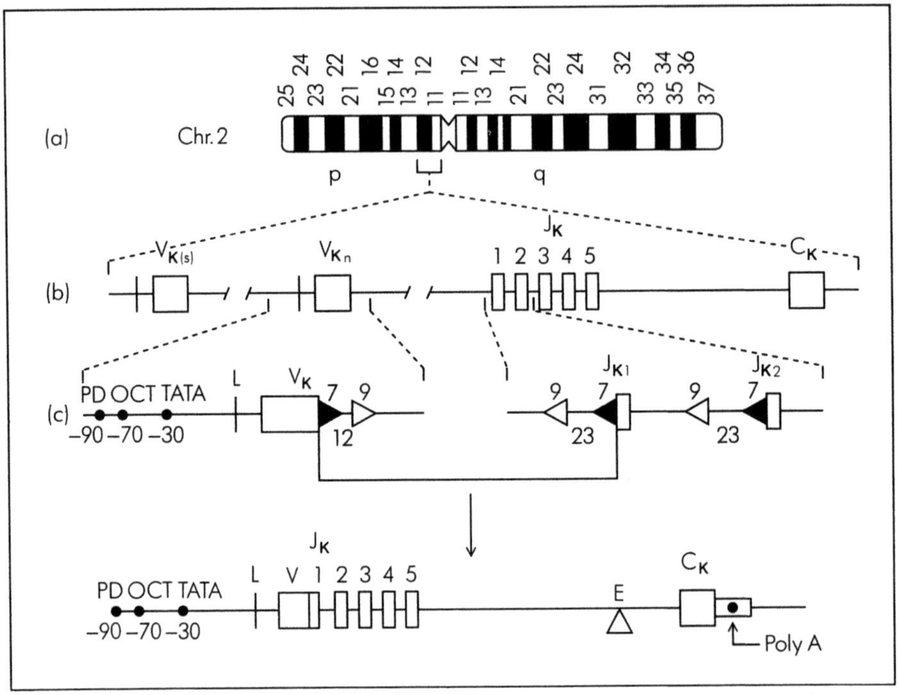

Figure 2.20. The location, organization and rearrangement of the κ light chain genes. The region on the short arm of chromosome 2 in which the genes are located (a) is depicted on a blown-up scale (b). The actual process of the rearrangement of the Vκ gene with the Jκ1 segment is shown in (c). The completed rearrangement is shown on the bottom line. PD = consensus pentadecamer, OCT = octamer, and TATA box located upstream of Vκ appear as dots. The figures beneath the dots indicate their position relative to the transcriptional initiation point. The open and filled triangles (c) represent the recombination sequences with spacers of either 12 or 23 base pairs. Recombination signals pointing towards each other can induce a recombination event.
The 3'-untranslated region is shown as a lowered box containing the poly(A)addition-RNA cleavage recognition site, represented by a dot.

diversity genes and six functional (plus 3 pseudo) J_H segments. The 3' portion of the gene cluster is occupied by 9 functional and two pseudogenes, coding for the constant parts of the various heavy chains. Each of the 100–200 V_H genes has two nucleotides sequences in its 5' flanking region, the TATA box at −30 base pairs and a "consensus octamer" at −70 base pairs. Again, these signals secure the appropriate transcription of the VH gene. The 12/23 base pair rule which we already learned about applies also to the recombination of heavy chain gene segments. Each V_H gene is flanked on its 3' end by the heptamer and the nonamer separated by the 23 bp spacer. The J_H segments which form the 3' end of the cluster of variable genes and also of each individual rearranged V_H gene carry the same signals, also separated by 23 bp with the opposite orientation. The diversity genes, which must be able to undergo recombination in both directions because they form the centre of each recombined chain, consequently have the 12 bp signals sequence in a down-stream orientation on their 3' end and in an upstream orientation on the 5' side. In this way the 12/23 bp rule applies to the recombination of V_H with D_H and of D_H with J_H *(Fig. 2.21)*.

After recombination of VD and J a transcript is made which contains these sequences plus the constant region of μ and/or δ. The necessary contiguity between VDJ and the C region is again produced by RNA splicing.

It is well established that the B-cell which started to synthesize IgM can "switch" to the production of another isotype. This is achieved by a recombinatorial event which brings the rearranged VDJ_H gene into the vicinity of another constant region gene (see *Fig. 2.22*). Each constant region gene except δ is preceded on its 5' end by a switch sequence. These sequences comprise approximately three kb and consist primarily of GAGACT and GGGGT motifs which are randomly interspersed and repeated. It is assumed that these sequences are recognized by a specific recombinase which is different from the multienzyme complex responsible for the VJ and VDJ recombinations. It is also possible that there is a specific enzyme for each isotype. However, this is still speculative.

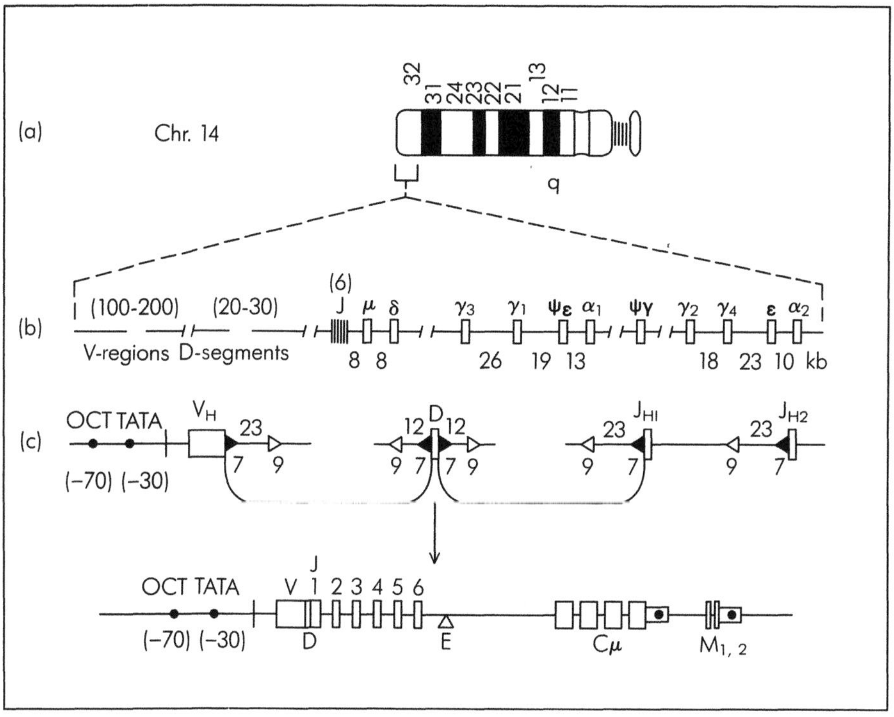

Figure 2.21. The location, organization and recombination of Ig heavy chain genes. The long arm of chromosome 14 and the region within which the genes are located is shown in (a). The overall organization of the genetic locus is shown in (b). The numbers in parenthesis give an idea of the estimated or known number of V-regions, D-segments or J-segments. The genetic information for the heavy chains is indicated by the Greek letters μ, δ, γ, α and ε; Ψ designates pseudo-genes. Transcriptional signals OTC and TATA are represented as dots, together with their distance from the initiation of transcription. The homologous heptamer-nonamer recombination signals flanking each gene are given in the direction of recombination: opposing directions indicate possible recombination events. At the bottom of the figure VDJ recombination has taken place. The triangle (E) indicates the location of the heavy chain enhancer sequence, a regulatory signal which enhances transcription of the rearranged gene.

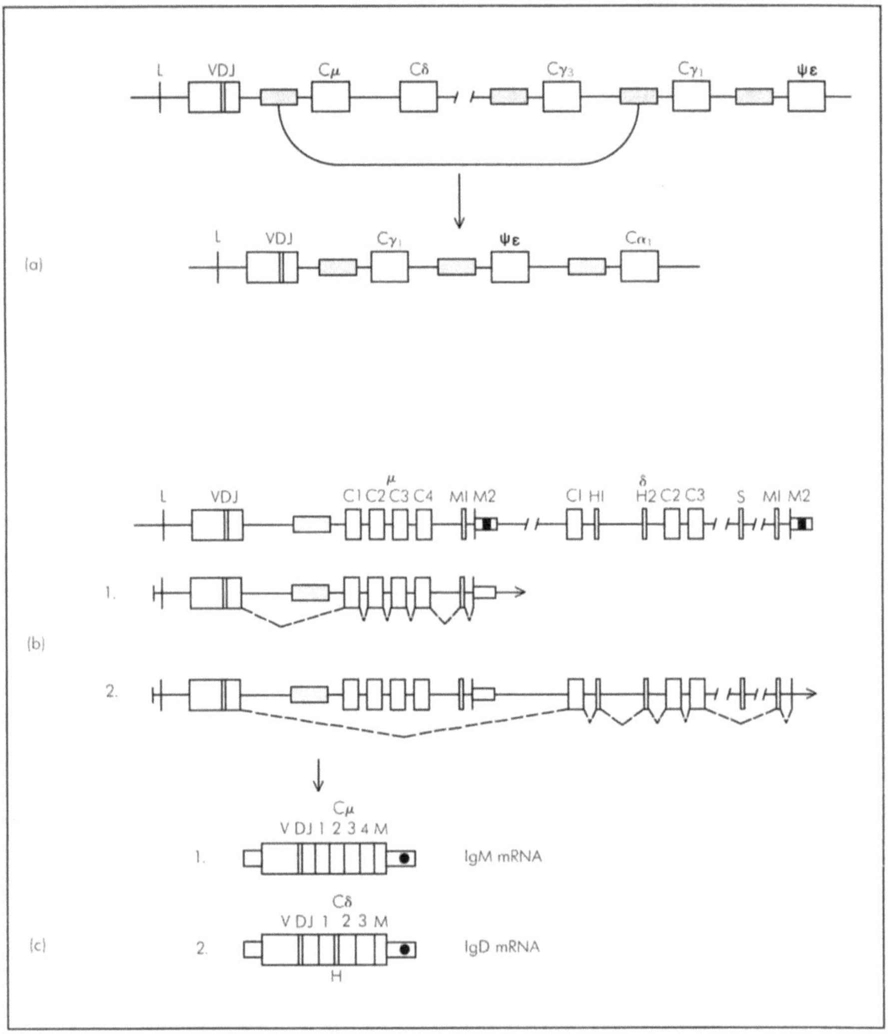

Figure 2.22. Scheme of the recombination events leading to isotype switch. The shaded boxes in front of every heavy-chain constant gene (ecxept Cδ) represent switch region sequences (see text). Through recombinational events the rearranged VDJ region can be brought into the vicinity of each of the heavy chain constant region genes (a). The structure of the primary transcripts is shown under (b). The dotted line indicates splicing events which lead to the formation of mature IgM and IgD messenger RNA molecules (c).

At any rate, switch recombinations result in the deletion of all constant region genes located upstream of the expressed constant region. It has been shown that B-cells which release IgG or IgA no longer contain genes for Cμ or Cδ. Another well-known phenomenon, the synthesis by a B-cell of two membrane-bound antibodies IgM and a second one, can be explained by the synthesis of long RNA transcripts followed by differential splicing.

With several hundred V_L genes and 4 J genes, the number of variable regions on κ-chains is about 1000. λ-Chains are created out of only 2 V_L chains and 1

J segment. The D genes raise the number of possible variable regions on heavy chains to approximately 10,000. If every light chain can combine with any heavy chain, this simple calculation means that $1000 \times 10{,}000 = 10^7$ variable regions can be synthesized. Furthermore, the joining of V and J genes is not absolutely guaranteed to take place at a given joint. A certain amount of "imprecision" in this process is yet another source of antibody variability. During B-cell differentiation, somatic mutations also occur in the V genes or their immediate vicinity. Even if many of these changes entail a loss of function, the combinatorial frequency of 10^7 would increase by a factor of 1 or 2 through accessory diversity generating mechanisms.

The term "allelic exclusion" indicates that a B-cell expresses only one allele of a given heavy or light chain, never both. This means that the pre-B-cell has to make a decision whether the paternal or the maternal allele of the heavy chain gene cluster should be expressed. The same decision has also to be made with the expression of the light chain. It is important to note that the paternal or maternal alternative has to be chosen for each of the three Ig loci, not for the antibody molecule as a whole. Heavy chains can be maternal or paternal in origin but never both. The same holds true for the κ and λ genes. The resulting antibody, however, can be a "hybrid" containing a paternal heavy chain and a maternal light chain or vice versa. Since the decision on allelic exclusion has to be arrived at for each B-cell separately, there are in reality many antibodies which contain only paternal or maternal sequences along with others in which one gene locus will be from maternal and the other from paternal origin *(Fig. 2.23)*.

2.2.1.2 Physico-chemical aspects of antibody binding

The binding of the antigen and antibody is reversible. This can be formulated as follows, according to the law of mass action:

$$\mathrm{Ag} + \mathrm{Ab} \rightleftarrows \mathrm{AgAb}$$

The strength of the binding between the antigen and antibody is reflected in the binding constant k

$$\mathrm{k} = \frac{\mathrm{AgAb}}{\mathrm{Ag} \times \mathrm{Ab}}$$

This constant can be determined by measuring the antigen concentration at which one half of all antibody-binding sites are occupied. The equation is then AgAb = Ab and k=1/Ag. The reciprocal value of the antigen concentration required to occupy half of all antibody-binding sites is therefore identical with the binding constant. This value is generally between 5×10^4 and 10^{12} l/mol. The binding constant reflects steric and electronic complementarity between the antigenic determinant and the binding site of the antibody; it has nothing to do with the number of binding sites.

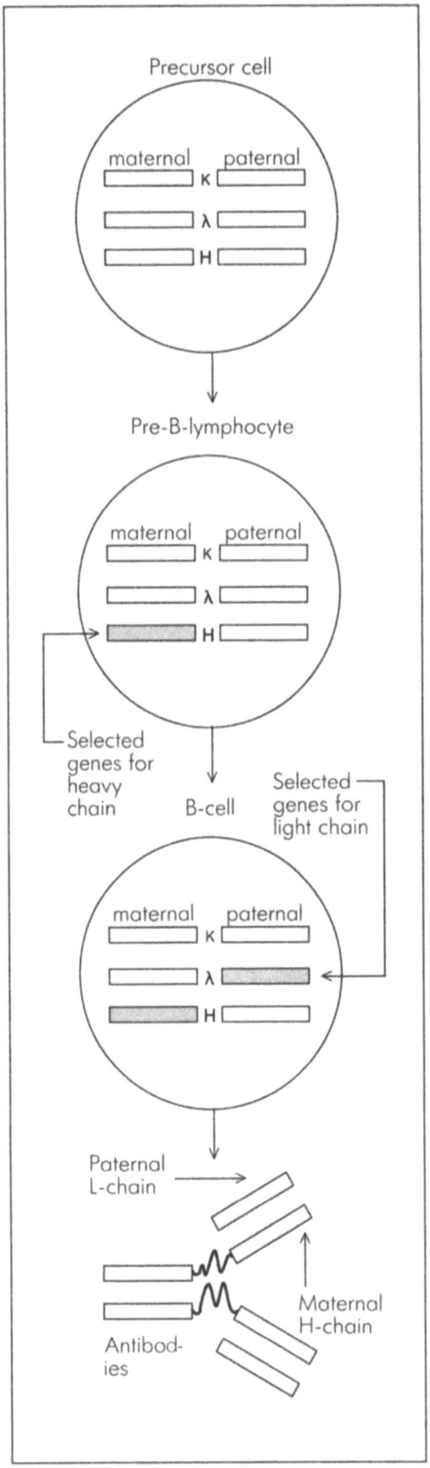

Figure 2.23. Allelic exclusion. Every cell has four groups of genes which code for light chains (κ and λ) and two groups which code for heavy immunoglobulin chains. In the course of cell development a precursor cell must first seek out and find a gene group for synthesis of a heavy chain (paternal or maternal). By this process the precursor becomes a B-cell that produces cytoplasmic heavy (μ) chains. After abundant proliferation the pre-B cell again has to make a "decision" with respect to the activation of a paternal or maternal κ-chain-gene. If the κ-gene rearrangement is not productive, a third "decision" has to be made with respect to the paternal or maternal λ-gene.

A precise match between the antigen and the antibody-binding site is a greater stimulus for cell division and antibody secretion than weak binding. That is why in a secondary immune reaction it is predominantly antibodies with a higher binding constant that are formed. In this connection we speak of "maturation adjustment".

In contrast to the binding constant, the avidity of an antibody for an antigen indicates the overall binding strength, which is also a function of the number of binding sites. An antigen with many antigenic determinants is more strongly bound by antibody than is an antigen which has relatively few such determinants. The frequency with which an antigenic determinant occurs on an antigen is known as valency. It is obvious that a multivalent antigen (i.e. an antigen on which the same antigenic determinant is repeated several times) can be bound more strongly by an antibody than the same antigen which carries only one or a few of these determinants.

Whether antigen-antibody binding gives rise to complex aggregates or not depends on the molar relation of the two components. In the event of gross antibody excess, every antigenic determinant will be occupied by another antibody. In the event of antigen excess, only a few antigen molecules will be interconnected with each other by antibodies. Only when the molar relation is approximately equivalent can the complexes become extensive, giving rise to large aggregates *(Fig. 2.24)*.

The interaction of antibodies with their antigens can be measured directly or indirectly. In direct measurement antibodies are added to radioactive antigen and the radio-labelled antibody-antigen complexes are precipitated by anti-IgG and measured.

Indirect measurement depends on secondary phenomena which occur after antibody-antigen interaction. These include precipitation, cell agglutination and complement utilization. This last reaction is based on the fact that complement combines with only one antibody molecule, which in turn has bound antigen. It is therefore possible to draw conclusions about the original antigen-antibody complex from complement activation which has been determined with a second complement-dependent immune reaction.

2.2.2. Lymphokines and cytokines

The immune system is composed of single cells, all capable of autonomous responses. In order to provide a functional advantage for the organism within which they are operating, immune cells have to respond to external stimuli as a system. A well orchestrated systemic response, on the other hand, requires the cells to communicate with one another. In the immune system, this communication is essentially achieved in two ways: by direct cell contact or by chemical signals. The presentation of antigen by a macrophage or B-cell to a T-cell, which involves the recognition of this antigen in the context of an MHC molecule via a T-cell receptor represents an example of communication through direct cell contact. There are, however, spatial limits to this form of communication between cells. Other means of signal transmission had therefore to be invented.

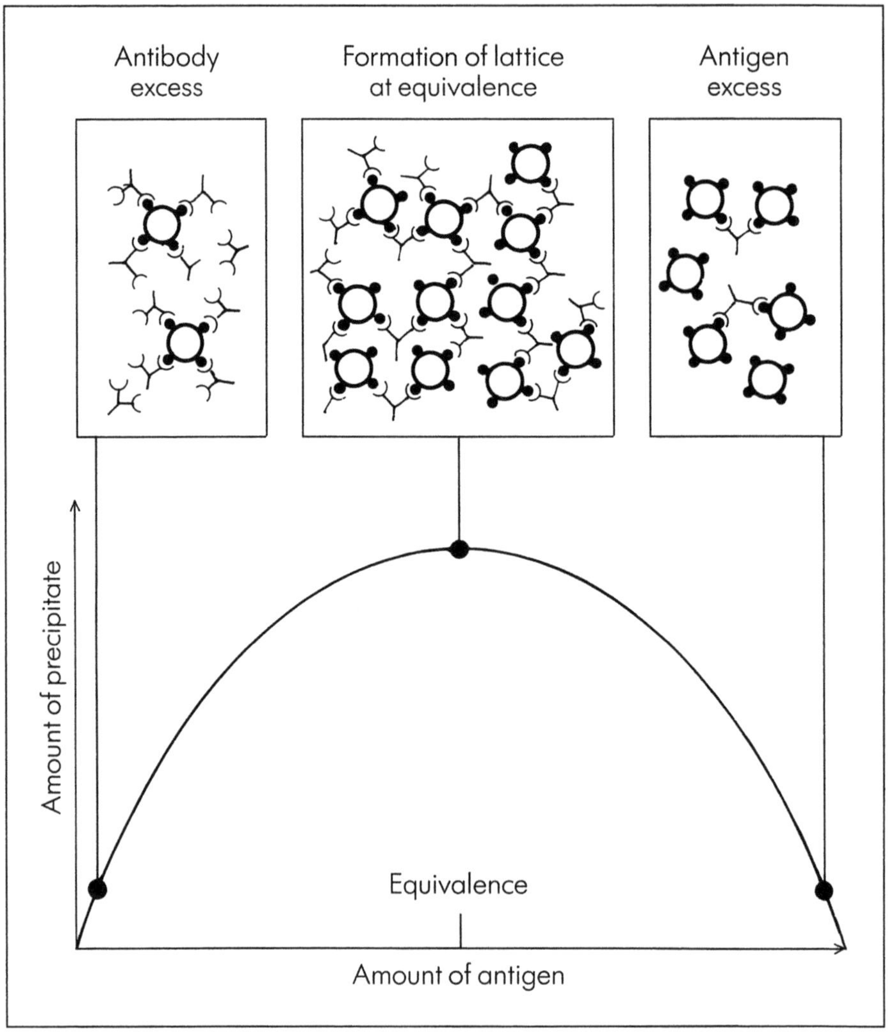

Figure 2.24. Effect of different antigen concentrations on the formation of antigen-antibody complexes. At equivalence, antigen and antibodies are present in about the same molar concentrations. The smallest complexes are obtained when antigen is greatly in excess. Antibody excess results in antibody-saturated though not extensively interconnected antigen. Large, multiply interconnected antigen-antibody complexes are obtained only at equivalence.

In the nervous system, which serves rapid coordination of functions over long distances, this problem was solved by the transmission of electric signals along a network of nerve fibres. In all other systems, chemical signals are used to orchestrate physiological responses.

Cytokines are chemical instruments of communication between cells. They are proteins or glycoproteins which are secreted by one cell type and recognized by virtue of specific receptors by the same and by other cells. In their signal function, cytokines resemble hormones. However, in general, cytokines are designed to secure communication at short distances. In contrast to hormones, which are secreted into the blood stream, cytokines are released into the local environment of a cell. Very often such topical cytokine secretion is not manifested by measurable cytokine concentrations in the blood. Cytokines were first discovered as products of lymphocytes and monocytes: accordingly, they were called lymphokines or monokines. When it became clear that the secretion of and the specific response to these proteins were the property of a much broader range of cells, the more general term cytokine was introduced.

Cytokines have three main functions. They are growth factors or stimulators of cell division. At the same time they induce differentiation, i.e. they bring about the proper development of a cell as seen in the sequential appearance of new morphological and functional parameters. Cytokines may also reinforce effector functions. An example is the enhancement of the NK function of large granular lymphocytes by interferon γ and interleukin 2. The three main elements of cytokine function are represented in a given protein to different degrees. They are rarely so clearly separated as to allow for a classification of cytokines on this basis. Colony stimulating factors, for instance, mediate both proliferation and differentiation. In addition, some of them also activate mature monocytes and granulocytes.

Cytokines are secreted by two different pathways. Most of them are synthesized on membrane bound ribosomes and subsequently transferred to the endoplasmic reticulum. In this process the leader sequences are removed from the native proteins. The cytokines are then oxidized (formation of disulfide bonds) and glycosylated before they leave the endoplasmic reticulum and are stored in the Golgi-apparatus from where they are transported to storage granules. The alternative pathway starts with synthesis of the protein on free cytoplasmic ribosomes. After their synthesis these cytokines remain in the cytoplasm and are not exposed to an oxidizing milieu. In the mechanisms which lead to the actual release of the cytokines, the two pathways may again converge: either the granules are brought into the vicinity of the cytoplasmic membrane and emptied by a mechanism which involves fusion of the granule and the plasma membrane, or the cytokines exist first as molecules anchored in the membrane through fatty acid residues or hydrophobic amino acid sequences, from which they are released by enzymatic cleavage (examples are CD23, M-CSF, Il-1, TNFα and others *(Fig. 2.25)*.

After secretion, cytokines can interact with extracellular matrix. This has been shown to be the case for Il-3 and GM-CSF and may also play a role for the chemotactic factors which all bind heparin. Such binding could have the purpose of localizing the action of a particular lymphokine.

Cytokines like hormones can also be complexed by carriers. The best known example of this mechanism is α2-macroglobulin, which binds Il-1, Il-6, PDGF and TGF-β. The carrier may or may not function as an inhibitor of receptor binding, and it can be covalent (as with Il-1) or not (Il-6). The biological significance of this attachment to carriers resides probably in the prevention of degradation of the cytokine.

In order to exert its physiological effect, a cytokine must interact with its specific receptor. The signal pathways which lead to cell activation, differentiation and proliferation are still largely undefined. Somehow the signals gener-

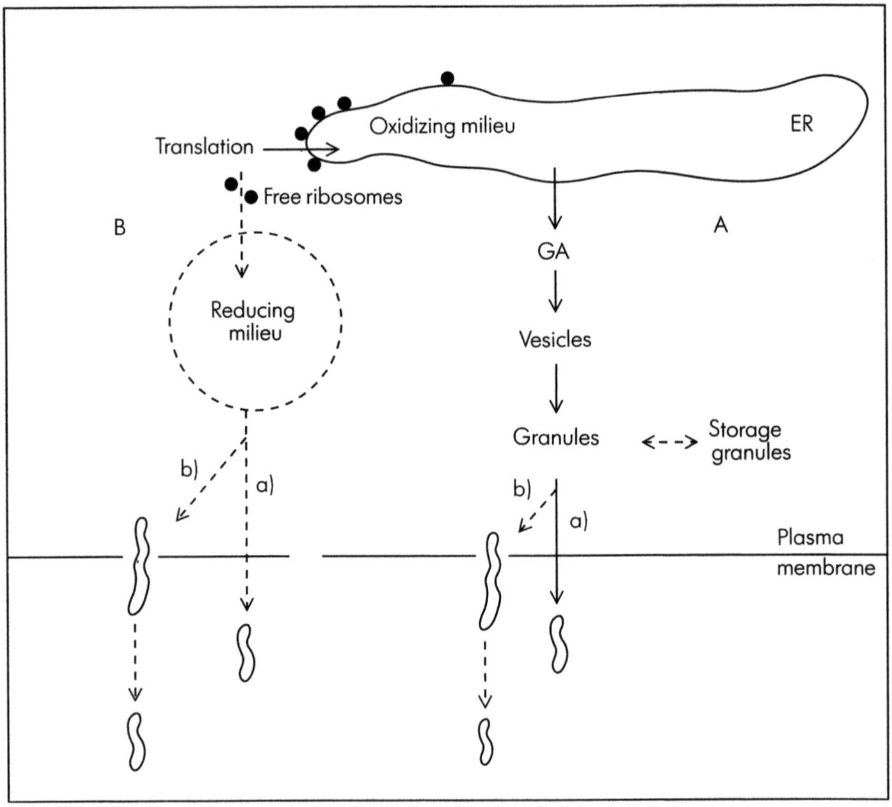

Figure 2.25. Pathways of cytokine secretion. Most cytokines are synthesized on ribosomes bound to the endoplasmic reticulum to which they are subsequently transferred. The leader sequence is usually cleaved off in the process. Within the endoplasmic reticulum an oxidizing milieu facilitates the formation of disulfide bridges and glycosylation. The correctly folded and glycosylated cytokines are then transported to the Golgi-apparatus where they are "packed" into vesicles and subsequently transferred to the storage granules. The granules are then emptied by a process called degranulation (see chapter 5). An alternative pathway of cytokine synthesis and secretion (B) starts with synthesis on free ribosomes and transport to the cell surface in a reducing milieu. The final steps of the two pathways may still be identical and involve either the degranulation of granules (a) or the anchoring of completed cytokines in the cell membrane via lipid molecules or hydrophobic amino acid sequences. Release from membrane attachment then occurs through proteolytic or lipolytic cleavage (b). Examples for cytokines which are primarily membrane attached and become released through enzymatic activity are: CD23, M-CSF, EGF, TGF-α, IL-1 and TNF.

ated through ligand-receptor interaction lead to an activation of transcription factors which subsequently 'switch on' certain genes. The first genes to be activated may again code for transcription factors which, in turn, activate further genes. This may then result in a cascade of gene activations, which produce the phenotypic changes that we can observe *(Fig. 2.26)*.

Many cytokines can be directly related to the purpose of defending the organism against viral or bacterial infections. The main 'organizers' of defenses against bacteria appear to include Il-1, Il-6 and TNF, while the interferons are specialized in organizing the antiviral defence. These cytokines, possibly 'old' from an evolutionary point of view, have some features in common: they are induced by the attacking microbes, they are self-inducers and also induce one another. They mediate acute phase responses which include parts of the complement system and the C-reactive protein and they also play a role in inducing the inhibitors of acute phase reactions like glucocorticoids, protease inhibitors and receptor antagonists (like the Il-1 inhibitor), in order to keep these potentially self-damaging reactions under control.

We are at present beginning to understand that there is a molecular basis for the coordinated regulation of the functionally related factors. The promotor regions of the genes coding for these antibacterial or antiviral cytokines contain certain common motifs (nucleotide sequences) which would enable a limited number of transcription factors to regulate their transcription in a coordinated fashion. In other words: at the transcriptional level many of these proteins are linked together by common modules which can react to one or at least to a very limited number of signals.

A great number of cytokines have already been discovered and characterized and most likely many more will be found. A fully convincing or logical way of

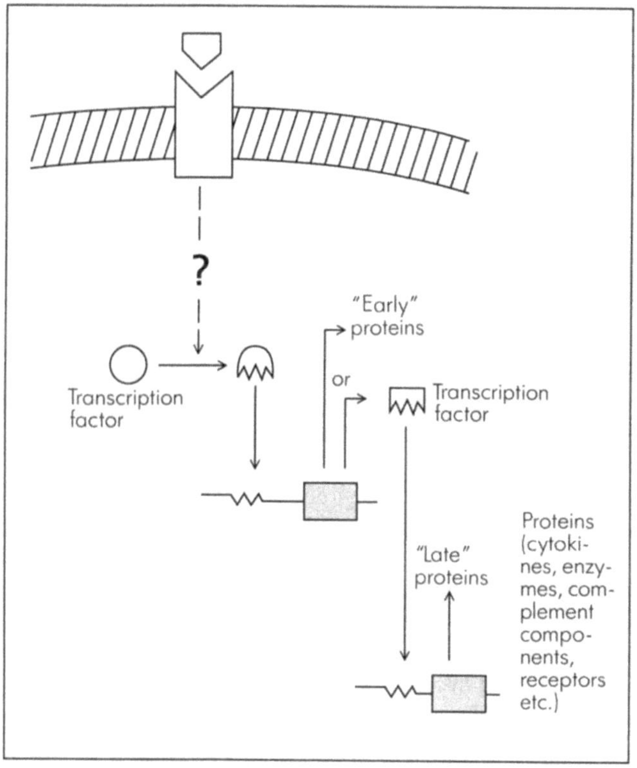

Figure 2.26. Biological effects of cytokines. A cytokine interacts with its receptor on the cell surface. This results in a conformational change of the receptor molecule. The chemical energy induced by this change is transmitted into the cell by largely undefined signal transduction pathways. Eventually the signals lead to the activation of transcription factors which activate the genes of "early" proteins. Some of these genes may again code for transcription factors which then induce the activation of "late" genes and proteins. The induced proteins may again be cytokines, cytokine receptors, antiviral proteins, such as Mx (see chapter 6) or any other functional protein.

classifying these substances does not exist. Neither their cellular origin nor their functional properties offer a reliable basis for classification. We will, therefore, follow a recent proposal of W. Haas to group the cytokines according to their evolutionary relatedness. This means that they will be ordered in agreement with their degrees of nucleotide sequence homology and the chromosomal location of the genes which specify their synthesis. While this procedure is not entirely satisfying, it is at least based on solid facts.

Applying this rule one arrives at five major groups of related cytokines and one additional group of individual substances with no apparent close relatives. The five families are: the interferon group, the interleukin family, the TNF family, the family of chemotactic factors and the chromosome-5 linkage group.

There are a number of additional cytokines or cytokine families like erythropoietin, transforming growth factors α and β, platelet-derived growth factors, fibroblast growth factor and epidermal growth factor which are not primarily regulating immune functions, although relations with the immune system exist. They will not be discussed here. Some of the cytokines to be mentioned in this section have gained prominence as therapeutic agents. These compounds (α-interferon, Il-2, the colony stimulating factors Il-3, GM-CSF, G-CSF and M-CSF) will be discussed in the context of their therapeutic applications and mentioned here only briefly. Table 2.8. gives an overview of the most common cytokines.

2.2.2.1. Interferons (see also Chapter 6)

In man as in other mammals, interferons are a multigene family. Three main groups of interferons can be distinguished, interferon α, β and γ. There is one gene for β and for γ interferons. In contrast, 23 α interferon genes have been found which code for 15 functional proteins. All of the α- and β-genes are clustered on the short arm of chromosome 9, while the interferon γ-gene lies on chromosome 12. γ-Interferon does not show any sequence homology with α- or β-interferon. Moreoever, the γ-interferon gene is located on another chromosome. Also in contrast to the α- and β-genes it contains three introns. γ-interferon should, therefore not be allocated to the interferon family.

α- and β-Interferons exert their action via the attachment to a receptor molecule which is encoded by a gene located on chromosome 21. The receptor protein itself has a molecular weight around 95 kd. The interferons are part of the humoral arm of the unspecific, 'old' immune system.

The main role of the interferons in evolution may have resided in their ability to protect against viral infections. However, other effects may also have contributed to the maintenance of these genes, effects which must not necessarily be reflected in the therapeutic roles which some of these substances play today. The synthesis of the interferons is regulated at the transcriptional level. The individual steps of this regulation have not yet been elucidated. From recent publications on the regulation of the interferon β-gene, however, a scheme can be derived which contains at least some key elements involved in the expression of the interferon β and probably other interferon genes. Upon entry of a virus

Table 2.8. Summary of cytokines

Cytokine	Chromosome	Source	Biological activity/Properties
IFNα1 (14) IFNα2 IFNβ	9	all	Inhibition of viral spread NK activation
Il-1α IL-1β	2	M, all?	Large variety of defensive/ destructive effects, mainly via induction of eicosanoids and other cytokines
TFNα TFNβ	6	M T	
Il-6	7	M	T-B-cell coactivator, APP inducer
G-CSF	17		N-coactivator
NAF(Il-8) IP-10 Gro PF4 PF4 type 1 PBP MCP-1 RANTES pID78	4 4	M(E) K(E, M, F) F(E, M) P P P M, T? T T	Similar 3-D structure Heparin binding Intracellular storage Not glycosylated N- and C-terminal processing Chemotaxis inflammation Tissue repair Control of cell proliferation
Il-3	5	T, Ma	Hemopoiesis, Eo-activator
GM-CSF		T, Ma, F, S	Hemopoiesis, M-, N-activator
Il-4		T, Ma	T-, B-, M-coactivator, IgE switch
Il-5		T, Ma	Eo-activator
M-CSF		M, T, B?	M-activator, placenta development
IFNγ	12	T, NK	M-activator, Il-4 antagonist
Il-2	4	T	T-, B-, M-, NK-coactivator
Il-7		S	Lymphopoiesis
CD23, IgE-BF		B, T, M	B-cell growth, IgE response
LIF		?	Inhibitor of stem cell differentiation
EPO	7	Ki, Hepatoma cells	Erythropoiesis
TGFβ1 TGFβ2 TGFβ3		P P P	Tissue repair Inhibitor of hemopoiesis and T-cell, resp. M-deactivator

Abbreviations:
N = neutrophils, M = monocytes, K = NK-cells, Eo = Eosinophils, APP = acute phase proteins, MA = macrophages, T = T-cells, B = B-cells, P = platelets, Ki = kidney, E = endothelium, F = fibroblasts, S = stroma cells, IP-10 = interferon γ-induced protein, Gro = MGSA (melanocyte growth stimulating activity), PF4 = platelet factor 4, PBF = human platelet basic protein, MCP-1 = human monocyte chemoattractant protein, LIF = leukemia inhibitory factor, TGF = Transforming growth factor

into a cell, double-stranded viral RNA induces a protein kinase which phosphorylates an inhibitory protein of a transcriptional regulator ($A_2 = NF_{\kappa}B$). The phosphorylation leads to a dissociation of the inhibitor from A_2 which in turn becomes activated and subsequently binds to a 'positive regulatory domain' (PRD) upstream of the interferon β-gene. A second transcription activating factor, A_1, is directly phosphorylated by a kinase which is activated as a consequence of viral infection. Through this event A_1 can bind to a second PRD even further upstream of the interferon gene. Thirdly the synthesis of A_2 ($NF_{\kappa}B$) is enhanced. All three events appear to result from virus infection. They can, however, also be triggered by other stimuli. Interestingly, the two PRDs which regulate the activity of the β interferon gene are also found in the promotor region of other cytokines which may play a role in the defense against viruses. The regulatory steps leading to interferon-β production are depicted in *Fig. 2.27.*

2.2.2.2. The interleukin family

This family comprises at least two well-characterized proteins, interleukin 1α and interleukin 1β. The genes for these proteins which can be traced back to a common ancestral gene are located on the long arm of chromosome 2. The family may be greater and include other more distantly related proteins like fibroblast growth factor. However, we will restrict ourselves to the description of Il-1α and β. The structure of the α- and β-genes are very similar. Each contains 7 exons and 6 introns. The first and part of the second exon, and the larger part of exon 7, remain untranslated. At the amino acid level, the sequence homology between the two proteins is only 26%. Both proteins have been crystallized: surprisingly, their 3-dimensional structures are very similar in spite of the rather low sequence homology.

Il-1 and the distantly related fibroblast growth factors have no typical leader sequences and are not exocytosed via the classical pathway through the endoplasmic reticulum, which means that they are not exposed to oxidation and glycosylation. They are synthesized as 31 kd precursors which are subsequently processed to smaller active forms. Pro-Il-1α and β are myristoylated through amide bonds in activated monocytes and probably in other cell types as well. The fatty acid chain may serve transient membrane attachment and/or other steps in the secretory process. 31 kd Il-1α and 22 kd Il-1β can be found attached to membranes. It has been claimed that Il-1α functions mainly as a membrane bound peptide while Il-1β is predominantly secreted. The secreted forms of both types of Il-1 have a molecular mass of 17 kd.

Both forms of Il-1 bind to one type of receptor which is expressed on a broad range of cells. The binding constants which have been reported in the literature for the interaction of Il-1α or β with the Il-1 receptor range between 10^{-10} and 10^{-12} M . It is therefore possible that several types of receptors exist, possibly low and high affinity forms analogous to the Il-2 receptor. A murine Il-1 receptor with a molecular weight of 80 kd has been cloned, its binding affinity is reported to be 4×10^{-9} M. Whether a second protein is needed to generate a 'high affinity' binding site is at present unknown.

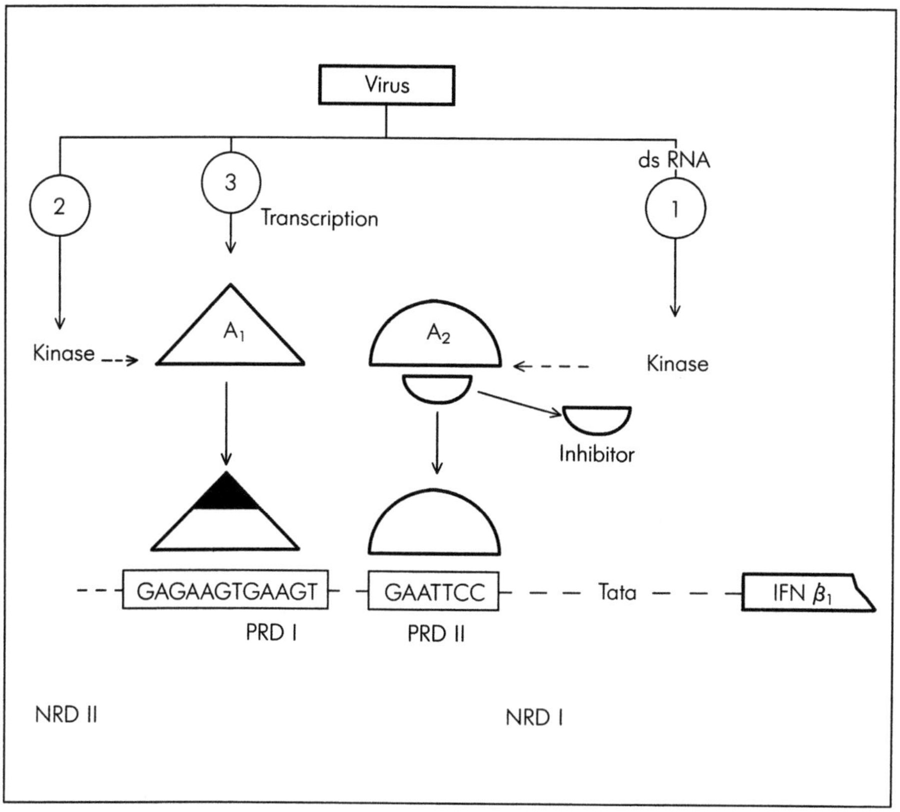

Figure 2.27. Regulation of human interferon β transcription. The promotor region of the interferon β gene contains two positive regulatory domains (PRD) and two less well-defined negative regulatory domains (NRD).
Transcription factors A1 and A2 bind to the PRD's and cooperate in promoting interferon transcription. In most cells three events are required for induction of interferon transcription:
1. activation of A2 (NFκB), phosphorylation of an inhibitor protein by protein kinase P1 (activated by double-stranded RNA) leads to the dissociation of the inhibitor and the binding of A2 to PRD II.
2. Activation of A1 by a protein kinase called casein kinase 2 and
3. Enhancement of transcription of A1. The A1 gene has a virus induceable promoter.
Infection of a cell with a virus may induce all three events. However, several other stimuli can lead to the same result. In particular IFN β itself can induce its own production. PRD I and II are found also in the promotor regions of other cytokines, complement factors and proteins which are involved in antiviral defences.

Interleukin 1α and β are pleiotropic factors which exert an even greater multitude of effects than other cytokines. Hardly any cell type in the body remains unaffected. *Table 2.9.* gives an overview of the most prominent actions of the Il-1 cytokines. Many cells which produce Il-1, like monocytes, T-lymphocytes, B-cells, eosinophils, neutrophils, fibroblasts and astrocytes, also react to it. Il-1 induces fever – as a matter of fact it is identical with the 'endogenous pyrogen' mentioned in the older literature. Il-1 stimulates T-lymphocytes which 'see' their antigen in the context of a particular MHC molecule: it represents the second signal which is delivered by the antigen presenting cell early in the

Table 2.9. Biological actions of Il-1
Local and systemic activation of host defence mechanisms by Il-1

Fever
Reduced food intake
Production of corticosteroids
Hypoferremia, hypozincemia
Synthesis of acute phase proteins in the liver
Stimulation of hemopoiesis; neutrophilia
Augmented immune responses
Increased antibacterial resistance (neutrophils!)
Altered endothelial cell function
Connective tissue repair

immune response. Il-1 induces the formation and secretion of acute phase proteins in the liver, it causes prostaglandin synthesis in a variety of cells; adhesion of neutrophils to endothelial cells is stimulated, monocytes and neutrophils are chemotactically attracted to the source of Il-1 formation, and muscle protein is wasted. In the brain stem the release of CRF is stimulated, and this effect leads to the secretion of ACTH and subsequently of glucocorticoids. At the same time, however, glucocorticoid receptors and gluconeogenesis are down-regulated by Il-1α and β. Il-1 has strong hematopoietic effects. Whether these effects are direct or the consequence of the secretion of other hematopoietic hormones is not yet clear. These are only some of the most prominent effects of Il-1.

Is there a common denominator of these effects? One could perhaps say that most, if not all, of these effects of Il-1 are either local or systemic manifestations of an acute inflammation and as such parts of a cascade of responses which aim at the elimination of bacteria on one hand, and at the mobilization of energy within the infected host organism on the other.

The stimuli which induce Il-1 production seem to support this general idea. Endotoxin, antigen-antibody complexes, complement components (C5a), leukotrienes all stimulate Il-1 secretion. So do other cytokines which also have a function in host defenses: interferon γ, interferon α, TNF, TGF β and even Il-1 itself can stimulate Il-1 secretion, while glucocorticoids and prostaglandins, but also inhibitors of 5-lipoxygenase, inhibit Il-1 formation and/or secretion. In particular PGE_2, which down-regulates several parameters of the immune response, also down-modulates Il-1 secretion. Most likely this is achieved through an intracellular increase in cAMP. This cyclic nucleotide seems to inhibit the translation of preformed Il-1 mRNA.

The central role which Il-1 plays in inflammation makes this cytokine, its synthesis, secretion or its interaction with the Il-1 receptor very attractive targets for potential antiinflammatory drugs. Indeed the strong antiinflammatory effects of glucocorticoids may at least in part be attributed to the steroid effect on Il-1 secretion. Moreover, there is at least preliminary evidence indicating that a naturally occurring Il-1 receptor antagonist displays strong antiinflammatory effects, which may be utilized therapeutically. On account of its interference with Il-1 during the activation of T-lymphocytes, this inhibitor may also have immunosuppressive properties. On the other hand, the hematopoietic effects of Il-1 -direct or indirect – make the two related cytokines Il-1α and β candidates for the treatment of myelosuppressive disorders. Il-1 can lead to faster recruitment of granulocytes in animals made neutropenic by chemotherapy or radiation and can synergize the actions of antibacterial drugs in experimental situations. It can also do this in healthy animals, though only to a limited extent (see Chapter 6, colony stimulating factors).

2.2.2.3. The tumour necrosis factor family

It has been known for many years that mice which are sensitized with BCG or *Corynebacterium parvum* and subsequently treated with LPS produce a factor which causes hemorrhagic necrosis in a number of transplanted tumours. This factor was subsequently called 'tumour necrosis factor'. It was shown to be elaborated by monocytes of sensitized mice. Later it was found that a very similar protein was produced by lymphocytes. This factor was called lymphotoxin or TNFβ.

The genes for human TNFα and β are located on the short arm of chromosome 6 within the HLA complex. Both genes have 4 exons and 3 introns. The sequence homology between TNFα and β at the amino acid level amounts to only 28 %. TNFα carries a long leader sequence which is not cleaved during the translocation of the protein into the endoplasmic reticulum. The 26 kd protein remains membrane-associated and is proteolytically cleaved to yield a soluble form of TNFα with a molecular weight of 17 kd. The 17 kd protein forms trimers, the three-dimensional structure of which has been elucidated.

Recent data seem to indicate that there are two types of TNF receptors, one with a molecular weight around 55 kd which is found on monocytic and promyelocytic cells and a second type which is expressed in epithelial cells and which displays molecular masses of 75 and 95 kd. Antibodies raised against the 55 kd receptor did not crossreact with the material extracted from epithelial cells and vice versa. Biologically the TNFs show certain parallels to Il-1. They also seem to be very general mediators of inflammatory responses at the local and the systemic level. TNFα may be the metabolic stimulus which induces cachexia in cancer patients but also in chronic infections. For this reason it has also been called 'cachectin'. TNFα or cachectin inhibits lipogenesis in adipocytes. Upon chronic application of TNFα to experimental animals the following symptoms were observed: anorexia, depletion of whole body protein and lipid stores, anemia, leukocytosis, subendothelial inflammation and periportal inflammation in the liver. TNFα represents the last common pathway of the pathophysiological events leading to gram-negative shock. In primates monoclonal neutralizing antibodies against TNFα can mitigate or prevent the shock inducing effects of lipopolysaccharides (LPS).

The TNFα gene seems to be constitutively transcribed in resting monocytes. Stimulation of the cells with LPS or mitogens increases the rate of transcription. In stimulated lymphocytes the TNFα gene is transcribed more heavily than the TNFβ gene which is not at all transcribed in monocytes. The synthesis of both TNFs, however, is also controlled at the translational level. LPS seems to be the most potent stimulus for the induction of TNS synthesis. However, viruses, fungi, mycobacteria and other cytokines, like Il-1, Il-2, colony-stimulating factors like GM-CSF and Il-3, interferon γ, type 1 interferons and complement components also stimulate TNF production. As in the case of Il-1, glucocorticoids and PGE_2 inhibit the synthesis of TNF.

Although monocytes and lymphocytes were first described as the main producers of TNFs, other cells can definitely synthesize TNFα; among them are B-cells, Kupffer cells, astrocytes, NK-cells, mast cells and certain tumour cell lines.

TNF can induce its own synthesis. It also stimulates the synthesis of other cytokines, most notably of Il-1, Il-6, the colony stimulating factors, interferon γ and PDGF.

TNF promotes a number of responses which can be interpreted as contributing to inflammation: it enhances pro-coagulant activity by down-regulating the expression of thrombomodulin by endothelial cells. It promotes the adhesion of neutrophils to endothelium. In addition TNF stimulates the phagocytic activity of neutrophils and up-regulates the expression of complement receptors on white blood cells. The effects of fat and protein metabolism have been mentioned.

TNF crosses the blood-brain barrier only in tiny amounts. However, the cytokine can be produced centrally by astrocytes. High levels of TNF in cerebrospinal fluid of patients with bacterial meningitis have been measured. TNF can induce a pyrogenic response and may – like Il-1 – also stimulate CRF and ACTH secretion.

The central role of TNF in the generation of cachectic states, and its role as a mediator of inflammatory reactions make pharmacological strategies directed at interference with TNF activities attractive. TNF receptor antagonists could be potent drugs for the treatment of chronic inflammation, perhaps even more so for the prevention of shock in gram-negative septic infections and of cachexia in cancer and in chronic inflammatory conditions. The use of TNFα or β as an antitumour agent seems to be severely limited by the pro-inflammatory, pro-cachectic and shock-inducing properties of these compounds. The most prominent biological activities of TNFα are summarized in *Fig. 2.28.*

2.2.2.4. Chemotactic factor family or 'small inducible gene' family

This group comprises a number of rather short proteins (70–75 amino acids) which were discovered only recently.

A number of common features suggest the classification of these novel factors as one family or group. All of the peptides in this group carry 4 cysteine residues in analogous positions. With respect to the first two cysteine positions one can distinguish between two subfamilies, a cysteine-x-cysteine family and a subfamily which is characterized by direct linkage of the first two cysteines. Members within each of these subfamilies display considerable sequence homology, which is, however, not found between the two groups. The genes specifying the synthesis of these factors appear to be located on chromosome 4; this statement is made with the reservation that not all of the genes in question have been

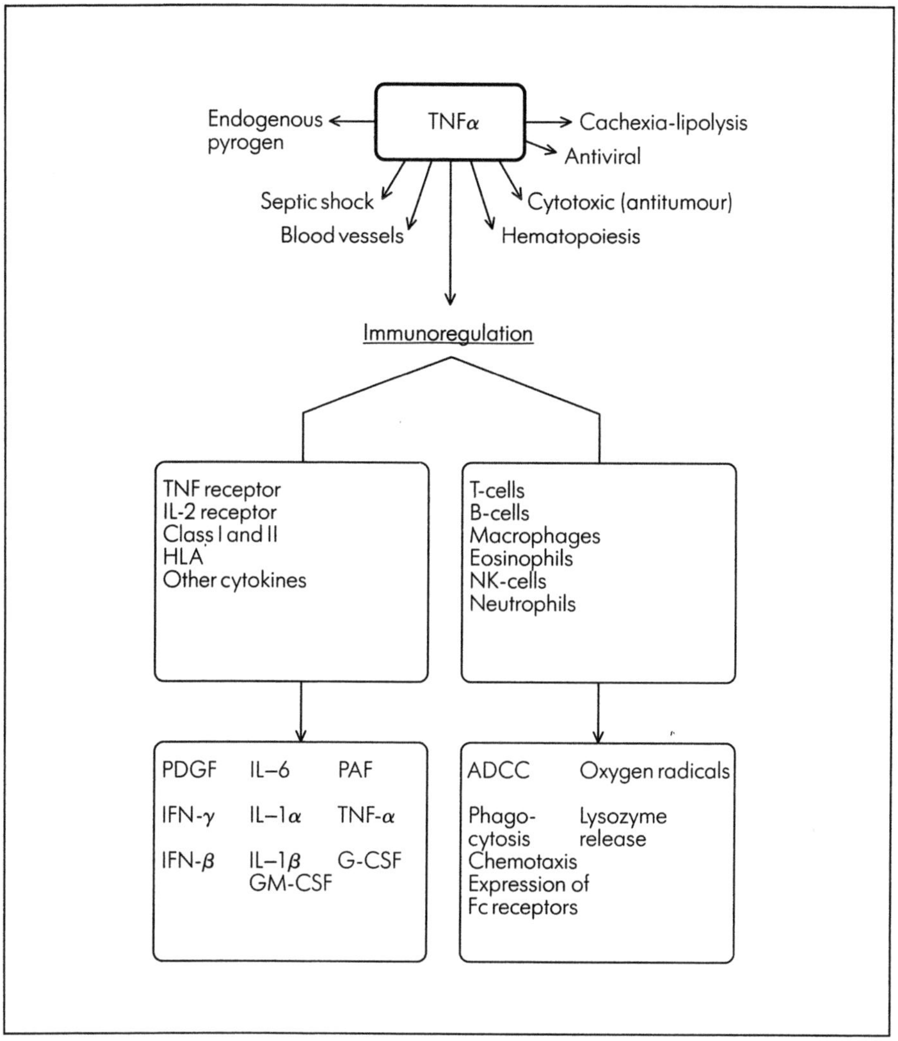

Figure 2.28. Actions of TNFα. TNFα exerts a large number of biological effects of which the most important ones are explained in the text. Of particular importance is the immunoregulatory effect of TNFα. It is characterized by a stimulation of the synthesis of several cytokines and of upregulating several receptors. On a more global scale, TNFα stimulates several cells of the immune system. The most important functional parameters of such activations are listed in the lower right box of the figure.

localized. All factors so far analysed carry three functional domains: a core region with the 4 cysteines connected by two disulfide bridges and 3 β-stranded sheets, an extended loop at the N-terminus and an α-helical domain at the C-terminus, which seems to be important for the chemotactic effects and for the binding of heparin or other glucose-aminoglycans. Both the N- and the C-termini are frequently modified by proteases. Adequate stimuli appear to induce the transcription of the factor genes within minutes. Such stimuli are represented by LPS, bacterial toxins, Il-α and β, TNFα and β, Il-3 and GM-CSF. Abundant production and intracellular storage appear to be further common features. The function of the chemotactic peptides is not at all clear. Their ability to attract neutrophils is prominent but some also support or suppress cell growth, induce a pro-coagulant state and activate inflammatory cells, notably neutrophils.

Table 2.10 summarizes some of the observations relating to this group of cytokines. The most prominent, though not necessarily the most important factor in this group has been reported under a large variety of different names: neutrophil activating factor (NAF), monocyte derived neutrophil activating peptide, monocyte derived neutrophil chemotactic factor and endothelial cell derived neutrophil activating peptide β (ENAP-β) are but a few of the names under which Il-8, as it is now called, has appeared in the literature. Monocytes

Table 2.10. Chemotactic factor family

Chemotactic factors	Produced by	Induced by	Biological effects
Interleukin 8 (Il-8) = Neutrophil activating peptide (NRF) = Monocyte derived neutrophil chemotactic factor (NCF)	Monocytes	LPS, Il-1, INF Staph. exotoxin Con A	In vitro: (chemotaxis for neutrophils) Neutrophil activation (respiratory burst degranulation) In vivo: Local skin reaction (redness, swelling 3 hours after s.c. injection) Transient leukocytosis
γ-IFN induced peptide (IP 10)	Keratinocytes Endothelial cells Monocytes Fibroblasts	γ-IFN	Mediator of inflammation
Melanocyte growth stimulating activity (MGSA) = gro protein (gro)	Fibroblasts Endothelial cells Epithelial cells Macrophages	LPS, IL-1, TNF PDGF, EGF, CSF-1 Thrombin, TPA STC-transformation MGSA (autocrine)	Positive growth regulator for mesenchymal cells (autocrine) Negative growth regulator for epithelial cells Mediator of inflammation Activation of endothelial cells? Control of melanocyte migration?
Platelet factor 4 (PF4) and variant 1 (PF4 var 1)	Megakaryocytes stored in α granules of platelets	Collagen, thrombin Epinephrine ADP	Chemotatic for leukocytes, fibroblasts Inhibits collagenase, neutralizes heparin
Platelet basic protein (PBP) connective tissue activating peptide (CTAP III) = low affinity PF4 (LA-PF4) β-thromboglobulin (β-TG)	Megakaryocytes stored in α-granules of platelets	Thrombin	Chemotaxis for leukocytes? Mitogenic for fibroblasts?
Monocyte chemoaatractant protein-1 (MCP-1)	Lymphocytes Monocytes? Glioma cells	PHA LPS, Il-1	Chemotaxis for monocytes
RANTES (cDNA)	Id4 and CD8 T cells	Mitogen, antigen	Function?
pLD78 (cDNA)	Lymphocytes	PHA, TPA	Function?

Other factors (not yet cloned) also belong to this family:
MCF (monocyte chemotactic factor): Matsushima et al. (1989) J. Exp. Med. 169, 1485
ENAPα (endothel cell derived neutrophil activating factor): Schröder and Christophers (1989) J. Imm. 142, 244

are its main source, but it is also formed in endothelial cells and perhaps even in lymphocytes. LPS, staphylococcal exotoxin and the cytokines mentioned above induce the synthesis of Il-8. Interferon γ seems to prime monocytes for an enhanced response to LPS, while glucocorticoids inhibit the induced synthesis of Il-8. If Il-8 is injected into the skin of rodents, granulocytes soon infiltrate the site of injection. Upon i.v. injections into rabbits (at doses of 2.5–10 ng) rapid leukocytosis ensues which peaks after one hour and disappears again within eight hours. The receptor for Il-8 is expressed on human neutrophils. The binding of Il-8 to its receptor is specific. Other cytokines do not interfere with it. Since relatively little is known about the specific actions of the other factors belonging to this group, they will only be listed here schematically *(Table 2.10)*.

2.2.2.5. The chromosome 5 linkage group

The long arm of chromosome 5 codes for a large number of genes which are functionally related to hematopoiesis but not restricted to it. GM-CSF, Il-3, Il-4 and Il-5 may be part of a related gene family. Their close linkage on chromosome 5, their similar gene structures, their joint expression in activated T-cells and the presence of conserved regulatory elements in the promotor regions of at least the GM-CSF and Il-5 genes would argue in favour of such a relationship. Also on the long arm of chromosome 5 are the genes for the M-CSF receptor and the genes for aFGF (acidic fibroblast growth factor) and M-CSF. It is, however, doubtful whether these latter two cytokines can be added to the chromosome 5 linkage family. The spatial location of the various genes on chromosome 5 is illustrated in *Fig. 2.29*.

Since the colony-stimulating factors Il-3, GM-CSF, M-CSF and G-CSF are discussed in some detail in Chapter 6 in connection with their therapeutic utilities, we will restrict ourselves here to a brief discussion of Il-4 and Il-5.

Il-4 is synthesized as a peptide comprising 153 amino acids. 24 amino acids at the NH_2-terminal end represent a leader sequence which is cleaved off. The protein contains two N-glycosylation sites and 6 cysteine residues.

The mature protein when it is fully glycosylated has a molecular mass of approximately 20 kd.

Il-4 was first described in 1982 as a cofactor in the proliferation of B-cells which had been stimulated by crosslinking their sIgG receptors by anti-IgG antibodies. It was shown to be synthesized by mitogen-stimulated T-cells. At first it was designated as BCGF (B-cell growth factor), later as B-cell stimulatory factor (BSF) and more recently as Il-4. The cytokine interacts with a receptor which is expressed on a large variety of cells. The kd of this interaction is put at 2×10^{-10} M.

Il-4 acts on resting B-cells which express low numbers of Il-4 receptors and on B-cells which are in late G_1-phase. It causes a striking increase on expression of HLA class II genes as well as an enhanced expression of the low affinity IgE receptor (Fc_ε II). In B-cells stimulated with LPS, Il-4 induces class-switching to IgG1 and IgE synthesis.

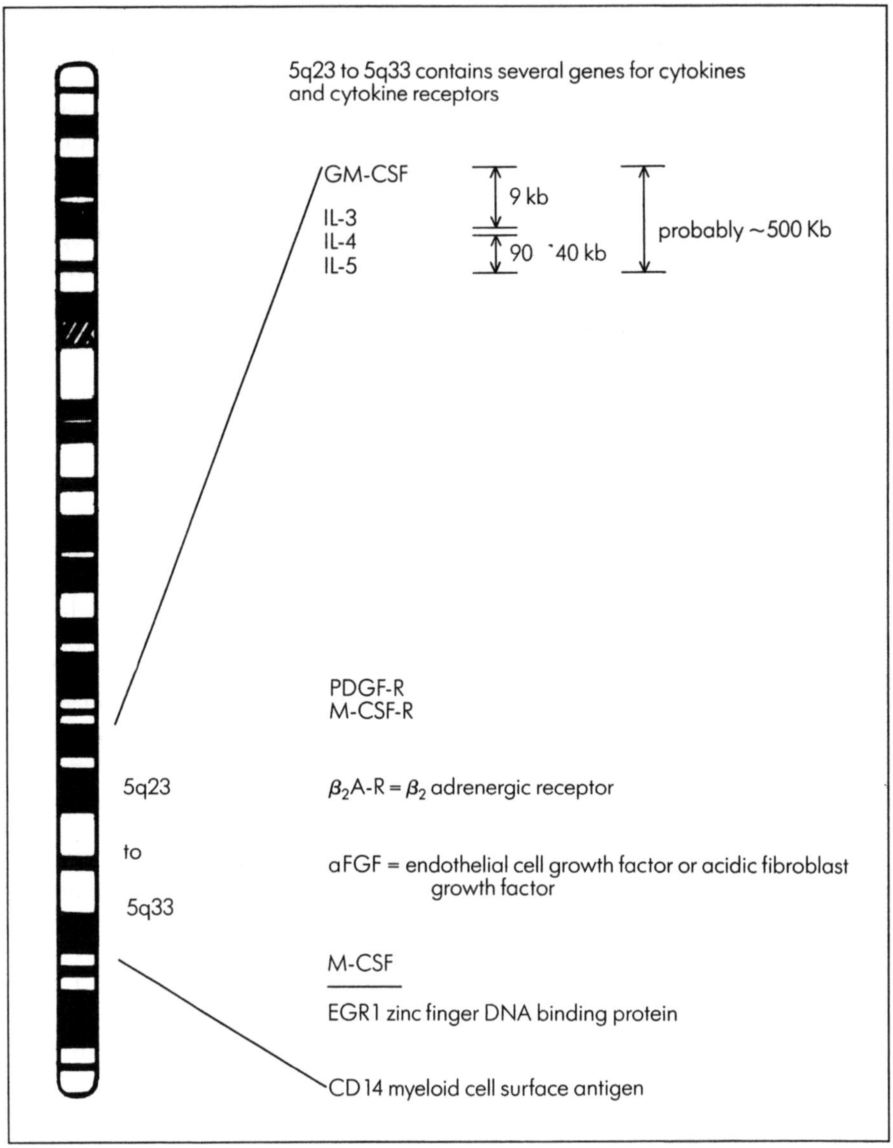

Figure 2.29. The long arm of chromosome 5. The genes for several cytokines, most of which have a role in hematopoiesis, are located on the long arm of chromosome 5 within the region indicated 5q23 to 5q33.

The precise order remains to be determined.
Physical close linkage has been shown (⟷) for some genes.

GM-CSF, IL-3, IL-4 and IL-5 may be part of a distantly related gene family
- close linkage at chromosome 5
- similar gene structure
- regions of low homology at the C-terminus (7)
- expression in activated T-cells
- conserved regulatory elements in promotor region at least of GM-CSF and IL-5 genes (7)

M-CSF and a FGF probably do not belong to this family.

Il-4 acts also on T cells. As a matter of fact, it can replace Il-2 in the stimulation of the so-called HT-2 cell line. Like Il-2, Il-4 acts on stimulated T-cells in the late G_1-phase. The range of cells on which Il-4 can act is quite broad. The cytokine was found to stimulate the proliferation of immature erythrocyte precursors, myelomonocytic precursors and megakaryocytic precursors. Its most important biological role besides its function as a B-cell stimulating factor resides in driving mast cell division. In this respect it cooperates with Il-3. This mast-cell augmenting property together with the enhancement of IgE and Fcε RII synthesis give Il-4 a pivotal role in the regulation of acute hypersensitivity reactions (see chapter 4). In mice the existence of two subsets of TH-cells has been demonstrated. The first subset, called TH_1, produces Il-2 and interferon γ but not Il-4. In contrast, the second subset, TH_2, secretes only Il-4 but not Il-2 or interferon γ. It has been speculated that the TH_1 subset is specialized in defending the organism against viral infections, while the TH_2 subset was designed to react to parasitic infections. Thus far, this dichotomy of T-helper cell functions has not been established for humans. It would, however, make sense. IgE antibodies, regulated by Il-4, can sensitize mast cells for the release of vasoactive amines and target cells (parasites) for antibody-dependent cytotoxicity reactions carried out by eosinophils.

In mice the synthesis of IgE antibodies critically depends on Il-4. This has been shown by infecting animals with larvae of the nematode *Nippostrongylus brasiliensis* and blocking Il-4 by neutralizing monoclonal antibodies.

From a therapeutic point of view the role of Il-4 can be viewed positively and negatively. In allergic diseases drugs which down-modulate the influence of Il-4 may be helpful: an Il-4 receptor antagonist could serve such a purpose. On the other hand, the therapeutic use of Il-4 itself may be desirable in certain parasitic infections, especially in connection with chemotherapy.

The gene for interleukin-5 (Il-5) comprises 4 exons and 3 introns. The protein is synthesized as a precursor containing a 19 amino acid signal peptide at the NH_2-terminal end. The mature protein comprises 115 amino acids. The molecule contains two potential N-glycosylation sites, as well as two cysteine residues.

Il-5 was first described as eosinophil differentiation factor (EDF). The role of these cells in the destruction of parasites in an IgE mediated cytotoxicity reaction, but also in tissue damage in diseases characterized by chronic hypersensitivity such as asthma, was mentioned above. In the mouse, Il-5 or EDF not only promotes the proliferation of eosinophils. In this species, it is also a B-cell growth factor. Actually, it was first described as T-cell replacing factor (TRF) and B-cell growth factor (BCGF II).

Il-5 was shown to enhance the production of IgA. In fact, Il-5 has even been proposed as an IgA specific switch factor. At the same time, however, it was shown that IgA secretion was stimulated in sIgA positive but not in sIgA negative cells. At least with respect to human B-cells, the role of Il-5 is not clear at present. Its main role in the human seems to be lineage specific stimulation of eosinophils. While GM-CSF has also been shown to stimulate eosinophil proliferation, this effect is part of a much broader support of hematopoiesis.

2.2.2.6. *Individual cytokines with no close relatives*

This group comprises a large number of proteins that are not easily associated with any of the previously listed families. Interferon γ belongs in this group (for lack of better reasons) as do Il-2, Il-6, Il-7, CD23 and LIF. Since CD23, interferon γ and Il-2 are discussed in Chapters 4 and 6, they will not be dealt with here any further. We will therefore restrict our discussion to Il-6 and Il-7.

Il-6 first became known as interferon $\beta 2$ because, like other interferons, it seemed to be capable of inducing an antiviral state. Structurally, however, Il-6 is quite different from the interferons. Moreover, the antiviral activity of Il-6 has not been generally confirmed. For these reasons, Il-6 is today regarded as an entity in itself. In fact, the Il-6 gene has a remote structural similarity to G-CSF. Il-6 has been identified and cloned several times, always in connection with another biological activity. After several years it became clear that all of these effects on B-cells, on T-cell activation in early stages of hematopoiesis, as well as on the synthesis of acute phase proteins, are caused by a single protein which seems to be almost as pleiotropic in its biological spectrum as Il-1.

The gene for Il-6 is located on chromosome 7. It comprises five exons, separated by one small, two medium sized and one large intron. The molecule is synthesized as a protein comprising 212 amino acids. After removal of a leader sequence of 28 amino acids, the mature protein contains 184 amino acids with four cysteine residues and two sites for N-glycosylation. The mature glycosylated protein has a molecular weight of 26 kd. The promotor region of the Il-6 gene contains a number of important regulatory elements which offer a clue to the ways in which the transcription of the gene is regulated: a cAMP responsive element (CRE: 5'-ACGTCA-3') provides responsiveness to this internal messenger: elevation of cAMP leads to gene expression. Two copies of short nucleotide sequences serve as binding sites for AP-1, a transcription activating protein which is activated by phorbol esters. A glucocorticoid responsive element (5'-AGAACA-3') occurs twice. Glucocorticoids are known to shut off Il-6 production at the transcriptional level. Additional elements are typical of genes inducible by interferons.

Il-6 is mostly produced by monocytes. Under appropriate circumstances, however, the cytokine is also elaborated by fibroblasts, endothelial cells, keratinocytes and perhaps also by B- and T-cells. Inducers of Il-6 transcription are phorbol myristate acetate (PMA) or signals from antigen receptors, agents which elevate cAMP levels, LPS, TNF, Il-1, viruses, interferon α, β, PDGF and poly-IC.

The Il-6 receptor (there may be several) has been cloned. It is a single polypeptide chain with 468 amino acids, 19 of which (NH_2-terminal end) function as a leader sequence. The extracellular part of the receptor contains eight cysteine residues and four sites for N-glycosylation.

The receptor has been found to be expressed on a large variety of cells in accordance with a multitude of biological effects which are exerted by Il-6. Resting T-cells carry the receptor, and it has been suggested that Il-6 may at least in some cases represent the second signal, which after antigen presentation to a T-cell, leads to the functional expression of the Il-2 receptor. This role, of course, is usually ascribed to Il-1! Il-6 has also been shown to induce the formation of cytotoxic lymphocytes from T-cell precursors. B-cells, once activated, also express the receptor, in line with the observation that activated B-cells require Il-6 for the production of immunoglobulins. The proliferation of plasmocytoma cells and hybridomas derived from them is stimulated by Il-6. In hepatocytes Il-6 induces the formation of acute phase proteins – similar to Il-1. In hematopoiesis Il-6 has been shown to stimulate the proliferation of the granulocyte and macrophage colonies in conjunction with Il-3 or GM-CSF. The cytokine is probably also involved in the expansion of an early committed precursor population in the bone marrow. Since many of the activities of Il-6 are so similar to those of Il-1 and, moreover, since Il-1 has been shown to induce the formation of Il-6 in fibroblast and endothelial cells, it is sometimes difficult to decide which effects must be attributed to either one of these two cytokines and which can be induced by both. Because of its hematopoietic effects Il-6 could become a drug which could be used alone or together with Il-1, Il-3 and the colony stimulating factors to support blood formation in the bone marrow. However, Il-6 has also been implicated in autoimmune disease: levels of Il-6 are clearly elevated in the synovial fluid of patients with rheumatoid arthritis. Moreover, paraneoplastic autoimmune conditions have been described: a patient with cervical cancer which produced Il-6 displayed symptoms of Sjögren's syndrome. It is also known that carriers of cardiac myxomas (benign tumours of the heart) often suffer from autoimmune phenomena and high titers of autoantibodies. These symptoms appear to correlate with the secretion of Il-6 by such tumours *(Fig. 2.30)*. It is therefore possible that agents interfering with the formation of Il-6 or with its action (receptor antagonists) could have therapeutic potential as antiinflammatory or immunosuppressive agents. The beneficial role of glucocorticoids in autoimmune diseases and chronic inflammatory disorders offers an interesting case in point, since glucocorticoids shut down Il-6 synthesis by virtue of a special regulatory element in the 5' promotor region of the corresponding gene.

The search for a factor which supports the growth of early B-cell precursors led to the discovery of a cytokine which was first called lymphopoietin and later received the name Il-7. The factor was found in stromal cells from bone marrow. Such stromal cells were needed as a "feeder layer" for the in-vitro growth of pro- and pre-B-cells. A cDNA library from these cells was generated in an *E. coli* expression vector. When transfected into CoS-7 cells, Il-7 was discovered as an active principle which supported the proliferation of pre-B-cells (B220-μ-) and of pro-B-cells (B220$^+$cytoplasmic μ^+). Mature B-cells which were also surface μ^+ did not respond to Il-7 any longer. Surprisingly, however, double negative T-cell precursors reacted to Il-7 with proliferation. The idea that Il-7 may also act on these cells became obvious when, after the cloning of Il-7, high levels of mRNA for the cytokine had been discovered in several lymphoid organs and also in the thymus.

Il-7 contains 152 amino acids. 25 amino acids serve as a leader sequence so that the mature protein comprises 127 amino acids. The protein contains two N-linked glycosylation sites and four cysteine residues. It has a molecular weight of 14.9 kd.

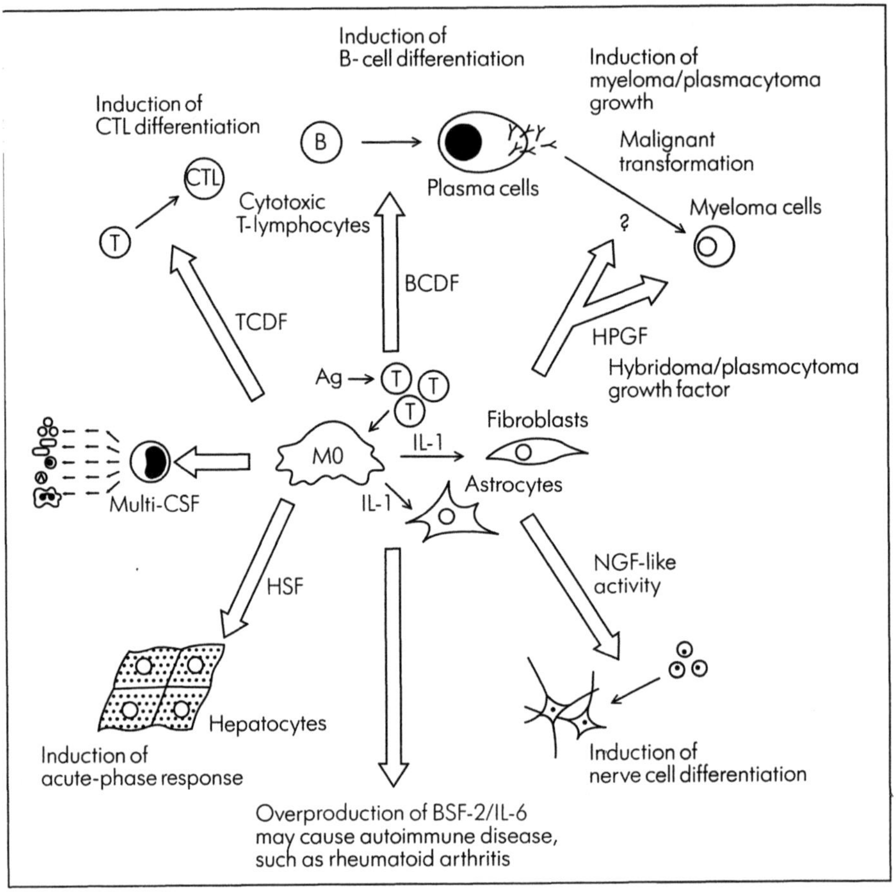

Figure 2.30. Biological actions of IL-6. The various biological actions of IL-6 are symbolized by the large open arrows. IL-6 stimulates hemopoiesis, induces cytotoxic lymphocytes, assists in the differentiation of B-cells to plasma cells and may also play a role in the malignant transformation of B-cells to myeloma cells. The overproduction of IL-6 may play a pathophysiological role in the generation of autoimmune disease, especially of rheumatoid arthritis. IL-6 also exerts an NGF-like activity and can induce the differentiation of nerve cells. Like IL-1 it induces hepatocytes to synthesize acute phase proteins.
HSF: hepatocyte stimulating factor.
NGF: nerve growth factor.
TCDF: T-cell differentiating factor.

Mature cells respond to Il-7 only when previously stimulated by a mitogen or antigen. There is at present no evidence that Il-7, apart from its proliferation inducing effects in young cells of the B- and T-cell lineages, exerts differentiating effects.

2.2.3 The complement system

Complement is a physiological constituent of blood plasma. It comprises a number of proteins, many of which are proteases which function like a cascade:

one enzyme splits and thereby activates a second enzyme, which in turn activates a third enzyme, and so forth. At the end of this cascade, several components of the complement system form a complex which can lyse cell membranes. The components of the complement system are all water-soluble and cover a wide range of molecular weights (between 24,000 and 400,000 daltons). The name 'complement' denotes the fact that this system functionally 'complements' antibodies. This complementation was described in connection with antibodies to erythrocytes. Antibodies which are directed against erythrocytes bind to these cells but do not lyse them. Lysis occurs only after the plasma proteins of the complement system are added. These proteins turned out to be present only in 'fresh' plasma but not in plasma which was inactivated by heating to 50 °C. Although the complementation of antibody function is perhaps the most important role that the complement system has to play, its overall function in the context of the immune system and in the organism is a much more general one. Certain fragments of complement proteins can stimulate cells to secrete mediators like histamine, serotonin, enzymes or prostaglandins. By way of binding components of the complement system, cell surfaces acquire the ability to bind other cells to become more active in phagocytosis. Recently it was found that fragments of the third component of complement like C3b inhibit the expression of MHC class II molecules on the surface of antigen presenting cells and that this effect can have a down-modulating influence on cellular immune responses. Another fragment of C3 (C3d) has even been shown to be a more general inhibitor of cell division.

In a narrow sense complement can be characterized as a humoral effector system which is a priori not antigen-specific but is frequently channelled to function in an antigen-specific manner through the cognitive properties of antibodies. In a wider sense, which embraces not only the soluble plasma proteins but also the proteins which react with complement constituents like inhibitors and receptors, complement would have to be defined as a system which regulates cellular functions by modifying cell surfaces. So far, the consequences of these cell surface modulations are particularly evident in the following physiological events:

1. Defence against infectious agents
2. Initiation of inflammatory reactions
3. Removal of immune complexes
4. Modulation of immune responses.

Activation pathways

Functionally, the pivotal component of the complement system is the C3 protein. It is composed of two chains, α and β, with molecular weights of 105 and 75 kd respectively. The two chains are bound to each other by two disulfide bridges. C3 is activated by an enzyme complex called C3 convertase, which removes a segment of 9 kd from the N-terminal end of the α chain. This small segment is called C3a; it has strong anaphylactic properties. The remaining structure,

C3b, has a strong affinity for cell surfaces and for the Fc portion of antibodies. It binds to these structures by virtue of a labile thioester group. The activation of C3 is the prerequisite for the cleavage and the activation of C5 and for the subsequent formation of the so-called 'lytic complex'.

Several pathways lead to the activation of C3. The antibody-mediated reaction sequence which was first studied in connection with the lysis of red cells is now called the classical pathway. There is one so-called alternative pathway which is also well defined. Besides these two reaction sequences, however, C3 can apparently be activated by proteases which are membrane-bound and become activated through tissue damage. In total, there are, therefore, several reaction sequences of which only the 'classical' and the 'alternative' pathway will be described in some detail *(Fig. 2.31)*.

The classical pathway starts with the formation of an immune complex. An antibody binds to its target. As a result of this event, the Fc portion of the antibody undergoes a conformational change which makes it recognizable for the first component of the complement cascade C1. This macromolecule is a conglomerate of three subunits which are called C1q, C1r and C1s. Clq is represented only once in this complex while C1r and C1s each contribute two copies to the C1 complex. Within the C1 structure, C1q is the recognition element. It has a molecular weight of 440,000 daltons and comprises 18 polypeptide chains of three types, called A, B and C. There are six chains of each type. The NH_2-terminal ends of the chains are characterized by a collagen-like structure (gly-x-y)n, while the C-terminal portions are non-collagen-like. The chains A-B and C form a triple-helical structure in which the A and B chains are held together by a disulfide bridge while the C chain of two neighbouring triple-helices are also linked together by an -S-S bridge. In this way six subunits are formed, each comprising an A, B and C chain. The total molecule has a structure somewhat reminiscent of a bouquet of flowers: the collagen-like strands are tightly held together by disulfide bridges and the C-terminal ends of each triple-helix form a globular structure like a flower. These globular parts of this molecule have a high affinity for the Fc parts of antibodies, which are engaged in antigen binding. If several such 'flowers' have bound to the Fc portions of antibodies, the C1q molecule undergoes a conformational change which 'activates' C1r *(Fig. 2.32)*. This molecule is a single chain or enzyme with a molecular weight of approximately 80,000 daltons. It represents the point where the conformational changes of the Fc part of the antibody and of C1q generate enzymatic activity, and more specifically, proteolytic cleavage. The substrate for this reaction is the proesterase C1s, also a single chain protein with a molecular weight of 80,000 daltons. Upon cleavage C1s becomes an active C1 esterase. This enzyme, which by virtue of its attachment to the Fc portion of an antibody is bound to the cell surface, then cleaves another soluble protein C4 into C4a and C4b, respectively.

C4 is synthesized as a single polypeptide chain of a molecular weight of 200,000 daltons. Prior to secretion it undergoes processing by proteolytic cleavage at four sites which are characterized by basic amino acid residues. This results in the formation of a three subunit structure (α, β and γ). The subunits are held together by disulfide bridges. C1 esterase cleaves a single bond in the

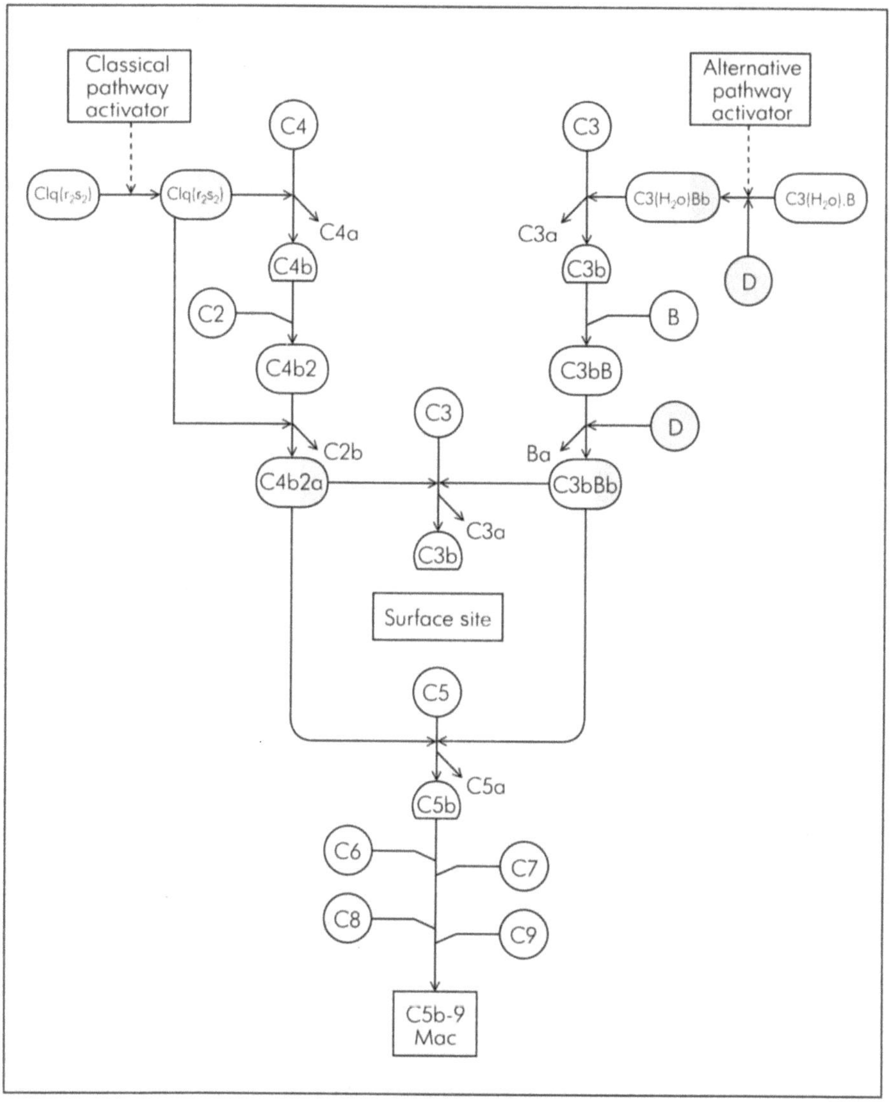

Figure 2.31. Schematic representation of the complement cascade. The classical and the alternative pathways are described more closely in the text. In accordance with its central role C3 is located in the centre of the scheme and the two C3 convertases generated by the classical and by the alternative pathway are on its left and right side (C4b2a and C3bBb).

a chain of the C4 molecule to yield the small C4a fragment of 9 kd and the large C4b fragment of 190 kd. C4b binds to the immune complex and forms the specific attachment site for native C2. Immediately after binding to C4b, C2, a single chain proenzyme is cleaved into C2a and C2b. The resulting C2b chain has a molecular weight of 30 kd and the catalytic C2a chain comprises 70 kd. C2a remains attached to C4b. Together these two proteins form the so-called C3 convertase which generates C3a and C3b as described above. C3b,

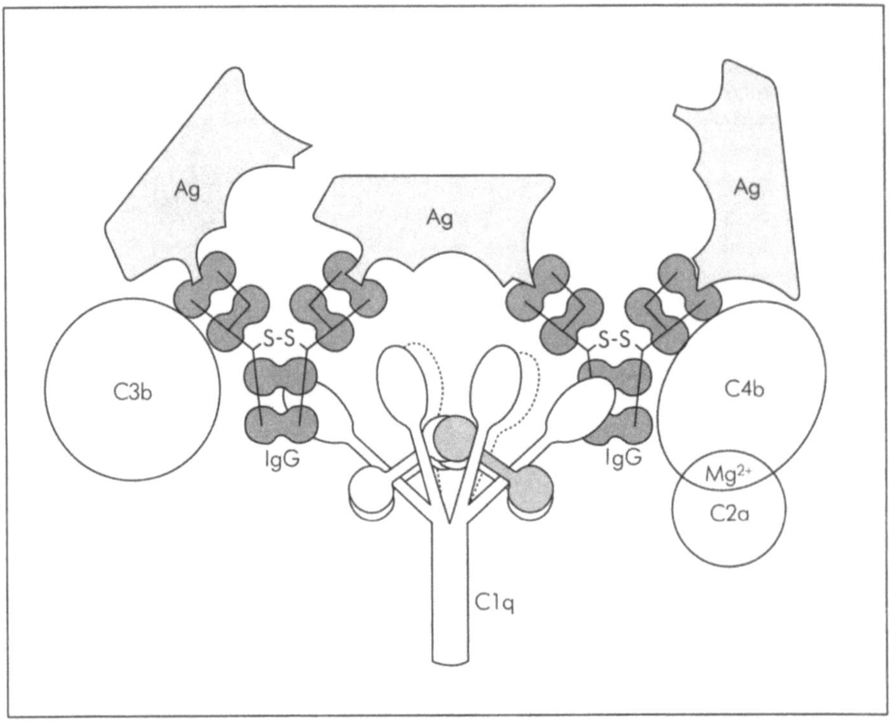

Figure 2.32. First step in the classical pathway of complement activation. The globular portions of the C1q molecule are attached to the Fc portions of two antibodies which, in turn, have reacted with antigen.

which remains covalently bound to the immune complex then cleaves C5 into C5a and C5b. The cleavage of C5, which is synthesized as a single polypeptide chain and then processed into a two-chain structure with an α- and β-chain, is quite analogous to the cleavage and activation of C3. The small NH2-terminal fragment which is removed from the α chain of native C5 is a potent anaphylotoxin, which, after binding to C5a receptors of granulocytes, promotes degranulation of these cells with consequent release of mediators of inflammation and anaphylaxis. The cleavage of C5 is the last enzymatic step in the complement cascade. C5b associates with C6 and C7. Both of these glycoproteins have a molecular weight of approximately 80,000 daltons. On account of its lipophilicity this trimolecular complex can insert itself into cellular membranes. A further component, C8, which comprises three chains (α-68 000, β-64,000, γ-22,000) reinforces the membrane attachment of the complex. At the same time it induces the association of C9 and the subsequent polymerization of this protein. C9 is a single chain protein of 537 amino acids. The final complex then contains C5b, C6, C7, C8 and C9 in a molar ratio of 1:1:1:1:12 −18! The complex forms a ring-shaped structure which acts as a pore in the membrane and destroys the osmotic gradient between the interior of the cell and its environment. Only one such lesion is sufficient to destroy an erythrocyte. Because nucleated cells have a membrane repair system, they can tolerate up to several thousand such lytic attacks before their capacity for membrane restoration is finally exhausted and the cell is destroyed.

In contrast to the classical pathway, the alternative pathway is based on the spontaneous hydrolysis of the thioester group in C3, which occurs permanently, though at a very slow rate. In this way C3 acquires the biological activity of C3b without cleavage of the α-chain. This 'activated' C3 binds a soluble protein, factor B. This factor is a single chain proenzyme of a molecular weight of 90 kd. Once bound to C3, factor B becomes the substrate for another soluble protease, factor D, which cleaves B into Ba and Bb. Bb can now cleave C3 as in the classical pathway. This then leads to the generation of a C3bBb complex which is a strong C3 convertase. Normally these spontaneous events are controlled by endogenous inhibitors. However, the substances that are known to induce the alternative pathway, LPS, dextranesulfate, polyanions, zymosan and $F(ab)_2$ fragments are strong stabilizers of the C3Bb enzyme. Therefore, more C3 is cleaved and complexes with the configuration of (C3b)nBb are formed which, in turn, have strong C5 convertase activity. C5 convertase produced by the classical pathway has the configuration C4bC2aC3b! With the conversion of C5 into C5a and C5b the alternative pathway joins the classical reaction sequence as described above.

Additional pathways which are initiated by proteases like trypsin start with the cleavage of C3: instead of the C3 convertases of the classical pathway C4bC2a or C3bBb, this reaction is now initiated directly by proteases which are activated by tissue injury. Apart from this different entry, the reaction cascade proceeds as described for the classical pathway.

Function of complement

We have already learned that the lytic complex which marks the final structure of the complement cascade represents one of the effector mechanisms by which cells can be destroyed after they have been recognized as foreign by antibodies. Another important function of the complement system resides in the removal of immune complexes from the organism. We know from genetic defects of those complement components that are involved in the clearance of immune complexes how important this 'cleaning up' function is. Defects in the genes coding for C1q, C1r, C1s, C4 and C2 are accompanied by clinical symptoms which resemble those found in systemic lupus erythematosus. Some of the components of the complement system which react with the immune complex or are cleaved while attached to it remain bound to the immune complex, on account of a high affinity for their target structure (C1q) or because their attachment is covalent (C4b and C3b). This 'loading' of immune complexes with complement components keeps these complexes in solution. It can even solubilize complexes which have already precipitated. These complexes can now react with cells which carry complement receptors. Erythrocytes carry complement receptor 1 (CR1), which binds C3b. These cells can therefore bind immune complexes which carry C3b and transport them into the liver and to the spleen where they can be taken up by sessile phagocytes. A physiological inactivator of C3b (factor H) can cleave the α chain of C3b, thereby depriving it of enzymatic activity. The conversion of C3b to inactive Cb3 (C3bi) makes this molecule recognizable by yet another complement receptor which is expressed on neutrophils (CR3). A final degradative step of C3bi to C3d makes the complex also recognizable by yet another receptor CR2. *Taken together, the removal of immune complexes which have reacted with complement again follows the pattern of a cascade. Immune complexes are bound to the surface of cells by virtue of C3b. This fragment is then degraded in a stepwise fashion. With each degradation step, the complex acquires affinity for a new receptor which adds to the total binding and 'elimination' capacity for the immune complexes. Finally they are eliminated in the spleen, together with white cells that have carried them there.*

It was already mentioned that C3a, C4a and C5a are potent anaphylotoxins. They bind to their respective receptors which are expressed on a large variety of cell types, such as thrombocytes, leucocytes, mast cells, macrophages and even smooth muscle cells. The large spectrum of cell types that can be stimulated by anaphylotoxins corresponds to a great variety of cellular responses which are induced by the anaphylotoxins. They include the release of mediators like histamine or serotonin, the provision of arachidonic acid, chemotactic stimuli, the contraction of muscle cells along capillary blood vessels and, subsequent to these effects, an increase in vascular permeability. In their totality these effects are all proinflammatory.

The modulatory effects of complement components on the immune response have already been mentioned. Interestingly, C3a may be able to activate T-suppressor cells which, in turn, can block T-helper cells from providing the necessary help to B-cells. In this way, antibody formation can be inhibited.

T- and B-lymphocytes carry receptors for C3b (CR1) and for the C3b derived cleavage product C3d which reacts with CR2. These findings provide a biochemical basis for the immune modulating effects of C3b which were mentioned above. Although the overall meaning of the effects of C3 fragments on immune parameters are not yet known, one might speculate that they represent a negative feedback loop by which complement components generated by antibody responses and by inflammatory reactions down-modulate earlier stages of those events that have led to their own generation: immune recognition, antibody formation and cell division.

2.3 Synopsis

With the description of the most important cellular and humoral components of the immune system, we now have created a basis for an understanding of the system itself. Since this is a textbook of immunopharmacology, we have to make sure that the reader is familiar with the major elements of the system and with the way these elements interact with each other. Only on this basis can therapeutic strategies be designed and understood. To conclude this chapter we would like to take a bird's eye view of the immune system. Perhaps the best way of doing this is to consider the immune system as the result of an evolutionary process.

Phagocytosis and intracellular killing and digestion – processes related to intake of food and creation of energy – are probably at the root of all endogenous defence mechanisms. As we have seen, the main mediators of these functions are cells of monocytic-myeloid lineage. The macrophage in all its manifestations is one of the best preserved cells in the evolution of higher forms of life. A certain distinction between "self" and "non-self", confined to rough molecular categories, was made at a very early stage by primitive multicellular organisms in confrontations with their environment.

The "spontaneous" increase in the aggressiveness of macrophages (which is manifested as "activation" and is not at first mediated by other cells) at the "sight" of bacterial antigens such as the lipopolysaccharides, β-1.3 or α-1.4 D-glucans, or the peptidoglucans illustrates the phylogenetic context. In this respect macrophages of the *Limulus polyphemus,* the horseshoe crab, react in exactly the same way as their mammalian descendants. As more and more forms of life came to be viewed as possible parasites, an increasing degree of specialization was needed to combat them. The development of effector cells which were specialized in combating bacteria can be understood in this way. The same applies to fungi and, in particular, to parasites of animal origin, which – in contrast to malignant tumours – were in evolutionary terms an effective threat to the development of multicellular, warm-blooded organisms. In this development of special defence mechanisms, as represented by specialized effector cells, a very important thread can be seen in the development of the immune system. The specificity of neutrophilic granulocytes for protection against bacterial infection has already been mentioned, and the same can be said of eosinophils as protection against helminths and schistosomes, or of mast cells as protection against primary toxic allergens, which are eliminated in an acute inflammatory reaction in which macrophages and neutrophils – brought in by extravasation – participate. In addition to this development of "immediate-type measures", a system later emerged – perhaps already at the earthworm level but more definitely in cartilaginous fish – which made it possible in the first place for biological individuality in the strict sense of the word to develop. Even cyclostomes are able to form antibodies. This system endowed the body's defences not only with a large number of more specific effector mechanisms such as antibodies and cytotoxic lymphocytes but also with the dimension of memory, the ability to store information. As a result, it came to dominate the more primitive mechanisms deriving from food intake and energy production; and made them much more efficacious by, for instance, selective recruitment of effector cells to the inflammatory foci. Conversely, it proved useful to evolve a system of humoral signals which could be directed by the older, immediate-type defence system at the more recent, "strategically" higher system. The secretion of interleukin-1 by activated and antigen-presenting macrophages is one such signal; it results in activation of lymphocytes and thus in improved regulation of defence processes (recruiting of inflammatory cells to a specific region), specification of defence mechanisms (formation of antibodies) and activation of the immunological "memory" cells.

The relative importance of the two phylogenetically different parts of the immune system is inadequately conveyed by the attributes "nonspecific" and "specific". It is of paramount importance for the survival of an individual that the effector mechanisms of the older system remain biochemically intact; this is demonstrated by many congenital disturbances which affect macrophage or neutrophil function.

The thymectomized nude mouse proves that a mammal can exist without thymus-dependent immune reactions. The absence of neutrophils or macrophages, on the other hand, would scarcely be compatible with life.

The various forms of endogenous defence mechanisms depend, however, on the manifold interactions between the "old" and the "new" immune systems. Macrophages and granulocytes can perform their tasks of phagocytosis and intracellular killing. But the existence of antibodies confers on these functions a new dimension of specificity and considerably boosts their efficiency. This improvement in function can be observed experimentally by investigating the effect opsonizing antibodies have on phagocytosis of bacteria by granulocytes.

Microbes such as *Listeria, Mycobacteria* or *Toxoplasma* which are not rapidly killed by phagocytosis or by the formation of intercellular oxygen radicals are localized by granuloma formation and thus prevented from spreading. This occurs within a functional system in which the presentation of microbial antigen by macrophages to T-lymphocytes and the secretion of interleukin-1 represent the *afferent* function while the release of γ-interferon, interleukin-2, and other cytokines represents the beginning of the *efferent* function. All these efferent signals at the site of microbial invasion result in influx of macrophages, granulocytes, NK cells and in further enhancement of their function. This is manifested as delayed-type hypersensitivity (DTH). Morphologically it is characterized by granuloma formation. "Intracellular" microbes, i.e. bacteria whose replication cycle can be accomplished within one cell and which are able to withstand the mechanisms of intracellular killing by macrophages or granulocytes in the first round, succumb to this concerted action by cells of the "immediate-type" defence and by the lymphocytes. Furthermore, the immunological memory provides a guarantee that the reaction to recurrence of an infection is more rapid and more intense – this also applies, of course, to the synthesis of antibodies.

All known forms of hypersensitivity are based on such interaction between primordial and phylogenetically more recent cellular and humoral mechanisms, the most important of which are summarized below:

Type I: Anaphylactic reaction. The antigen reacts with homocytotropic antibodies (IgG or, more often, IgE), which occupy the cell surfaces of basophilic granulocytes or mast cells through Fc receptors. The "bridging" of two or more antibodies by one or several antibody molecules results in a conformation change in the Fc region of the antibodies, influx of calcium into the cell, degranulation, and secretion of serotonin (in rodents) or histamine. Depending on the amount and site of the antigen involved, the clinical correlates of these disturbances are: hay fever, bronchial asthma, urticarial reactions, and generalized anaphylactic shock.

Type II: Antibody-dependent cytotoxicity. This defence or hypersensitivity mechanism is based on antibody-mediated killing of bacteria, parasites, virally infected cells or tumour cells by neutrophilic granulocytes, macrophages or NK-cells. The reaction involves either phagocytosis and intracellular destruction of the infecting organism, or killing by an extracellular mechanism, and is known as antibody-dependent cell-mediated cytotoxicity or ADCC. This category of reaction also includes antibody-mediated activation of the complement cascade, and destruction of parasitic cells by the formation of the membrane-attack complex.

Type III: This form of hypersensitivity is observed in the antibody-antigen reaction. Soluble antigen-antibody complexes are formed which activate complement and bring about platelet aggregation. Activation of complement results in chemotactic mobilization of granulocytes by C5a and in degranulation of these cells (see section on eosinophils and neutrophils). Platelet aggregation results in the formation of microthrombi and provides a source of vasoactive amines (serotonin, histamine). The clinical course of such reactions depends on the ratio of antigen to antibody: with antibody excess the immune complexes are rapidly precipitated and tend to be localized to the site of introduction of antigen (Arthus reaction) *(Fig. 2.33)*. Gross antigen excess and intravenous administration of incompatible donor blood or xenogeneic immunoglobulins lead to generalized complement utilization, and deposit of antigen-antibody

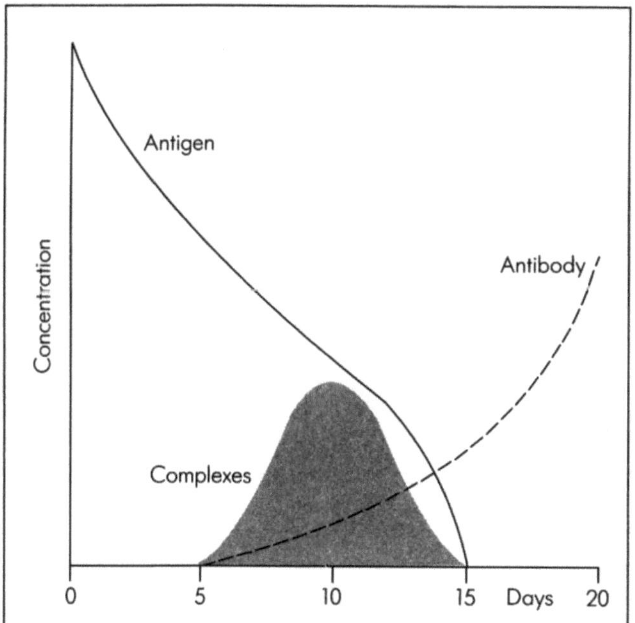

Figure 2.33. Formation of soluble antigen-antibody complexes after injection of a large amount of antigen (e.g. serum of another species). From about the 7th day, the antigen gives rise to the formation of antibodies; between the 5th and the 15th day soluble antigen-antibody complexes may be formed (see dotted line). These complexes can cause serum sickness (cf. Figure 2.24).

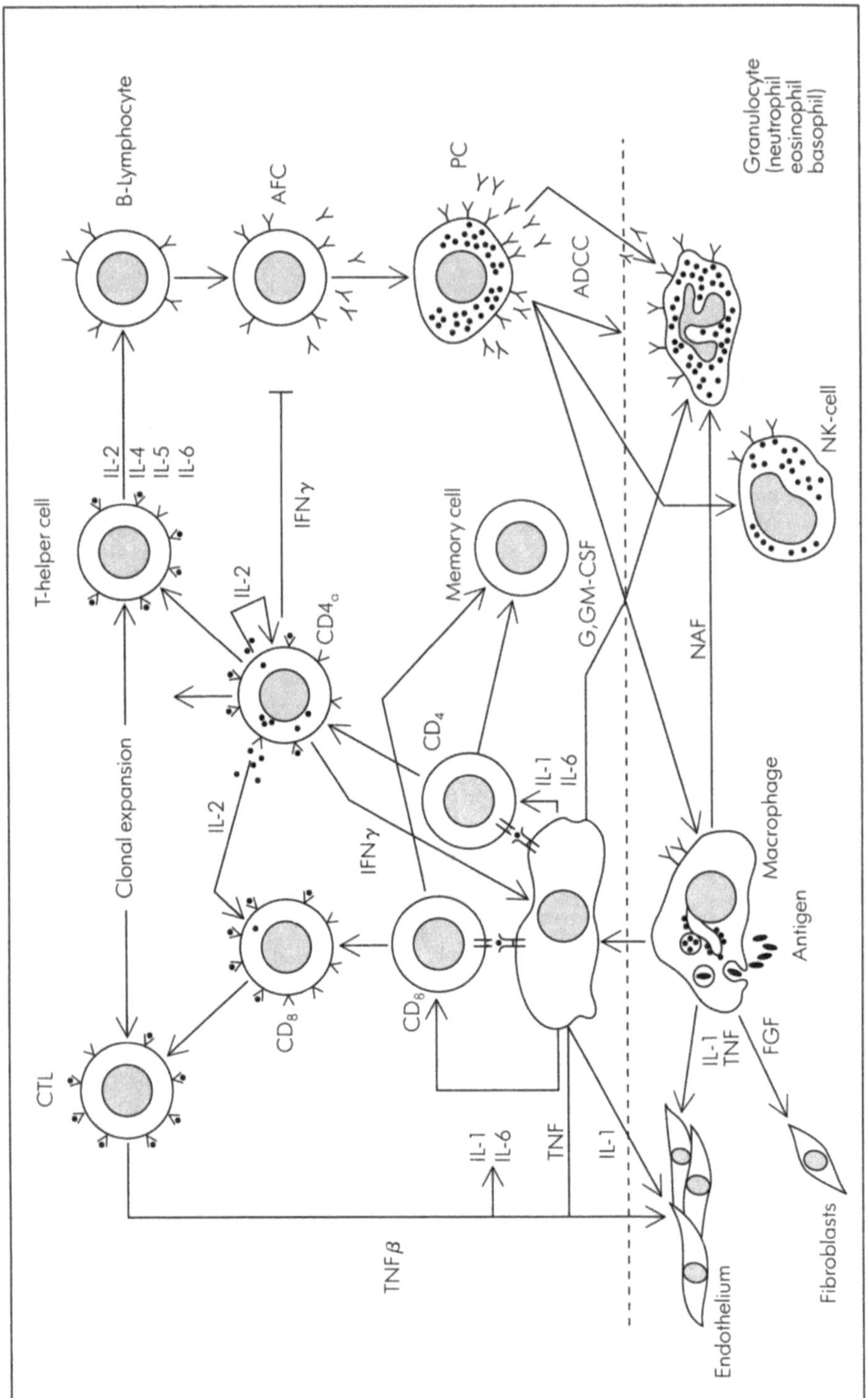
B-Lymphocyte
AFC
PC
Granulocyte (neutrophil eosinophil basophil)
ADCC
T-helper cell
IL-2
IL-4
IL-5
IL-6
IFNγ
NK-cell
Memory cell
CD4a
G,GM-CSF
NAF
Clonal expansion
CD4
IL-1
IL-6
Macrophage
Antigen
CTL
CD8
CD8
FGF
IL-1
TNF
TNF
TNFβ
Endothelium
Fibroblasts

complexes in the peripheral tissue and the capillaries of the skin, kidneys and joints. The generalized activation of complement is followed by release of histamine from the mast cells and generalized urticaria. Increased discharge of pyrogens from the leucocytes gives rise to fever. The clinical designation for this condition is "serum sickness".

Type IV: Delayed-type hypersensitivity has already been described. *Fig. 2.34* provides a schematic outline of the main elements.

Some authors refer to a fifth type of hypersensitivity, "stimulatory hypersensitivity" or hypersensitivity stimulated by antibodies. This type is not in fact a model reaction of defence but, rather, a special pathological or pathophysiological phenomenon. An antibody to a receptor or to a region adjacent to the receptor exerts a similar stimulatory effect on the cell as the binding of the actual receptor ligand. Hyperthyroidism, for instance, can develop as a result of autoantibodies, which have the same triggering function for the active endocrine cell as thyroid-stimulating hormone (TSH). This phenomenon could be of interest in relation to the pharmaceutical use of antibodies (see relevant chapter).

Figure 2.34. Simplified synopsis of main interactions within the immune system.
The dotted line marks the "border" between the "old" defence system and the "new" immune system capable of cognitive functions.
Abbreviations: CTL = cytotoxic lymphocyte, NAF = neutrophil activating factor, FGF = fibroblast growth factor, AFC = antibody forming cell, PC = plasma cell, a = activated.

3. Antibodies as Immunopharmacological Agents

Approximately a century ago, xenogeneic antibodies against diphtheria toxin were first used by Emil von Behring and his Japanese colleague Shibasaburo Kitasato to treat children who were suffering from the life-threatening complications of diphtheria. Although not all of these early therapeutic attempts were successful, "serum therapy" or "passive immunization" proved to be a highly effective approach to the prophylaxis and treatment of many infectious diseases. In 1901 Emil von Behring was awarded the first Nobel Prize in Medicine for this ground-breaking achievement which in the words of the Nobel Committee had "opened a new road in the domain of medical science and thereby placed in the hands of the physicians a victorious weapon against illness and death". In the decades to come, however, progress in this field was slow. Several major hurdles had to be overcome: xenogeneic sera caused disturbing side effects, such as anaphylactic shock, which seriously limited their use. When human antibodies finally became available, they could only be applied intramuscularly. The first antibody preparations for intravenous administration had a very short biological half-life and were functionally unreliable. Many avenues of experimentation had to be probed before human antibody preparations became widely available which could be applied intravenously, were well tolerated and retained all the important biological properties of native antibodies. These new preparations have furnished many new opportunities for the treatment of infectious diseases and other disorders.

Another vigorous impulse for the use of antibodies was generated by the monoclonal antibody technique.

Today antibodies are used therapeutically in an ever growing number of pathological conditions. They are successfully applied as substitutes for the lack of natural antibodies in congenital or acquired immunoglobulin deficiencies. Antibodies are incorporated today into therapeutic concepts aiming not only at the solution of the old and new problems associated with infectious diseases but also at the treatment of cancer and the prevention or suppression of undesired immune responses which cause graft rejections and autoimmune diseases. Some new applications of antibodies have already proven to be highly successful. In this context, the almost complete elimination of morbus hemolyticus neonatorum deserves special comment. In order to prevent the immunological reaction of Rhesus (Rh)-negative mothers to the red cells of their Rh-positive fetuses, mothers are given antibodies to the Rhesus factor during the birth of the child. These antibodies bind to the child's erythrocytes which have entered the mother's blood stream and in this way prevent an immune reaction to Rhesus antigen. The concept of using antibodies as "magic bullets" first put forward by Paul Ehrlich has seen an impressive revival: in particular, monoclonal antibodies are targeted at onco-fetal antigens on cancer cells and at a great number of surface antigens on T-lymphocytes. The effects of antibodies directed at specific cellular structures can be enhanced by attaching toxic substances, drugs or sources of radiation to the antibodies. These clearly "artificial" applications of antibodies are currently under extensive preclinical and clinical investigation. Even if not all of these novel concepts are eventually successful, they illustrate that antibodies as therapeutic and diagnostic tools have come of age and form an integral part of modern medicine.

3.1 Polyclonal animal immunoglobulins

After protective humoral "substances" had been discovered in the sera of both humans and animals and serum therapy had become an obvious and attractive possibility, the pioneering immunologists turned to large animals as antitoxin donors from which they could obtain sufficient quantities of immune serum. Heterologous antibodies from these large animals proved to be highly efficient against certain infections, particularly when they were applied at early stages of the disease. In many parts of the world they are still used to treat patients who are suspected of having acquired life-threatening pathogens such as rabies virus, *Clostridium tetani* or animal toxins. Even today, antisera from animals are the only agents available for the in-vivo neutralization of certain snake or spider venoms. Heterologous antibodies function well as antitoxins but their therapeutic value is severely limited by their foreignness in human hosts. They can cause acute adverse reactions and induce immune responses. They might also fail to interact appropriately with complement components, Fc-receptors or other host factors, since these interactions are to some extent species-specific. With the spectacular success of vaccination and antibiotics on the one hand and with the availability of human IgG preparations on the other, heterologous antibodies against microbial antigens have virtually disappeared from today's clinical scene.

Apart from the use against snake and spider venoms, heterologous sera have found only one important additional application: In the 1960s the use of heterologous antibodies directed against non-microbial antigens emerged as a result of the fast progress which was then being made in cellular immunology. Antisera against lymphocytes were found to be potent immunosuppressive agents. Subsequently such antisera were widely used for the treatment of rejection episodes after organ transplantation and to some extent for the treatment of aplastic anemia.

3.1.1 Anti-lymphocyte (ALG) and anti-thymocyte (ATG) globulins

Antisera against human lymphocytes are produced in a variety of animal species such as horses, goats or rabbits and with a variety of human cells or cell extracts as immunogens. The preferred animals are horses, which serve as donors of anti-lymphocyte globulins (ALG) after immunization with lymphatic cell lines or thoracic duct lymphocytes from patients undergoing therapeutic thoracic duct drainage. Anti-thymocyte globulins (ATG) are usually obtained through immunization of horses with homogenized emulsions of thymocytes from thymus glands which were routinely removed from children undergoing thoracic surgery. The crude immune plasma obtained from one horse (up to 90 l) is partially purified by serial absorptions with red cells and insolubilized human plasma proteins, then precipitated by acrinol and further purified by ion exchange chromatography to remove β-globulins. The final product is adapted to 50 mg protein/ml. Standard preparations contain more than 90 to 95% IgG with small amounts of other Ig classes and unknown contaminants.

Before they are clinically used, ATG or ALG preparations have to be tested for pyrogens and sterility as well as for the presence of hepatitis B surface antigens, and for IgG content. Aggregate formation and fragmentation of antibodies as well as anti-complementary activity and the presence of antibodies directed against human cells and serum proteins must be excluded before use.

The content of polyclonal immunoglobulins in antibodies of particular specificities can be analysed by testing the ability of such preparations to block the binding of monoclonal antibodies to known antigens. ATG and ALG preparations were found to inhibit the binding of monoclonal antibodies to resting T-lymphocytes (CD2, CD3, CD4, CD5, CD8, T-200) and activated T-lymphocytes (HLA-DR, Il-2 receptor: CD25) but failed to block the binding of anti-Leu7 antibodies to large granular lymphocytes (NK-cells). ATG and ALG preparations both induce cell proliferation in short term cultures of peripheral blood mononuclear cells and the production of hematopoietic growth and differentiation factors in bone marrow cultures. Besides the dominating anti-lymphocyte-antibodies, ALG and ATG preparations contain antibodies against many other hematopoietic cells and against a large variety of non-hematopoietic cells. Quantitative differences between clinically active and some inactive lots were observed. However, the question, as to which of the components of ALG and ATG preparations are responsible for their therapeutic effects cannot yet be answered satisfactorily.

3.1.2 ATG/ALG can suppress transplantation immunity

ALT or ATG preparations have been used for more than ten years in many transplantation centres for immunosuppression of allogeneic kidney or bone marrow transplant recipients. Encouraging results in kidney transplants were first reported by Najarian and co-workers in 1969. With a daily dose of 20–40 mg ALG/kg body weight, they achieved a one year transplant survival rate of 80%, as supposed to 50% for the low dosage of 10 mg/kg. Subsequent controlled clinical trials gave variable results but a large randomized Canadian multicentre study reported in 1976 strongly supported the use of ALG. 179 renal allograft recipients participated in the trial. Following kidney transplantation, two groups were formed according to strict randomization principles. One group was placed on "conventional" therapy consisting of azathioprine, prednisone, actinomycin D or local radiotherapy, while the other group received ALG in addition. The dosage was 20 mg/kg body weight i.v. for ten days following the organ transplant. One year after surgery, the transplant survival rate of the ALG treated patients on this study was markedly better *(Fig. 3.1)* than that of the control group.

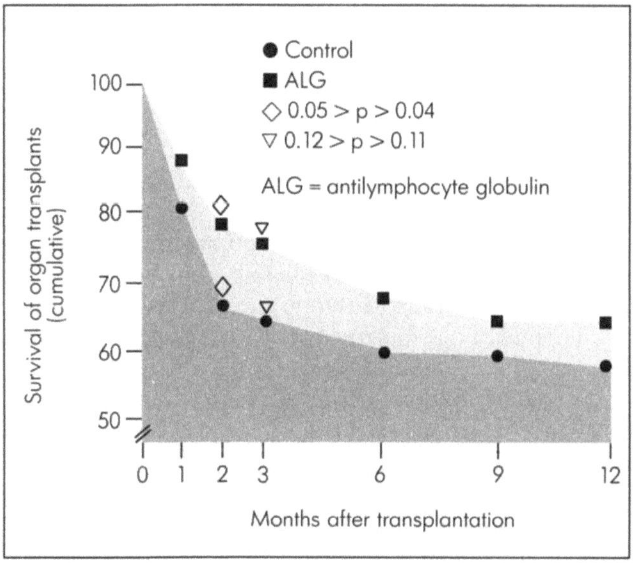

Figure 3.1. Cumulative survival of kidney transplants in patients receiving only drug therapy (azathioprine, actinomycin D and prednisone) or additional treatment with antilymphocyte globulin (ALG). Size of group: ALG n = 87; control group n = 92.
p = thresholds of significance.

Organ function in the ALG group, measured by serum creatinine, was also better. Other parameters such as the effect of prednisone on the incidence of severe rejection reactions in the first three months were also more favourable for the ALG group. These findings clearly argue in favour of the use of ALG in organ transplant surgery.

ALG/ATG preparations which were initially employed prophylactically as a temporary supplement to azathioprine and steroids in the first two to three weeks after transplantation were later found to be also useful in the treatment of acute rejection episodes. Approximately 40% of the rejection episodes cannot be reversed by an increase in steroid dosage alone. These cases can be treated successfully with ATG or ALG, in particular when histological examinations of biopsies reveal mononuclear focal infiltrates in the graft.

With a combination of azathioprine and steroids in the induction and maintenance phase and with the application of ATG/ALG in the immediate post-transplant period and during acute rejection episodes, one-year graft survival rates of up to 100% have been achieved in recent studies in Germany and in the United States.

The clinically active components of ATG and ALG preparations are probably antibodies against one or several T-cell surface antigens. This assumption is supported by the recent finding that host versus graft reactions could be suppressed or inhibited in many renal allograft recipients with murine monoclonal antibodies directed at single T-cell surface antigens (see below).

3.1.3 ALG/ATG can facilitate hematopoietic recovery in patients with aplastic anemia

Aplastic anemia is a life-threatening hematological disorder characterized by peripheral pancytopenia and an acellular or hypocellular bone marrow. Spontaneous recovery occurs rarely. Without bone marrow transplantation less than 25% of patients with severe bone marrow failure survive despite improved supportive care. On the other hand, transplantation with HLA compatible bone marrow has been successful in up to 80% of newly diagnosed patients who did not receive blood transfusions prior to transplantation. It is surprising that not only the transplantation of allogeneic bone marrow but also of syngeneic marrow which comes from an identical twin requires immunosuppression. This observation as well as a number of experimental findings support the common assumption that an immunological mechanism is responsible for the hematopoietic suppression in these patients. Thus immunosuppressive therapy is increasingly being used to treat patients with aplastic anemia who are not eligible for allogeneic bone marrow transplantation. Immunosuppression with ATG/ALG has been successful in a large number of clinical trials: transfusion independence could be achieved in 30 to 75% of the cases. One possible explanation for this rather wide variability in success rates may reside in differences between the antibody preparations which were used. Occasional ALG preparations have been found to be completely inactive. Differences in the stage of the disease or in the pathophysiological mechanism leading to bone marrow failure might be another reason for the variability of the results. Most investigators assume that a particular subset of T-cells is responsible for the suppression of hematopoietic activity, possibly through an overproduction of interferon. These putative T-cells may be reduced or even eliminated by ALG or ATG treatment. Thus the "brakes" on blood cell formation would be removed with the consequence of a restoration of hematopoiesis to normal. Once the mode of action of ATG or ALG in aplastic anemia has been outlined in greater detail, more selective monoclonal antibodies could be employed to substitute for ATG/ALG. Preliminary attempts with combinations of two or three monoclonal antibodies against pan T-cell antigens were unsuccessful.

3.1.4. ALG/ATG can cause serum sickness

Intravenous infusion of ATG/ALG preparations is surprisingly well tolerated. Acute adverse reactions appear to be rarely severe. However, despite their immunosuppressive activity, ATG/ALG preparations do induce immune responses in the host: after the usual ten-day treatment course, serum sickness occurs in practically all cases. In a recent study, for example, 11 of the 12 patients with aplastic anemia who were treated for ten days with daily i.v. infusions of only 15 mg ATG/kg body weight, developed serum sickness in spite of additional treatment with methyl-prednisolone (1 to 1.5 mg/kg/day). Typical symptoms which occur eight to fourteen days after the initiation of ATG/ALG therapy are fever, lymphadenopathy, gastrointestinal disturbances, cutaneous eruptions and arthralgias, often in association with proteinuria but without any additional evidence of glomerulonephritis. The same symptoms were already observed in the very early clinical trials with equine diphtheria antitoxins. They were described in great detail by Pirquet and Schick as early as 1905, but it was only 50 years later that animal experiments revealed the persistence of antigen, circulating immune complexes and complement components as likely pathogenic factors. The host response to heterologous antibodies is the major disadvantage of their clinical application, not only because of the pathological reactions associated with it but also because host antibodies can abrogate the therapeutic effect. With monoclonal antibodies which can be used in much smaller doses than ATG/ALG, serum sickness can be largely avoided. The problem of the induction of neutralizing anti-idiotypic antibodies, however, is aggravated (see below).

Unfortunately serum sickness and induction of host immunity are not the only disadvantages connected with ALG/ATG treatment. The predisposition to viral and bacterial infections which is a side-effect of all immunosuppressive treatment modalities seems to be more pronounced with ALG/ATG than with other immunosuppressive agents.

3.2. Polyclonal human immunoglobulins

In the early 1930s, human IgG which was isolated by ammonium sulfate precipitation from placental serum extracts was successfully used for both the prophylaxis and treatment of measle infections. However, only after Cohn and his colleagues at Harvard Medical School had introduced their procedure of precipitating serum fractions with cold ethanol, the large-scale isolation and purification of human immunoglobulins became feasible. Fraction II was the main source of the human IgG preparations which became known as standard γ-globulins (SGG) or immune serum globulins (ISG). For a long time the Cohn method, which uses only alcohol for fractional precipitation, remained the method of choice at least in the United States. One modification which was introduced by Kistler and Nitschmann during the early 1950s at the Swiss Red Cross Blood Transfusion Centre in Berne combines fractional precipitation and extraction. This method, which is frequently used in Europe, reduces working times, volumes and alcohol consumption and gives a better yield of IgG, but the final product is less pure than that obtained with the classical Cohn method. SSG or ISG was quite satisfactory in the treatment of patients suffering from IgG deficiencies. It could also replace heterologous antibody preparations in the prophylaxis of certain infections. However, ISG preparations have one major disadvantage: when given intravenously, they can lead to devastating vasomotor reactions. Therefore, SGG can only be given by the intramuscular route, which is painful and therefore does not always allow for the application of adequate doses. Furthermore, the slow absorption rate limits the therapeutic value of SSG or ISG preparation in advanced disease states. In particular, patients with IgG deficiencies suffered from the regular i.m. injections. Therefore, i.v. infusion of fresh plasma, which is normally well tolerated and causes only mild systemic effects, in some individuals was preferred by many physicians for antibody replacement therapy. Again, this was not the ideal solution. Plasma transfusions carry the risk of transmitting infectious agents like hepatitis B, even when the samples are pooled from small numbers of carefully selected donors (buddy system). Moreover, elderly patients and children under the age of six years did not tolerate the large plasma volumes which were required to keep IgG levels from falling below the minimum level which provided safety from infections. The need for preparations of concentrated human IgG which could be applied intravenously remained a major challenge to experimental workers. Eventually, a group of investigators at the Swiss Red Cross Agency in Berne solved the problem in principle. They found that mild acid treatment combined with exposure to low concentrations of pepsin resulted in preparations which met the basic requirements. Since the early 1960s, several enzymatically or chemically modified IgG preparations suitable for intravenous use (IGIV) have been described. Initially, these preparations were not optimal because important biological functions of the antibodies were affected by the modifications. In recent years, however, a number of different IGIV preparations with only minor modifications and long biological half-lives became available, first in Europe and in Japan and finally also in the United States.

Since the biological functions of γ-globulins are associated with certain domains of the antibody molecule, one must aim at preserving the intactness of these domains during the preparation of IgGs. As will be described in the following section this goal is not always attained ideally.

Table 3.1 describes biological functions residing in the various domains of the antibody molecule.

Table 3.1. The biological functions of the individual domains of the IgG molecule

Domain	Function
$V_H + V_L$	– specific antigen binding – noncovalent binding of heavy and light chains
$C_H1 + C_L$	– noncovalent and covalent binding of heavy and light chains – "spacer" between antigen binding and effector functions
C_H2	– binding of C1 (activation of complement system) – regulation of catabolism
C_H3	– interaction with the Fc receptor on macrophages, monocytes, and other cells – noncovalent binding of heavy chains
$C_H2 + C_H3$	– interaction with the Fc receptor on neutrophils, cytotoxic K-cells and syncytiotrophoblasts

3.2.1 Human IgG preparations

Human γ-globulins are purified from pooled plasma of up to 5000 donors and thus contain a large antibody repertoire which reflects the immune status of the normal population. There are, however, also preparations which are obtained from a limited number of convalescent patients or from vaccinated individuals and which are enriched with antibodies against a specific pathogen.

These preparations are known as hyperimmunoglobulins. The differences between polyvalent preparations and hyperimmunoglobulin preparations are quantitative, not qualitative.

In recent years a number of different immunoglobulin preparations have been developed. In principle they are all obtained by cold ethanol fractionation of plasma with cold ethanol and through a subsequent modification step which is either chemical or enzymatic. The most important ones which are currently available will be briefly described below.

3.2.1.1 Standard γ-globulin (SGG)

Standard γ-globulin, obtained by the classic Cohn alcohol fractionation method, is still used frequently. The 16% polyvalent concentrate (at least 2000 donors) contains predominantly IgG, while IgA and IgM antibodies are present in only very small quantities.

The preparation has some obvious advantages. With the exception of the aggregated material, the IgG immunoglobulins are native and thus possess all the biological functions of humoral antibodies, in particular a normal biological half-life, normal complement activation in the presence of antigen, and the ability to opsonize antigens.

In a polyvalent immunoglobulin preparation obtained from 2,000–5,000 donors, there are about one million different antibodies. Given this broad donor basis, the relative amount of antibodies remains very constant from one batch to another.

Besides the monomers sedimenting at 7S and dimers (8–10S) the SGG preparation also contains polymer aggregates (30–40S) which are created as artefacts by surface denaturation in the course of plasma fractionation. These IgG aggregates possess the property of activating the complement system even in the absence of antigen (anticomplementary activity). If SGG is administered intravenously, it may cause life-threatening anaphylactoid reactions, particularly in immunocompromised patients. For this reason the preparation may be given only by the intramuscular route. Of course, this has certain drawbacks. Firstly, no more than 1.5–3 g in 10 or 20 ml can be administered at a time and even these doses cause pain at the site of injection. Secondly, the preparation is absorbed relatively slowly from the muscle depot, and peak blood levels are measured only four to six days after administration. Thirdly, even intramuscular injection may produce shock in immunocompromised patients. Thus, SGG can only be administered for prophylaxis. It is not possible to achieve adequate therapeutic doses with this compound.

3.2.2 Intravenously applicable IgG preparations (IGIV)

Low-risk immunosubstitution which ensures sufficiently high dosage levels requires intravenous antibody concentrates which contain no aggregates and do not carry the risk of anticomplementary activity which causes shock.

A number of different approaches have been employed in order to obtain such preparations:

1. Proteolytic cleavage of the Fc fragment from the IgG molecule.
2. Chemical modification of the Ig molecule so that spontaneous complement activation is prevented.
3. Prevention of aggregation during fractionation (e.g. by the addition of polyethylene glycol, albumin or other substances).
4. Selective elimination of the aggregates which are formed (precipitation with polyethylene glycol, treatment with adsorbants, pH4 treatment in the presence of low concentrations of pepsin).

The fact that so many different approaches have been employed to discover effective and well tolerated preparations throws some light on the dilemma facing investigators. The more the immunoglobulins are modified or fragmented, the better they are tolerated. However, chemical modification and splitting of antibodies deprives them of their biological effector functions. With unmodified, i.e. native antibodies, there is always the danger of spontaneous

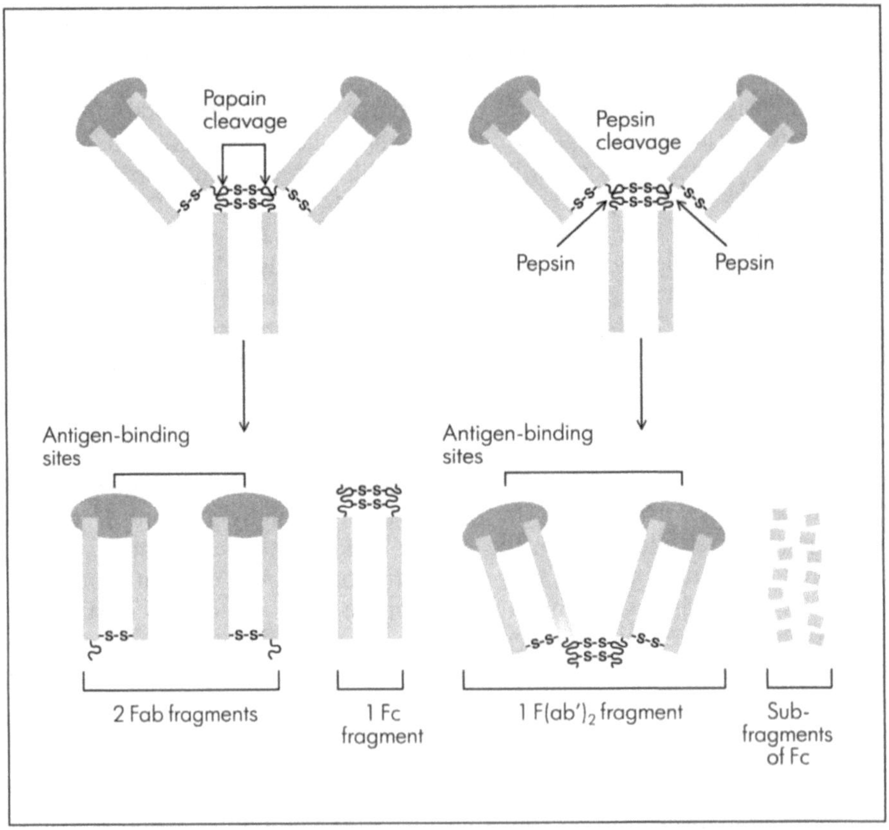

Figure 3.2. Development of antibody fragments by papain and pepsin digestion. In the case of papain, two individual Fab fragments and one Fc fragment develop. Cleavage with pepsin results in one F(ab')$_2$ fragment, while the Fc fragment is entirely split up into subfragments.

aggregation during fractionation and thus the risk of anaphylactic reactions, particularly in agammaglobulinemic patients.

3.2.2.1 Enzymatically split immunoglobulin preparations

Treatment with pepsin

By treating SGG with pepsin, the IgG molecule cleaves at a position immediately behind, i.e. on the C-terminal side of the disulphide bonds which bind the two heavy chains. This gives rise to a product, over 80% of which consists of the bivalent $F(ab')_2$, and which is well tolerated on intravenous injection *(Fig. 3.2)*. This bivalent fragment is able to form antigen-antibody complexes and thus to neutralize viruses and toxins. Lacking the Fc fragment, however, it cannot exert the nonspecific effector functions that belong to this part of the molecule. Thus it cannot activate complement by the classical pathway, it does not speed up phagocytosis, and, what is more, it has the disadvantage of being eliminated from the bloodstream within a short time (half-life: one to two days) *(Fig. 3.3)*. For these preparations, their 'so-called' tissue diffusion therefore depends on rapid elimination of the fragmented antibodies from the blood-

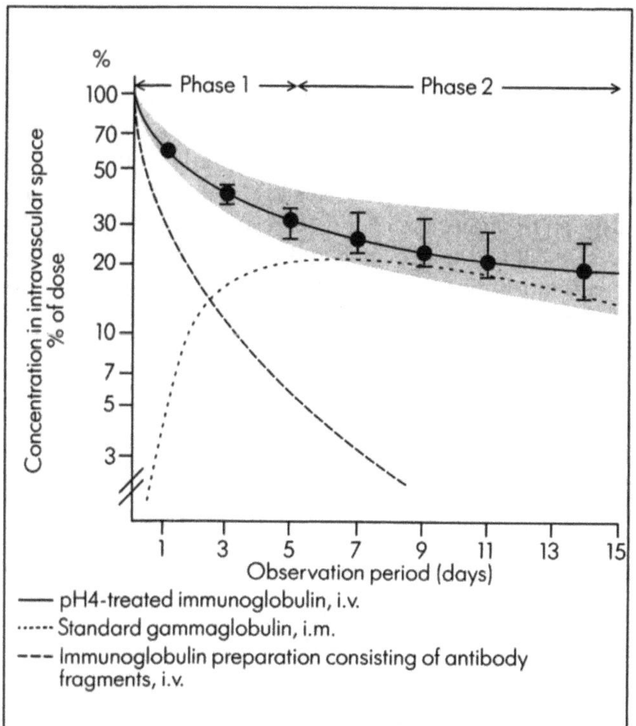

Figure 3.3. Blood levels of two intravenously administered IgG preparations compared with that of SGG given i.m.

stream and not on specific accumulation of the antibodies at the site of infection. Unfortunately, the rapid elimination of these preparations from the bloodstream is not due to a specific accumulation of the antibodies at infection sites as is sometimes claimed. Rather, it reflects a high distribution volume and rapid excretion through the kidney.

Treatment with plasmin

In contrast to pepsin, plasmin (and papain) cleaves the IgG molecule immediately in front, i.e. on the N-terminal side, of the disulfide bonds of the γ-globulin molecule (see *Fig 3.2*). Three fragments of approximately equal size result from this action: two identical monovalent Fab fragments and one Fc piece. The two monovalent Fab fragments can react with their antigen without any ensuing interconnections. These Fab fragments can neutralize toxins, e.g. digoxin, and – at least in vitro – viruses. The therapeutic effect of this preparation is, however, solely due to the fact that 30–40% of the IgG molecules cannot be split by plasmin. Biologically, this plasmin-resistant IgG fraction is active in every respect. The intravenous tolerance of the whole preparation is very good.

3.2.2.2 Chemically modified γ-globulins

Treatment with beta-propiolactone

Cohn's fraction II is virtually identical with standard γ-globulin. If this fraction is treated with beta-propiolactone, which possesses both alkylating and acylating properties, certain structures of the IgG molecules (particularly of the Fc fragment) are modified in such a way that IgG aggregates lose the ability to activate complement spontaneously. In the presence of the corresponding antigen, however, it is thought to be still able, though in a reduced fashion, to activate complement. The biological half-life of this preparation is slightly shorter than that of unchanged SGG. Other effector functions such as binding of protein A from staphylococci are also impaired.

Sulphonated or reduced and alkylated γ-globulins

This is also basically an SGG which has subsequently been reduced, thereby dissolving the disulfide bonds between the heavy and the light chains. The molecule loses part of its anticomplement properties, but activation of the complement system is still possible by the classical pathway.

3.2.2.3 Largely intact immunoglobulins

These preparations are also slightly modified chemically. The changes are, however, so discrete that both the structure and the function of the γ-globulin are almost completely intact.

Treatment with polyethylene glycol

Here we are concerned basically with an unmodified γ-globulin that has been treated by the addition of polyethylene glycol alone or polyethylene glycol and hydroxyethyl-starch with the aim of preventing aggregation of IgG molecules and of precipitating already existing aggregates. In fact, only traces of aggregates are found in these preparations. However, γ-globulins treated in this way still display spontaneous anticomplement effects and can therefore trigger adverse reactions in agammaglobulinemic patients. These preparations are biologically equivalent to standard γ-globulin.

Treatment with pH 4

This preparation is obtained by modification of Cohn's alcohol fractionation procedure, which includes gentle acid treatment at pH 4 and minimal addition of pepsin (1:10,000). This procedure eliminates any aggregates that are present.

The preparation no longer displays spontaneous anticomplement activity and is therefore tolerated by agammaglobulinemic patients, even in very high doses. Furthermore, the preparation has the same specific and non-specific effector properties of native γ-globulin as standard γ-globulin.

Recent studies have shown that pepsin treatment is superfluous if the IgG preparation is formulated at pH 4 (IGIV pH 4.25). Contrary to earlier observations, IgG was found to be stable at pH 4, whereas at pH 5, near its isoelectric point, it is unstable, like most other globular proteins. IGIV pH 4.25 contains only traces of aggregates, has a very low anticomplementary activity and is well tolerated after i.v. application. The low pH of the preparation represents no problem. With a dose of 28 g of protein given to a 70 kg patient the total acid burden introduced is at most one third of that which is contained in one unit of fresh citrate-phosphate-dextrose plasma.

"Intact" γ-globulin preparations that are only slightly modified chemically have biological half-lives close to that of native γ-globulin.

Fig. 3.4 gives an overview over the properties of γ-globulin preparations which are intravenously applicable.

3.2.3 The subclass composition of IgG preparations

For the optimal use of γ-globulins in the clinic it is important to determine the IgG subclass composition of both the patient's serum and the preparation that is administered. Preparations enriched in a particular subclass or even in specific antibodies of a particular subclass may be selected for treatment according to the patient's immune state.

IgG subclasses differ in amino acid sequences of the heavy chain constant regions, in the number of inter-heavy chain disulfide bonds and in the points at which light chains are linked to the heavy chains. Our knowledge of the biological significance of these structural differences is still incomplete.

Preparation	Structure (IgG)	Production	Absorbance profile	Clinically relvant components
Standard GG	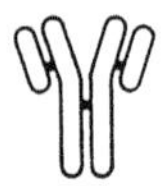	ETOH	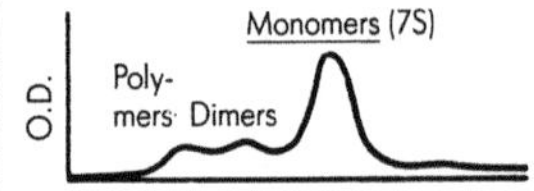	7S-IgG
Gammavenin F (ab')$_2$	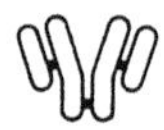	Pepsin	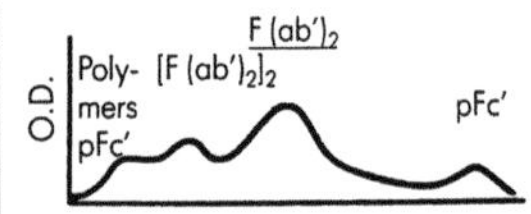	F (ab')$_2$
Veinoglobuline	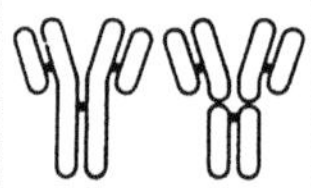	Plasmin	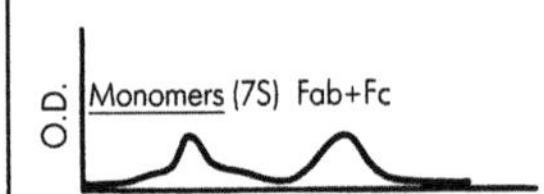	PRG-7S
Intraglobin	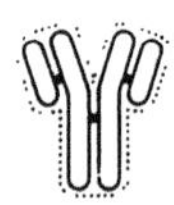	Beta-propiolactone	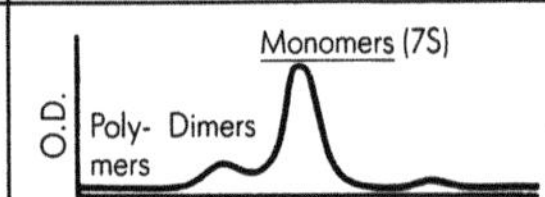	7S-IgG
Sulphonated GG	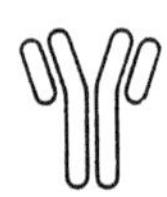	Sulphite + tetrathionate	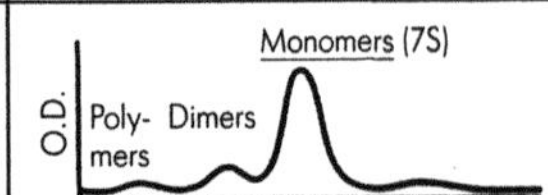	7S-IgG
Immunoglobulin human 7S	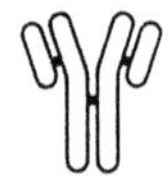	PEG/HES	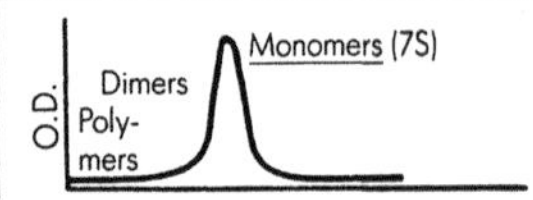	7S-IgG
Acid-treated immunoglobulin	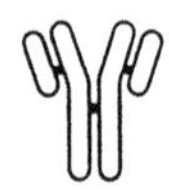	pH 4	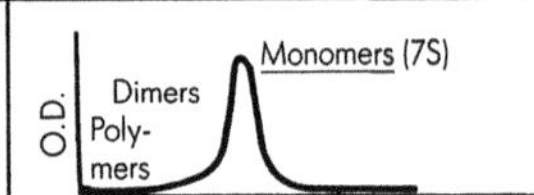	7S-IgG

Figure 3.4. Schematic diagram of the properties of some commercially available, intravenous gamma globulin preparations. The absorbance profiles, measured at 280 nm after gel filtration, indicate the proportions of monomer, dimer and polymer antibodies.

IgG_1 is the predominant subclass in the serum of normal individuals. It amounts to approximately two thirds of total IgG and plays the major role in humoral antibody responses to proteins. In patients with chronic purulent otitis media it is often undetectable. In contrast, elevated levels can be found in patients with IgG_4 deficiency.

IgG_2, which represents about 25% of total IgG, is relatively stable to proteolytic digestion and binds complement less well than IgG_1 and IgG_3. It is often the predominant subclass in responses to polysaccharide antigens and present at low levels in patients with systemic lupus erythematosus, diabetes mellitus or in young children with recurrent otitis media. A combined IgG_2–IgG_4 deficiency is found in patients with ataxia-telangiectasia and is frequently associated with a deficit in IgA.

IgG_3 represents on average 6% of total IgG but the normal range varies widely. The molecule has several unique features: the heavy chains are linked by five disulfide bridges, the angle between the Fab arms is narrow, it does not bind staphylococcal protein A, it is most susceptible to denaturation, it binds strongly to Fc-receptors of lymphocytes (IgG_1, IgG_2 and IgG_4 bind strongly only to cells treated with neuraminidase or stimulated by lectins) and it has the shortest half-life (six to ten days) among the IgG subclasses. Its complete absence is compatible with perfect health, although humoral antiviral activity has been claimed to reside exclusively in the IgG_3 subclass.

IgG_4 accounts for about 2–3% of total IgG. The normal range of plasma concentrations, however, can vary from 10 to 800 $\mu g/ml$. Like IgE this subclass is functionally univalent and appears to bind to Fc receptors of basophils and mast cells. It is not yet known whether IgG_4 has a pathogenic or a protective role in allergic subjects [illegible] whether it plays neither of these two roles. The biological significance of two varieties, IgG_{4a} and IgG_{4b}, is unknown. IgG_4 is relatively stable to proteolytic digestion. Compared with the subclass composition of serum, IgG_4 is enriched in breast milk and bronchial secretions. Its absence is correlated with frequent pyogenic infections, particularly of the respiratory tract. IgG_4 seems to be decreased or absent in ataxia-telangiectasia and idiopathic bronchiectasis and elevated in atopic dermatitis, asthma, cystitis fibrosis, schistosomiasis and in patients with advanced malignant melanoma. Curiously, the majority of autoantibodies to factor VIII in patients with bleeding disorders belong to the IgG_4 subclass.

IgG subclasses are differently affected by various purification procedures. Particularly IgG_3 is often found at very low levels and may even be undetectable in chemically modified IgG preparations. It is not necessarily lost during the fractionation process but, rather, denatured in such a way that its reactivity with anti-IgG_3 monoclonal antibodies or antisera is lost. IgG_4 tends to be concentrated in Cohn fraction III and is therefore depleted in IgG preparations which are derived exclusively from Cohn fraction II. IgG_4, which during isoelectric focusing bands in a narrow acidic pH-region, appears to be also eliminated by DEAE-Sephadex treatment, which is used by some manufacturers as the final purification step.

IgG_1 and IgG_2 are the least variable subclasses in IgG preparations. They are usually present in concentrations which reflect their relative abundance in normal serum.

Table 3.2 gives an overview of the properties and subclass composition of a number of widely used immunoglobulin preparations.

3.2.4 Contaminants of IgG preparations which can cause adverse reactions

Adverse reactions to SGG or IGIV preparations have been associated with protein contaminants such as IgG aggregates, excess in IgA, vasoactive enzymes or antibodies against recipient serum proteins or cells.

Table 3.2. Characteristics of various immunoglobulin preparations

Preparation	IgG subclass distribution	Biological function Fab	Fc	t/2	Ac activity	Indi-cation
Standard GG	Normal	Intact	Intact	18–22 d	++	P
Gammavenin	Not ascertainable	Intact	Absent	Short	0	Th
Veinoglobuline	PRG: G_2 enriched G_1 reduced G_3 lacking	Intact	PRG: intact	PRG: normal	0	P+Th
Intraglobulin	G_3 Not ascertainable	Intact	Reduced	Slightly shortened	0 +	P+Th P+Th
Sulfonated GG	G_3 Not ascertainable	Intact	Reduced	Slightly shortened	+	P+Th
Immunoglobulin Human 7S	Normal	Intact	Intact	Normal	+(+)	P+Th
Immunoglobulin Swiss Red Cross	Normal	Intact	Intact	Normal	0	P+Th

Abbreviations:
GG = gamma-globulin
PRG = plasmin-resistant gamma-globulin
t/2 = biol. half-life (d = days)
Ac activity = anticomplementary activity (shock risk in agammaglobulinemia)
P = prophylaxis
Th = therapy
Biol. function:
Fab specific antigen binding
Fc = nonspecific effector functions

IgG aggregates can fix complement and cause serious side effects when infused i.v. The typical reactions are flushing of the face, feeling of oppression in the chest, lumbar pain, tachycardia, shortage of breath and, one to two hours after infusion, a slight rise in temperature and chills. More violent reactions, reminiscent of anaphylactic shock, are characterized by the sudden onset of symptoms which, in addition to those already mentioned, include nausea, vomiting and eventually circulatory collapse with loss of consciousness. Interestingly, severe adverse reactions have been observed almost exclusively in patients with impaired Ig synthesis. In patients with secondary hypogammaglobulinemia such reactions are rare and – if they occur at all – rather mild.

It has already been mentioned that preparations which are to be given i.v. should not have high levels of aggregates and anti-complementary activity. However, even products which do fulfil these requirements may occasionally cause adverse reactions. The causes are not always understood. Complement activation as the only or main cause of side effects has perhaps been overemphasized in the literature.

Practically all commercially available IgG preparations contain low amounts of IgA. The clinical significance of this contaminant lies not so much in a potential benefit (which is questionable since serum IgA is not associated with the secretory piece) but rather in the fact that traces of IgA can cause severe side effects in IgA deficient patients.

Cohn fraction II is known to contain components of the contact activation system such as factor XII, prekallikrein activator (PKA), kallikrein and kinins. Especially after rapid infusion the presence of these contaminants can lead to a whole range of vascular complications – from mild hypotension to complete circulatory collapse. Guidelines which limit the concentration of these contaminants in commercially available preparations have therefore been established by the 'Bureau of Biologics'. Drastically elevated PKA levels have been found in some preparations treated with PEG.

Alloimmune antibody titers are generally so low in IgG preparations that even massive doses are not expected to cause side effects. Anti-Al and anti-B isoagglutinins are found in variable, but generally low, titers in most preparations. They have not been reported as causing hemolytic reactions. However, IgG preparations should not contain any irregular antibodies against rhesus antigen. Surprisingly, no adverse reactions have been reported yet which might be caused by immune responses of the recipients of human IgG preparations against allotypic immunoglobulin determinants.

IgG preparations should of course be free of microbial pathogens. The risk of transmission of hepatitis has been considered to be negligible or nonexistent. However, the use of alcohol in the fractionation procedure does not guarantee that the preparation will not transmit an infectious agent. Recently, cases of non-A-non-B (NANB) hepatitis were observed after IGIV treatment. In contrast to the situation with pooled factor VIII concentrates or factor IX complex, IgG preparations have never been reported as transmitting the acquired immune deficiency virus. Since it is unlikely that HIV-positive individuals were never included in IgG donor pools, we may assume that the alcohol treatment used during the fractionation of IgG eliminates the virus.

3.3 Therapeutic applications of human immunoglobulins

3.3.1 Animal experiments with γ-globulins in infections

Besides the standard indications for immunoglobulins, i.e. prevention of certain viral and toxic diseases, and substitution therapy in antibody deficiency states, polyvalent preparations are now being increasingly recommended for the management of severe systemic infections in patients without manifest impairment of humoral defence mechanisms. Since the results of controlled clinical studies are not yet entirely conclusive, however, opinions understandably differ on the value of treating such patients with immunoglobulins. The planning and performance of appropriate randomized double-blind studies in man is, in fact, particularly difficult. In order to provide relevant information these studies have to be carried out on as homogeneous a patient population as possible. What is more, ethical reasons necessitate concurrent administration of optimal chemotherapy. Since the benefit to be expected from treatment with γ-globulins could well be limited in these circumstances, a large cohort of patients will eventually be needed for statistical confirmation of the results.

In animal experiments, on the other hand, virtually uniform conditions can be created with regard to the immune status of the animals, mode of infection, the infectious dose, the environmental conditions, and duration. Animal experiments have therefore often been used in the past to test the efficacy of immunoglobulin preparations. It has been repeatedly demonstrated in small rodents that the administration of large doses of γ-globulins enhances the therapeutic effect of suboptimal antibiotic therapy in septic infections. These findings are remarkable since most antibody effector mechanisms are likely to be suboptimal in foreign hosts. However, the results obtainable with high doses of an effective antibiotic on its own can be improved by the additional administration of γ-globulins only in infection models in which multiresistant bacteria have been used.

More impressive results can be obtained in newborn piglets. Because γ-globulin does not cross the placenta of the pig, these animals are born agammaglobulinemic. They receive the γ-globulin needed for the first weeks of life orally by ingestion of colostrum. Piglets that were fed with colostrum containing human IgG instead of maternal IgG showed protective concentrations of γ-globulins of the range of 500–700 mg% in the blood only 24 hours after the first feed. Animals pretreated in this way and then infected by intraperitoneal injection with various human pathogens proved to be completely protected against the majority of infectious agents, whereas, conversely, almost all non-pretreated agammaglobulinemic animals succumbed to infection.

Because of the fact that enterobacteriaceae have identical or nearly identical lipopolysaccharide core structures, several laboratories have explored the possibility of using antisera containing high titers against lipid A or the glycolipid core structures as 'broad-spectrum' agents against gram-negative infections. Antilipid A sera were repeatedly shown to be ineffective in protecting experimental animals against infections with wild-type enterobacteriaceae pathogens or against their endotoxins. In contrast, anti-core antibodies have been consistently reported as conferring protection against challenges with gram-negative organisms and their endotoxins. These results, which seemed to be corroborated by clinical findings, have recently been called into question. In a series of very well controlled experiments, workers at the University of Maryland showed that rabbit antisera directed at the E. coli J 5 and the Salmonella minnesota Re 595 core glycolipids were ineffective against gram-negative infections while – as expected – antisera against the O-antigens were fully protective. It appears possible that many of the positive results previously obtained were in fact due to antibodies directed at O-antigens of the infectious agents used in experimental models or occurring in clinical infections. The exclusion of this possibility would require rigorous controls and – in clinical situations – the serological analysis of the infectious bacterial agent(s), in other words, conditions which have hardly been met in previous experiments. The prospects of developing anti-glycolipid antibodies of the J 5 or Re 595 type as broad spectrum antibacterial agents must, therefore, be judged with scepticism.

Experimental infections with herpes viruses and cytomegalovirus have helped to demonstrate the feasibility of using antibodies against these agents for the prophylaxis or treatment of human infections. They have also been instrumental in delineating the mechanisms through which antibodies eliminate different viral agents. In experimental mouse encephalitis induced by intranasal application of herpes 2 virus, homologous or heterologous antiserum containing high titres against herpes 2 antigens was effective prophylactically: the survival of the infected animals depended entirely on the timing of the initial dose of antibody. There is evidence that antibody dependent cellular cytotoxicity (ADCC) is an important mechanism in the elimination of primary herpes infections. Neonatal mice are not capable of mounting an ADCC reaction. To the degree to which the animals develop this ability, they become resistant to herpes virus. During the early vulnerable period, the animals are not protected by lymphocytes or by antiserum alone. A combination of both of these constituents, however, is highly effective in preventing disease induced by herpes virus.

3.3.2 Clinical applications of human γ-globulins

3.3.2.1 Prophylaxis

The establishment of highly successful vaccination programmes and the introduction of sulfonamides and antibiotics has limited the need for a prophylactic application of IgG preparations in healthy individuals. However, passive immunization with antibodies is still indicated in individuals who have been exposed to a dangerous infectious agent and may have been infected and who show no evidence of immunity against the agent in question. Prophylaxis with antibodies may also be justified for individuals (e.g. health professionals) who are about to expose themselves to a potential source of infection. The absence of specific immunity must be assumed or demonstrated in such situations by a negative history of infection or vaccination or – in cases of herpes zoster or rubella – by negative serodiagnosis of specific serum antibodies. Relatively low doses of special IgG preparations (hyperimmunoglobulins) given i.m. provide protection against Clostridium tetani, rabies or hepatitis A. In cases of endemic infections such as herpes zoster, measles or hepatitis B, protection can be provided by the i.v. application of high doses of polyvalent IgG preparations, which usually do contain the appropriate antibodies in sufficiently high titres.

An important indication for the prophylactic use of human γ-globulins has recently been documented. Individuals who received organ transplants are at risk of acquiring cytomegalovirus infections. There are two possible causes for this: first, the virus is present in 60–70% of individuals in the European or North American populations and can be 'reactivated' by the immunosuppressive modalities surrounding the transplantation. Secondly, the virus can be transferred with the transplant or with blood transfusions from infected donors. A recent study from the University of Heidelberg has shown that two intramuscular applications of CMV-immunoglobulin immediately before and after the transplantation can drastically reduce the number of patients experiencing an increase in their CMV titres and, more importantly, of those patients who actually come down with clinical infections. Without specific prophylaxis, up to 60% of the seronegative and up to 90% of seropositive patients who receive a kidney transplant can acquire a CMV infection. 2% of transplant recipients die of severe disease manifestations. In the recent study mentioned above, only 12.2% of the transplant recipients experienced a 'reactivation' of their latent infection and only 2% acquired a primary infection. The corresponding figures for an untreated control group observed in parallel were 24% reactivations and 10% primary infections. In the group which received prophylactic γ-globulins only 16% of those who had experienced a reactivation of their latent infection and none of the patients who had acquired a primary infection fell ill. In the control group the rate of clinical manifestations was higher: 58% of the patients with secondary infections and 50% of those with primary infections actually showed disease symptoms.

In view of the fact that chemotherapy of cytomegalovirus infections is still unsatisfactory, the possibility of preventing and/or mitigating the disease through the use of γ-globulins has considerable merit.

3.3.2.2 Replacement of immunoglobulin

Congenital immunoglobulin deficiency syndromes represent the most straightforward indication for IgG treatment. A variety of genetic defects, only a few of which have been characterized at the DNA level, can result in reductions (hypogammaglobulinemia) or the complete lack (agammaglobulinemia) or all IgG classes or of particular subclasses. Patients with such genetic defects can be protected from acute infections by the regular application of polyvalent IgG preparations. This has been well documented in several controlled trials. One such study involved 13 patients with congential agammaglobulinemia who were observed for two years. In the first year the patients were treated only occasionally with small doses (10–20 ml) of SGG i.m. or with modified i.v. preparations. In the second year they received 9 to 12 g of an intact immunoglobulin i.v. at regular three-weekly intervals. The mean serum IgG level was 125 mg % in the first year and 450 mg % in the second year. The number of days on which the patients could not go to work, on which they had fever over 38°C and on which they had to be treated with antibiotics were recorded over both years as parameters of susceptibility to infection. In the first year, the average number of days on which temperature rose to about 38°C in the population was 23; antimicrobials had to be given on an average of 117 days; 65 working days were lost. In the second year of treatment, temperatures over 38°C were measured only on one day on average; antibacterials had to be given on 6 days and only 13 working days were lost.

The results of this trial show, therefore, that the high, and in some cases disabling, susceptibility to infection in this cohort was greatly reduced by substitution with γ-globulins.

In this and in similar studies a good correlation was found between the serum IgG levels and the degree of protection. Today application of about 0.3 g IGIV/kg body weight once every month is recommended to keep the serum IgG levels above 200 mg %, which, according to most experts, is the minimum level that provides protection. In contrast to acute infections, chronic local inflammatory processes such as sinusitis, bronchitis or arthritis are generally more difficult to control in patients with IgG deficiencies.

In cases of selective defects, the IgG preparation used should of course contain appropriate amounts of the IgG class or classes which are lacking. As mentioned above, problems can arise in patients with IgA deficiencies. Almost half of the patients with selective IgA deficiencies and some patients with hypogammaglobulinemias can be sensitized to IgA and have anti-IgA antibodies in their serum. This is a major problem, particularly for those patients who have a combined IgA-IgG_2 deficiency, since they need IgG replacement. Recently an IGIV preparation especially depleted in IgA (<2 mg/ml) has been used successfully in such a case.

IgG replacement should also be considered in some cases of so-called secondary antibody deficiency syndromes. These can be iatrogenic (extensive surgery, x-irradiation, chemotherapy) or a consequence of extensive injuries (particularly burns), infections, neoplastic diseases (particularly myelomas and acute leukemias), malnutrition or extensive protein loss through the kidney or the gut. IGIV treatment has been reported as preventing or at least ameliorating herpes zoster and cytomegaly virus infections in immunocompromised transplant patients. An overview of the most important causes of antibody deficiencies is given in *Table 3.3*.

Table 3.3. Antibody deficiency syndromes (ADS)

		Serum concentration	
		Antibody[a]	IgG[b]
Physiological:	Premature birth	↓	↓
	Newborn infants	↓	○
	Advanced age	↓	○↑
Congenital:	Humoral immune defects	↓	↓
Acquired: (symptomatic)	Lympho-reticular neoplasma	↓	○↓↑
	Protein-losing enteropathy	○	↓
	Antibody consumption	↓	○↑
Iatrogenic:	Irradiation	↓	○↑
	Immunosuppression	↓	○
	Chemotherapy	↓	○
	Plasmapheresis	○	↓

○ normal ↓ reduced ↑ elevated

[a] Determination by means of corresponding antigen
[b] Determination by immunochemical methods

3.3.2.3 Therapy

The therapeutic value of special or polyclonal IgG preparations in patients with severe, generalized infections who have no apparent defect in the humoral immune system is still controversial. In fact, it is very difficult to demonstrate the efficacy of immunoglobulins in clinical trials involving such patients. For ethical reasons chemotherapy cannot be omitted. Therefore, a beneficial effect of IgG, which might be expected from the results of the extensive animal experiments mentioned abbove, is difficult to demonstrate. Controlled randomized clinical trials with large numbers of carefully selected individuals are required in order to provide conclusive evidence for or against the efficacy of immunoglobulins in such situations. However, a number of recent studies have indicated that i.v. γ-globulins may have a role as a complement to antibiotics in the treatment of severe infections. In one such study Just and his colleagues at the University of Freiburg in Germany have shown that 50 patients in an intensive care unit who received i.v. immunoglobulin combined with antibiotics did better than 54 control patients who received antibiotics alone. The prevailing infections in these patients were pneumonia, septicemia, peritonitis and wound sepsis. In the patients receiving immunoglobulins, infections were significantly more rarely the cause of death than in the control group. Likewise, ventilation time in the high risk surgery group amounted to only 5.5 days for those receiving immunoglobulins as opposed to 12.7 days in the controls. While the average duration of intensive care was 21.5 days in the control group, patients who received IgG stayed only 14.8 days. The differences were statistically significant at a level of $p < 0.01$. This study and similar ones which have been carried out provide tentative evidence for the usefulness of IgG treatment in severe infections. More substantial proof, however, is still needed.

Patients with generalized infectious diseases often lack protective antibodies because these antibodies are "consumed" by the excessive amounts of antigen which they carry in their circulation. This situation is defined by the term "consumptive" or "selective" normogammaglobulinemic antibody deficiency. In this condition, the IgG serum levels are normal or even elevated. Diagnosis is based on the isolation of the pathogen and on the demonstration that antibodies against this pathogen are lacking. This is a time-consuming procedure. Moreover, it has therapeutic consequences only if IGIV preparations with high titres of the appropriate antibodies are available.

Neonates, particularly those born before term, are highly susceptible to bacterial infections. Group B streptococci are a major cause of neonatal sepsis and meningitis. In a Swiss study combination therapy with antibacterials and immunoglobulins in neonates suffering from septic infections proved markedly superior to therapy with antibacterials alone. 82 neonates were admitted to the trial; 35 had bacteriologically confirmed septicemia, while 47 had only the clinical signs of an infection. 20 of the neonates with proven septic infection received, in addition to treatment with an antibacterial, 0.5 g (preterm infants) or 1 g (term birth) polyvalent γ-globulin i.v. for six days. In the group only treated with antibacterials, 4 of the 15 neonates died, whereas in the group treated with antibacterials and γ-globulins only 2 out of 20 died. This difference is not statistically significant. If, however, we specifically consider the preterm infants in both groups, the difference is significant. Of the 9 preterm infants without immunoglobulin substitution, 4 died of their infection; of the 13 comparable preterm children treated with immunoglobulin only one child died.

Of the children whose bacteremia was not bacteriologically proven, the group treated with immunoglobulins and antibacterials did better than the group treated only with antibacterials. Mortality in the group which received immunoglobulin substitution was 2 out of 21 (10%), as compared with 4 out of 26 (15%) for the neonates treated only with antimicrobials.

Follow-up of the surviving children two and a half years later showed that those treated with immunoglobulins had completely normal immunoglobulin concentrations and normal antibody titres to tetanus toxoid, with which they had been immunized in the meantime. Assay of antibodies to polyvalent IgG by passive hemagglutination yielded normal results for all children. The tuberculin reaction was also the same in the two groups: 16 of 18 IgG-treated children and 9 of 11 children in the control group were tuberculin-positive. It is probably justified to conclude from these data that the administration of high doses of γ-globulins to preterm or normal term infants neither suppresses humoral immunity nor leads to abnormal sensitization to polyclonal IgG. Cell-mediated immune reactions also appeared unimpaired.

The results of this study are consistent with animal experiments and many other clinical trials which indicate that beneficial, therapeutic effects of IGIV therapy are largely restricted to the immunocompromised host. However, antibodies might eventually make a significant contribution to the treatment of life-threatening infections if a greater number of IGIV preparations become available that are enriched in antibodies of the appropriate class and specificity. The most suitable targets for antibody therapy are toxins like tetanus or botulinus toxin, staphylococcal exotoxin, endotoxins from gram-negative bacteria or even endogenous toxins such as tumour necrosis factor which is the main mediator of endotoxin shock. Since these toxins have conserved structures monoclonal antibodies may be particularly suited for therapy. Also, IgM antibodies might neutralize toxins in the blood-stream more efficiently than IgG antibodies.

3.3.2.4 Morbus hemolyticus neonatorum is largely prevented by anti-D IgG prophylaxis

Another major field of application for γ-globulins is Rhesus incompatibility. In this disease, a mother with an Rh-negative blood group develops antibodies to the Rh-positive erythrocytes of the fetus. In later pregnancies, these antibodies may cause severe hemolytic anemia of the newborn with hyperbilirubinemia and damage to the basal ganglia ("kernicterus"). In a number of controlled trials it has been demonstrated that by giving anti-Rh-(D)-γ-globulin to expectant Rh-negative mothers carrying an Rh-positive child, the baby's erythrocytes which are released into the mother's bloodstream during birth can be intercepted and lysed. Immunization of the mother to Rhesus factor is thereby prevented. In a Canadian multicentre study, 216 Rhesus-negative women were given a single intramuscular injection of an anti-Rh-immunoglobulin (435 μg specific antibody) within 72 hours of delivery. Not a single one of these patients was immunized against Rhesus factor. 18 (8.9%) of 203 untreated primiparas and 18 (6.1%) of 279 untreated multiparas exhibited Rhesus antibodies. These figures, confirmed by other studies, have resulted in the installation of anti-Rh prophylaxis after every Rh incompatible pregnancy. Consistent prophylaxis is expected to soon eliminate Rh-related hemolytic anemia from pediatric and obstetric practice completely.

This successful prophylactic strategy was developed on the basis of two observations: it was first noticed in 1909 by T. Smith that active immunization against diphtheria toxin was often not successful if an excess of anti-toxin antibodies was given at the same time. Second, Levine in 1943 and later others noticed that a Rhesus-negative mother giving birth to a Rhesus-positive child was at a lower risk of becoming sensitized to D-antigen if the child was also incompatible with the mother's AB0 blood group system. This was interpreted to mean that sensitization to the D antigen was prevented because the child's red cells which entered the circulation of the mother were eliminated by isoagglutinins in the mother's serum. Later this explanation was shown to be wrong, but it led to a successful trial with male volunteers at Sing Sing prison and finally to what can be considered the conquest of hemolytic disease due to Rh-incompatibility. The mechanism by which anti-Rh(D) antibodies prevent sensitization is still not clear.

3.3.2.4 IgG in the treatment of diseases caused by autoantibodies

The first antibody mediated disease to be treated with IGIV was idiopathic thrombocytopenic purpura (ITP). In children, acute ITP is generally a benign disorder with a spontaneous recovery rate of about 80% occurring within a few weeks. A chronic form of the disease, however, develops in about 10% of children and in adolescents. In both the acute and the chronic forms, platelet production is increased but the newly formed platelets are quickly removed from the circulation. The increased amount of platelet-associated IgG (immunocomplexes bound to platelet Fc-receptorps or specific antiplatelet autoantibodies) is probably responsible for the accelerated clearance rate of platelets by Fc-receptor bearing cells, particularly in the liver and spleen. Following the observation that platelet and hemoglobin levels rose again in 2 agammaglobulinemic children suffering from severe thrombocytopenia and hemolytic anemia after they had received replacement therapy with i.v. γ-globulin, this therapeutic modality was also tested in idiopathic thrombocytopenic purpura (ITP). Repeated doses of 0.4 IgG/kg body weight on five consecutive days had a dramatic effect on platelet counts of 6 children with acute, 4 with intermittent and 3 with steroid-resistant chronic ITP. Platelet counts started to rise within 24–48 hours in all patients up to normal levels. In 4 of the 6 children with acute ITP and in one of 4 children with intermittent disease, a single five-day treatment course was sufficient to induce prolonged, if not permanent, remissions. In the other patients repeated maintenance doses have since been required. In 3 patients who had previously been treated unsuccessfully with steroids and splenectomy, prolonged remissions could not be achieved with IGIV treatment despite good initial responses. Subsequently, beneficial effects have been obtained also in adult patients with ITP after treatment with a variety of γ-globulin preparations. In a British study, good results were obtained in adults between 14 and 62 years of age with a dosage of 0.4 g per kg bodyweight if the patients had been suffering from their disease for less than sixteen weeks. Those individuals who had been ill for a longer period of time also reacted to γ-globulin therapy with initial normalization of their platelet count. In contrast to those patients with relatively acute disease, however, in whom the success of therapy was maintained for the entire observation period of 173 days, the platelet count of patients who had been ill for more than sixteen weeks fell again to pathological levels within a few weeks. Positive findings have also been reported with IgG therapy in pregnant women with acute ITP.

The following mechanisms have been postulated for the short- and medium-term effects of γ-globulins in ITP:

1. The disease may be an autoimmune reaction to antigens of the patient's own platelets. Raised concentrations of antibodies directed against platelets are in fact found in some patients. It is thought that such antibodies opsonize the platelets, thus accelerating their elimination via the mononuclear-phagocytic system. The administration of large quantities of native IgG molecules might inhibit the accelerated elimination of opsonized platelets by blocking the Fc receptors on macrophages.
2. The illness may result from an as yet unidentified microbial (?) antigen forming immune complexes with autoantibodies. On account of relative antigen excess, these complexes remain water-soluble, bind to platelets and either accelerate lysis (through complement) or speed up elimination through macrophages. High-dose γ-globulin completely saturates the circulating antigens; they no longer bind to platelets and no longer affect their viability.
3. The recently administered antibodies occupy the Fc receptors of the platelets and thereby prevent adsorption of soluble immune complexes to these receptors.

The three possible mechanisms are illustrated in the diagram in Fig. 3.5. Experimental evidence supports the first hypothesis. If patients with ITP receive an injection of labelled erythrocytes or erythrocytes opsonized with anti-D-IgG (i.e. with antirhesus factor IgG), these cells very quickly disappear from circulation. If, however, before administration of the erythrocytes, the patients receive an injection of high-dose IgG, the erythrocytes stay in the bloodstream for a very long time. At the same time platelet counts rise. To employ a popular expression which used to be current, this mechanism might be called a blockade of the reticuloendothelial system or, even better, of the mononuclear-phagocytic system.

Permanent remissions of ITP induced by the administration of IgG are rare but they do occur. How can they be explained? As early as 1974 Niels Jerne had postulated that the immune system functions like a network. Every immune reaction gives rise to antibodies with a certain antigen specificity. The idiotypes of these antibodies, i.e. those portions of the variable regions of the heavy and light chains responsible for antigen binding, now in turn act as antigens and induce the synthesis of antibodies directed against these idiotypes (anti-idiotypic antibodies). By an analogous process, the anti-idiotypic antibodies trigger the synthesis of anti-antiidiotypic antibodies.

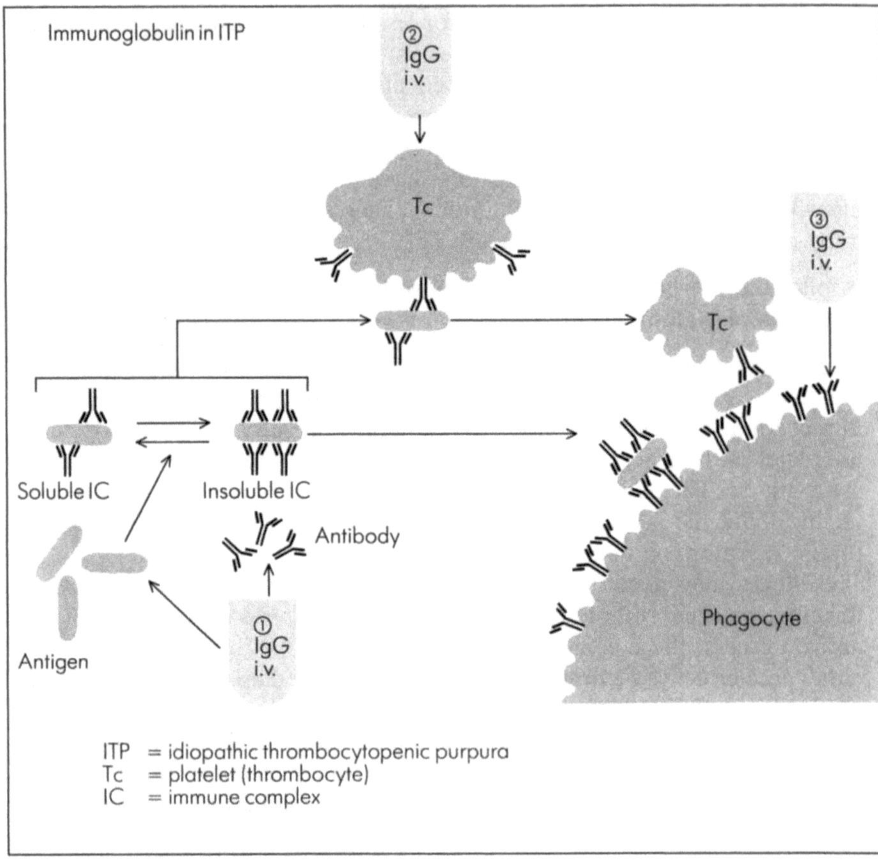

Figure 3.5 Diagram of the hypothetical mechanisms of action of i.v. gamma globulins in idiopathic thrombocytopenic purpura.

1. Monomeric IgG can eliminate circulating immune complexes and/or microbial antigens.
2. Monomeric IgG can prevent binding of immune complexes to platelets, thereby protecting the platelets against the effects of complement.
3. Monomeric IgG can block the Fc receptors of macrophages and thus prevent an antibody-mediated cytotoxic reaction of the macrophages with platelets or interaction between macrophages and platelets by way of antigen-antibody complexes.

The experimental evidence so far obtained appears to confirm this hypothesis. The anti-idiotypic antibodies seem to play a regulatory role in this process. In simple terms, they ensure that “things don’t get out of hand”, in other words, that an appropriate humoral immune response is stopped once it reaches an adequate level. In newborn mice, the injection of anti-idiotypic antibodies can suppress synthesis of the corresponding idiotype for a life-time. Attempts have been made to interpret these data in order to explain the long-term remissions in patients with ITP managed with high-dose IgG. If the antibodies responsible for ITP carry idiotypes which are not regulated by anti-idiotypic antibodies, the disease could be fuelled by this absence of regulation. The administration of large quantities of polyvalent antibodies might, fortuitously, contain the anti-idiotypic antibodies necessary to rectify the imbalance and to stop, permanently or for a period of time, the synthesis of the antibodies causing the pathological process. This model provides at least a hypothetical explanation of how intravenous γ-globulin brings about permanent remission of ITP.

Recently beneficial effects of high doses of IGIV have also been reported for a number of other disorders in which antibodies appear to play a major pathogenic role. Examples are immune complex glomerulonephritis, Kawasaki syndrome of children, myasthenia gravis, autoimmune neutropenia and autoimmune hemophilia associated with anti-factor VIII antibodies.

Autoantibodies have been implicated in all of these diseases, although low levels of autoantibodies directed towards host antigens are considered by many researchers to be normal. The levels of autoantibodies associated with disease, however, appear to be elevated above normal. What is more important, clinical improvement caused by IgG is followed in most patients by a fall in autoantibody titres.

Quite often, the remissions induced in autoimmune disorders by IGIV last longer than two to three months, which is the time needed for a complete breakdown of the infused antibodies. At present, there are two possible explanations for this phenomenon. First, many preparations of IGIV seem to contain antibodies directed against Fc-γ receptors on blood lymphocytes. There is at least tentative evidence from clinical and experimental observations that such antibodies are immunosuppressive. The second explanation reverts to what has been said in connection with ITP: anti-idiotypic antibodies contained in IGIV preparations could react with the corresponding surface bound idiotypic receptors and thus specifically switch off B-cells which produce autoantibodies. As recently shown, the cross-linking of surface-attached IgM molecules may be the appropriate signal for the inhibition of B-cell maturation.

3.4 Monoclonal antibodies

3.4.1 Methods of monoclonal antibody production

The standard antibody preparations currently used in therapy are polyclonal, i.e. they contain a large number of different antibodies each of which goes back to a specific B-cell clone. In contrast, monoclonal antibody preparations represent only one such clone. Lymphocytes can be fused with other cells to form hybrid cells. Clones of single hybrid cells can subsequently be obtained by diluting suspensions in which hybrid cells were formed. For a long time, however, these clones were short-lived and were therefore not a feasible source of large amounts of monoclonal antibodies. This problem was not solved until 1975, when George Köhler and César Milstein succeeded for the first time in fusing antibody-forming lymphocytes with myeloma cells, which are tumour cells also derived from B-cells. The resulting hybridoma cells could form stable cell lines with an almost unlimited capacity for division and for the synthesis of large amounts of monoclonal antibodies. Since then, the techniques of hybridoma formation and monoclonal antibody production have been further developed *(Fig. 3.6)*.

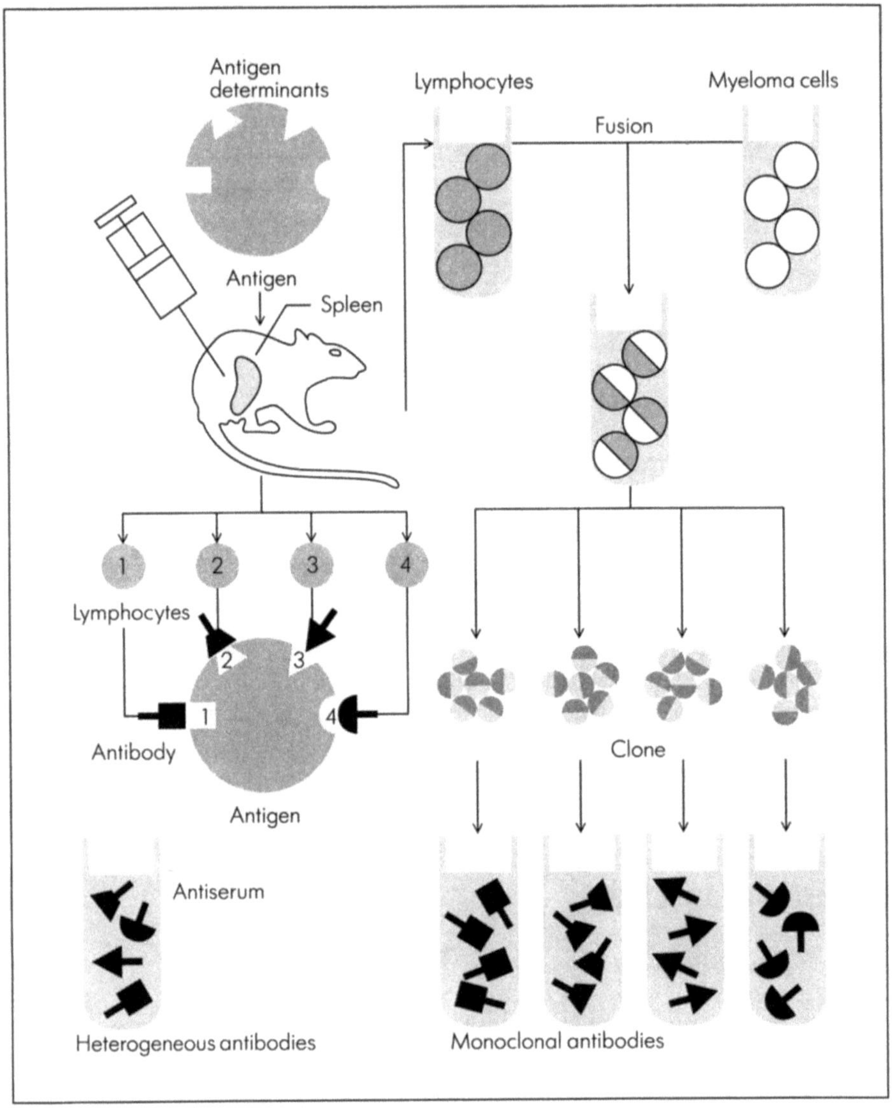

Figure 3.6. Schematic diagram of hybridoma formation and the production of monoclonal antibodies.

The advantage of the hybridoma technology is that it provides permanent cellular sources of homogenous antibody populations, and makes it possible to produce antibodies against antigenic determinants (epitopes) that are not available in pure form. Fusions with spleen cells of mice immunized, for example, with human cells can yield many different monoclonal antibodies with specificities for a large variety of cellular antigens. Moreover, with functional screening tests it is possible to select antibodies against structures (epitopes) on molecules or cells that are involved in a particular function. One can, for example, raise antibodies which are directed at various epitopes of a cellular receptor like that for interleukin 2 (Il-2) or acetylcholine. These antibodies can then serve as sensitive probes in the functional dissection of the receptor molecule.

Within the last ten years the generation, selection and establishment of B-cell hybridomas became routine procedures in a large number of laboratories. Several thousand hybridomas have been described in the literature and this number is steadily increasing.

Some antibodies are required in large quantities, especially for therapeutic purposes. Ascites of mice which were inoculated intraperitoneally with hybridoma clones is the richest source of monoclonal antibodies: one ml of fluid contains up to 20 mg antibodies. Monoclonal antibodies thus obtained can be used for in-vitro diagnostic procedures. But murine monoclonals are also used for in-vivo diagnosis and therapy. Such techniques, however, are not without their risks since the human immune system reacts to mouse antibodies by forming antibodies of its own. As already described, this process will lead to sensitization within a very short period of time. If at all possible, human monoclonal antibodies should be used for therapeutic purposes and also for repetition of an in-vivo diagnostic procedure. Such antibodies are, however, still difficult to obtain. To find human B-cells with a desired specificity for a particular antigen is comparable to searching for a needle in a haystack – at least if one looks at B-cells from the blood. The situation is somewhat more favourable if draining lymph nodes which are obtained during surgery are used as a source for specific B-cells. The occurrence of B-cells which are reacting against a particular microbial or onco-fetal antigen is higher in lymph nodes from an area afflicted by infection or tumour growth than in the peripheral blood or in unaffected lymphatic tissue. Establishing human myeloma cells which are suitable partners for the fusion of B-cells presents another difficulty. In principle these problems have been solved but the number of human hybridomas and monoclonal antibodies which can be considered for therapeutic use is still much smaller than the corresponding figure for murine material.

Some antibodies are required in large quantities, especially for therapeutic purposes. Ascites of mice which have been inoculated intraperitoneally with hybridoma clones is the richest source of monoclonal antibodies: one ml contains up to 20 mg of material. However, this production method has obvious disadvantages. It is unacceptable for ethical reasons, it creates hazards with respect to the transmission of pathogenic agents into material which is destined for use in man and it cannot be used for the growth of human hybridomas. Fortunately, in-vitro methods which allow antibody mass production either by very large suspension cultures in fermenters or in reactors containing immobilized cells and perfusion systems have been developed over the past few years and are constantly being improved upon.

Some recent developments have extended the potential spectrum of "artificial" antibodies which can be produced. The fusion of two hybridomas leads to the formation of so-called hybrid-hybridomas in which the four parental Ig chains can be assembled into ten different antibody molecules. Six of these possible structures are "hetero-bispecific": this means that their antigen specificity is different in each of the two arms. Such antibodies have potential applications in diagnostics but also in therapy (*Fig. 3.7;* see below). More extensive

Heavy \ Light	rr	rg	gg
RR	RrRr	RrRg*	RgRg
RG	RrGr*	RrGg* / RgGr*	RgGg*
GG	GrGr	GrGg*	GgGg

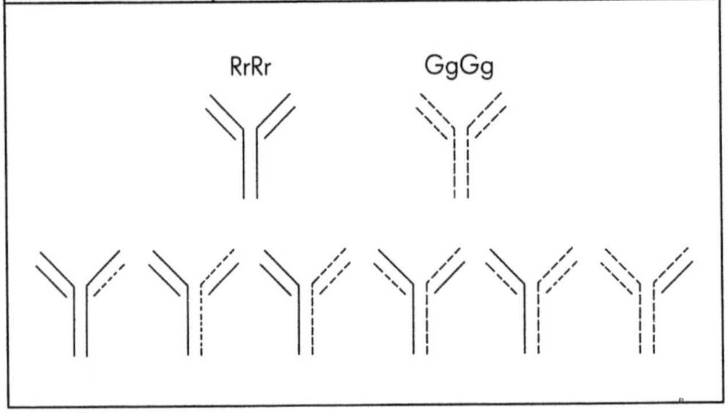

Figure 3.7. Formation of heterobispecific antibodies.
Two hybridomas synthesizing antibodies RrRr and GgGg are fused. The new cells now synthesize two types of heavy chains and two types of light chains which can be recombined in ten different ways to result in new antibodies. Six of the new antibodies (marked with an asterisk) are heterobispecific: they can bind two different epitopes with each of their arms.

alterations of antibody molecules are made possible by the application of recombinant DNA methods. Messenger RNA specifying the synthesis of heavy and light chains of antibodies can be isolated from hybridoma cells, transcribed into DNA, inserted into expression vectors and transfected back into myeloma cells. The resulting transfected cell lines which are often referred to as "transfectomas" produce the same antibodies as the hybridomas from which the genes were isolated. Engineering of the genes before the transfection step allows the production of recombinant molecules such as mouse-human hybrid antibodies which contain only the variable or even the hypervariable regions of a murine antibody, while the rest of the molecule is of human origin. Moreover various parts of antibodies can be deleted or recombined with other proteins by DNA recombinant techniques. In this way, novel molecules which have the specificity of antibodies and at the same time carry properties of other molecules can be designed for many experimental and eventually even therapeutic applications.

3.4.2 The use of monoclonal antibodies in neoplastic diseases

Malignant tumours are a major cause of death in the human population. However, they do not threaten the existence of the human race, or for that matter, of any other species since they occur with sufficiently low frequency and predominantly after the reproductive period in life. Therefore, there was no need in evolution for the development of a special defence system against cancer cells. Immune surveillance, as envisaged by Burnet, does not exist. Thus it is hardly surprising that neither active nor passive immunization procedures have been successful against cancer. In many experimental systems it has however been shown that tumour cells can be eliminated by the cellular and humoral mechanisms that normally kill microbial pathogens or parasites. This finding, together with the fact that there is a continuing lack of sufficiently specific drugs against cancer, has been a strong motivation for many investigators to search for possible applications of highly specific immunological tool in particular of antibodies to treat cancer. The advent of the monoclonal antibody technique was a major step forward. On the one hand it facilitated the identification of many tumour-associated antigens, and on the other, it allowed the production of specific antibodies specifically directed against these antigens.

3.4.2.1 Tumour-associated antigens

Tumour-specific surface antigens that are not expressed by normal cells would be the ideal target antigens for therapeutic antibodies. However, despite extensive search such antigens have never been found. Many antigens which were initially thought to be unique products of tumour cells were later also detected in normal tissues. However, many so-called tumour-associated antigens (TAA) are nevertheless considered to be suitable targets for antibody therapy since their expression on normal cells is restricted to fetal tissues or to cells that are either dispensable or replaceable. And even if TAAs are expressed in normal cells, their density in these cells is often much lower than in tumour tissue. Therefore, tumour-associated antigens can provide at least partial selectivity for an antibody-based therapeutical approach. The majority of these TAAs are oligosaccharide side-chains which are associated with glycolipids or glycoproteins in the plasma membrane. Their aberrant expression probably contributes to the unsocial behaviour of cancer cells but is apparently not directly related to the initial events of transformation.

The genes and gene products which are primarily involved in transforming cells to the malignant state were discovered through the analysis of transforming retroviruses and through gene transfection experiments. Four of the more than 30 cellular protooncogenes encode tyrosine kinases which are also potential targets for antibody therapy. They are plasma membrane-associated receptors for external ligands: c-erbB1 codes for receptors that bind epidermal growth factor (EGF) and the transforming growth factor TGF-α, c-erbB2 and c-ros specify receptors for unknown ligands and c-fms encodes receptors for the colony-stimulating factor CSF-1. C-erbB1, c-erbB2 and c-fms are quite frequently expressed by a variety of human tumours. These oncogene-encoded TAAs would be obvious targets for an attack by antibodies if it should turn out that their continued expression on the cell surface is required for the maintenance of the transformed phenotype.

3.4.2.2 Strategies for the use of antibodies in cancer treatment

There are two principal approaches to the use of antibodies in cancer therapy: the first builds on the normal functions of unmodified antibodies while the other uses antibodies as targeting devices for anti-tumour agents which by themselves are limited by their lack of specificity.

3.4.2.2.1 In vivo use of unmodified antibodies

Several anti-TAA antibodies have been shown to inhibit growth or to induce the differentiation of neoplastic cells in vitro. These antibodies bind to plasma membrane receptors for hormones or cytokines which normally control cell growth and differentiation. Whether their in vitro effects on cancer cells can be exploited in vivo for therapeutic purposes remains to be seen.

Antibody dependent lysis of tumour cells is initiated by activation of C1q and subsequent triggering of the complement cascade. The degree to which C1q is activated depends on the class of cell-bound antibodies. Artificial monovalent antibodies can be more efficient activators of C1q than the corresponding bivalent antibodies, and combinations of different antibodies can be more efficient than each single type of antibody. In vivo, inflammatory reactions are induced by several complement components which are generated as a consequence of the C1q activation. Some of the murine and human anti-TAA antibodies currently used in clinical trials fix human complement. Whether this has any therapeutic effects with tumour cell lysis or through the induction of inflammatory reactions is still an open question.

Antibody-dependent cell-mediated cytotoxicity (ADCC) can be mediated by a variety of Fc-receptor-bearing leucocytes. The efficiency of ADCC depends on the concentration, the affinity and the class of the antibodies involved, as well as on the molecular nature and the density of the target antigen on the surface of the cancer cell. Human effector cells mediate ADCC with murine IgG_{2a} and rat IgG_{2b} but also with some antibodies that belong to other classes. Those antibodies which are the best mediators of ADCC in vitro are also the most efficient inhibitors of human tumour xenografts in nude mice. In several recent clinical trials murine anti-TAA antibodies or autologous ADCC effector cells loaded in vitro with anti-TAA antibodies were given to cancer patients by infusion. Tumour regression was observed in a few cases. However, a reliable assessment of this strategy is not yet possible.

Active immunization with anti-idiotypic antibodies directed against the antigen-binding site of anti-TAA antibodies has recently been initiated in cancer patients with the hope of inducing anti-TAA immune responses. The rationale of this approach is the following: antibodies directed against a particular antigen, have a particular idiotype, which complements a particular structure of the antigen (epitope). If antibodies of a particular idiotype are injected into another individual, anti-idiotypic antibodies against the injected idiotype are formed. A proportion of these anti-idiotypic antibodies carry an 'internal image' of the original antigen in their own idiotype. If these anti-idiotypic antibodies are injected into yet another individual, they trigger the formation of antibodies that are directed against the original antigen. Whether this strategy will be more successful than immunization with tumour cell extracts remains to be seen *(Fig. 3.8)*.

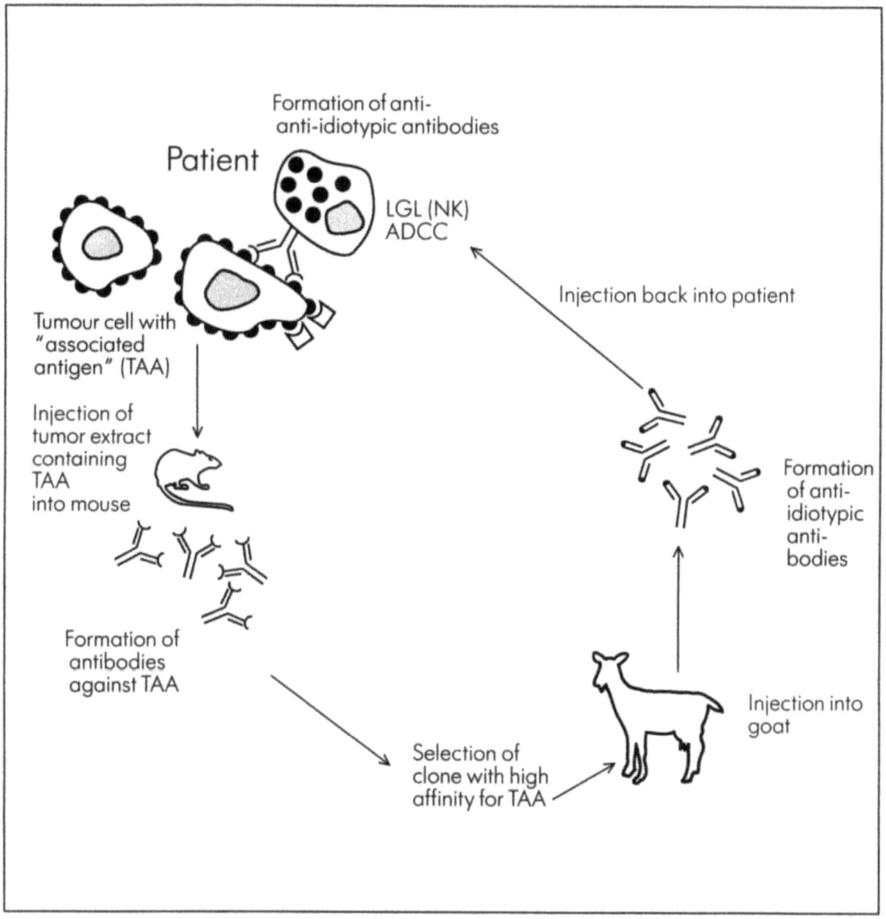

Figure 3.8. Production of anti-anti-idiotypic antibodies for the immune therapy of tumours. Inactivated tumour cells or cell homogenates with tumor associated antigen are injected into mice which form a large spectrum of antibodies. These antibodies can be recovered as monoclonals. A clone with high affinity for the tumour associated antigen is selected and the corresponding antibodies injected into a goat. Among many other antibodies this animal will now form anti-idiotypic antibodies. When anti-idiotypic antibodies are injected back into the patient, they serve as an antigen which contains an "internal image" of the tumour associated antigen. This antigen now elicits the formation of anti-anti-idiotypic antibodies. These antibodies can then react with tumour associated antigen in the context of an ADCC reaction.

3.4.2.2.2 In vivo use of modified antibodies

Radiolabelled antibodies can be used for the in vivo localization of tumours by external scintigraphy (tumour imaging) and eventually for cancer therapy. Tumour imaging methods were developed in preclinical studies with nude mice bearing human tumour xenografts. γ-Emission with energies ranging from 120 to 350 KeV is optimal for external scintigraphy. Iodine isotopes are γ-emitters which can be readily coupled to antibodies by a variety of methods. So far, iodine-131 has been used most frequently for imaging, although its γ-emission is too strong for optimal scintigraphy. Iodine-123 has an optimal γ-emission but is not as readily available as iodine-131. Indium 111, which can be coupled to antibodies via chelating agents has a γ-emission that is well suited for tumour imaging. However, it has the disadvantage of being transmitted to transferrin in exchange with iron and that it tends to accumulate in the liver for unknown reasons. Technetium-99m is an excellent imaging isotope which is frequently used in radiology. Recently, it has also been used for antibody-guided tumour imaging. Unfortunately, the coupling of Te-99m to antibodies is difficult. Furthermore, the isotope has a half-life of only six hours. Radiolabelled Fab (F(ab)2 fragments have advantages over complete antibodies for tumor imaging: they are quickly eliminated from the circulation, they do not unspecifically bind to Fc-receptor-bearing cells and they do not sensitize the host against the constant regions of mouse immunoglobulins.

Therapy with radiolabelled antibodies has two principal advantages over the use of drug-or toxin-antibody conjugates. First, there is no need for the internalization of radiolabelled antibodies by the tumour cells. Second, the antibody does not have to bind to every tumour cell, since killer isotopes (α- and β-emitters) can destroy cells at distances of up to 50 cell diameters. Iodine-131 has been used in animal experiments and in a few clinical pilot studies although it is far from being an optimal therapeutic isotope: it has a high energy γ-emission that is of minor therapeutic importance but adds to the damage of normal tissues and it can be split from the antibodies in vivo by dehalogenation. Several other killer isotopes have been used in preclinical studies. Bismuth-121, which can be coupled to antibodies via chelating agents has an α-emission with a therapeutically useful highly linear energy transfer but it has a very short half-life and is not readily available. The use of Bor-10 is limited by the fact that its α-emission needs to be induced by slow neutrons that cannot penetrate far into tissues. Little is known so far about the α-emitter astatine-211 and the β-emitter yttrium-90, both of which are considered to be promising candidates for antibody-guided radiotherapy. The pharmakokinetic data which are available so far from clinical trials with cancer patients indicate that the radiation dose which can be delivered to solid tumours by radiolabelled anti-TAA antibodies is still far below the critical limit of 50 to 100 Gy (grey) which would be required for therapeutic effects on tumour tissues.

Hetero-bispecific antibodies express two distinct antigen-binding sites. Such antibodies can be obtained from hybrid-hybridomas (see above) or by the dissociation and recoupling of two monoclonal antibody populations with the aid of hetero-bifunctional agents *(Fig. 3.7)*. Bispecific antibodies can be used to focus onto tumour cells, toxins, drugs, radionuclides, or cells such as cytotoxic T-lymphocytes or monocytes which bear Fc-receptors. The most encouraging results were obtained with cytotoxic T-cells and bispecific antibodies which recognize a TAA with one arm and the T-cell receptor/T3 complex with the other arm. Unfortunately, this strategy has not been readily applicable to cancer patients. In the first place, the selective targeting to activate a cytotoxic T-cell is not simple in the human host. Second, the common tumour-associated antigens which are expressed in low density on some normal cells are, of course, recognized by these antibodies. Since a very low antigen density on cell surfaces was found to be sufficient for lysis to occur, normal tissues can easily be damaged by this approach. Third, the mass production of heterobispecific antibodies is still a very difficult task.

Cancer chemotherapy is limited by the toxicity of currently available anticancer drugs to normal tissues. A more selective delivery of cytotoxic drugs to cancer cells has been attempted by conjugating cytotoxic drugs to anti-TAA antibodies. The success of this approach depends on three factors: the retention of the functions of the drug, the antigen-binding capacity of the antibody when antibody and drug are linked together and finally the uptake and the appropriate processing of the conjugates by the cancer cell. Up to 40 mol of various cytotoxic drugs could be coupled to one mole of anti-TAA antibody via intermediate carriers such as human serum albumin, dextrane or poly-L-glutaminic acid. In preclinical studies some of the antibody drug conjugates have given encouraging results, but very little is known so far about the effects in the human host.

Attempts to deliver larger doses of drugs to tumour tissues led to the development of drug-containing liposomes *(chemo-immunoliposomes)*. Although the trapping of such liposomes by phagocytes could be limited by using liposomes of a neutral charge, some technical problems remain to be solved. So far this approach suffers most from the leakiness of the liposomes and the insufficient uptake of the liposomal contents by the target cells.

In a cancer drug which can be targeted selectively, even high cytotoxicity may be acceptable. Therefore, the coupling of highly toxic substances to monoclonal antibodies which specifically address tumour-associated antigens may be a viable therapeutic strategy.

Several bacterial and plant toxins are highly efficient inhibitors of protein synthesis in eukaryotic cells. After entering a cell, diphtheria toxin (DT) has been shown to catalyze the binding of ADP-ribose to elongation factor 2 (EF-2). As a consequence of adenosyl-ribosylation, the factor loses its catalytic function which is essential for protein synthesis. Since DT as well as plant toxins which show a similar structure, such as ricin, abrin and others, act as enzymes, only a few molecules have to gain access to a cell in order to kill it. While most cytotoxic drugs affect only cells in divisional cycle, these protein synthesis inhibitors also kill resting cells. Ricin, the most extensively studied plant toxin, is formed by two disulfide bonded polypeptide chains. In this respect, it is similar to some other plant toxins and to diphtheria toxin. The A chain is the toxic part, while the B chain is a lectin with galactose-binding sites on both ends of the chain. Both peptides carry oligosaccharide side chains with terminal mannose residues. Via the galactose binding site, the toxin can bind to practically all cells in the body. The terminal mannose residue mediates attachment to cells which bear the asialoglycoprotein receptor, i.e. liver cells. With the aid of coupling reagents, the toxins can be bound to antibodies which are specific for the cell surface antigens of particular target cells. These conjugates are often referred to as 'immunotoxins'. The nonspecific uptake of immunotoxins by asialoglycoprotein receptor bearing cells can be prevented by the use of deglycosylated toxins. It is more difficult to avoid the nonspecific binding of immunotoxin molecules to galactose residues on cell surfaces via the B-chain. In vitro, this unspecific absorption can be prevented by lactose. However, this is not a viable strategy for the in vivo situation. Therefore, conjugates were made which contain only the A-chains. Under these conditions, A-chain delivery to the cytoplasm is not optimal. It can, however, be enhanced by lysosomotropic substances (NH_4Cl, chloroquine, methylamine) or carboxylic ionophores (monensin, grisorexin, lasalocid) or by the simultaneous application of B chains from which the galactose-binding sites were removed. Immunotoxins have been shown to be highly specific in vitro. They are increasingly used for the purging of bone marrow before transplantation (see below). So far their in vivo use has been limited by the rather fast uncoupling of the toxins from the antibodies which would result in unacceptable toxicity. However, more suitable coupling procedures have recently been developed and first clinical trials with ITs could be initiated. Since the genes encoding the diphtheria toxin and ricin have been cloned, it is conceivable that novel immunotoxins which are fusion proteins of heavy globulin chains with the subunits of toxins which carry the toxicity will be generated soon by recombinant DNA technology.

3.4.2.2.3 In vitro use of unmodified or modified antibodies

Because of the toxic side effects, radio- and chemotherapy of cancer patients must be limited to doses which, in most cases, are not sufficient to eliminate the tumour. The organ which is most sensitive to cancer chemotherapy is the hematopoietic system. The possibility to reconstitute a lethally damaged hematopoietic system by bone marrow transplantation has somewhat extended the applicability of radiation or chemotherapy to malignant diseases. Since, however, very high doses of radiation or cytotoxic drugs are not only damaging to hematopoietic but also to non-hematopoietic tissues, this strategy is limited to tumours which are relatively sensitive to chemo- and radiotherapy, such as acute and chronic myeloid leukemias, acute lymphatic leukemias, non-Hodgkin lymphomas, Hodgkin lymphomas, germ cell tumours, Ewing sarcomas, small-cell lung cancers or neuroblastomas. Hematopoietic reconstitution can be achieved with bone marrow cells from allogeneic donors or with autologous bone marrow cells which were explanted before the high-dose treatment of the cancer patient. Allogeneic bone marrow transplantations are often complicated by immune responses of donor T-cells against minor or major histocompatibility antigens of the recipient. Clinically these events become apparent as acute or chronic graft-versus-host disease. Autologous bone marrow transplantations, on the other hand, carry the risk that tumour relapses might originate from tumour cells which were present in the explanted bone marrow sample. Attempts have therefore been made to overcome these difficulties by *in vitro* treatment of the bone marrow transplants with monoclonal antibodies, the aim being the elimination of T-cells from allogeneic bone marrow grafts or the purging of autologous bone marrow from tumour cells. The elimination of the undesired cells has been achieved with a variety of methods, such as treatment with antibodies and complement, treatment with immunotoxins or by adsorption of target cells to antibody-coated particles. Graft-versus-host disease can be almost completely prevented by T-cell depletion of allogeneic bone marrow grafts. Unfortunately, T-cell depletion is often associated with a higher relapse rate (lack of graft-versus-tumour effect) and a higher graft rejection rate. It has not yet been shown that the elimination of tumour cells from autologous grafts reduces relapse rates. The in vitro use of antibodies in bone marrow transplantation could make a major contribution to the treatment of some malignancies. However, the following three conditions will have to be satisfied before this can happen: First, more efficient treatment protocols must be developed for the *in vivo* elimination of tumour cells by radio- and chemotherapy. Second, the rejection rate of allogeneic bone marrow grafts must be further reduced by more rigorous immunosuppression of the recipient and third, more effective measures for the prevention of infections in the post-transplantation period must be developed.

3.4.2.3 Prospects of cancer therapy with monoclonal antibodies

There can be no doubt that the concept of cancer therapy with antibodies directed against surface antigens of tumour cells has considerable aesthetic appeal. However, there are also some reservations to be made. The fact that tumour-associated antigens are never absolutely specific for tumour cells has already been mentioned. Though important, the lack of specificity is perhaps the least serious argument against this strategy, because certain antigens which are rather scarcely represented on healthy adult cells are indeed expressed on tumour cells in high density. So, at least, one can build on the existence of considerable quantitative differences in the expression of onco-fetal and other tumour-associated antigens. Another problem, perhaps a more serious one, resides in the genetic instability of tumour cell populations. Tumours tend to escape the attack by antibodies through variants which have lost the target antigen. This phenomenon has been observed in preclinical as well as in clinical studies. Well-documented examples are the *in vitro* selection of variants lacking the transferrin receptor or the *in vivo* selection of idiotype-negative variants of B lymphoma cells in patients who were treated with anti-idiotypic antibodies.

A related problem lies in the shedding of antigens. Some surface structures of tumour cells are released into the environment, or, for that matter, into the bloodstream. In such cases, antibodies directed against these antigens would form soluble complexes which would be ineffective therapeutically but could cause side effects. The number of antibodies which could be expected to actually reach the tumour would, under these conditions, be reduced. Finally, antibodies are in themselves antigens. Preliminary results of a clinical trial conducted with human antibodies indicate that even these molecules are very effective in eliciting the formation of anti-idiotypic antibodies in the recipient. Such anti-idiotypic antibodies can undoubtedly detract from the therapeutic effect of antibodies directed against tumour antigens.

In summary, the use of monoclonal antibodies in the treatment of malignancies represents an intriguing concept. In view of the fundamental difficulties inherent in this concept, some of which have been touched upon, one cannot expect this approach to become a generally applicable treatment modality. In contrast to the use of drugs which, despite their shortcomings, are distinguished by a rather general applicability in cancer, antibodies are likely to remain very specific tools which will be helpful in certain segments of the therapeutic spectrum. Undoubtedly, many antibodies will be developed. Each of them, however, will be capable of addressing only a narrow, well-defined therapeutic problem. A general applicability of one or even a small number of antibody preparations to a large number of malignancies appears out of question. In spite of claims to the contrary, therefore, the use of monoclonal antibodies will bring an increase in quality but not a revolution to cancer therapy.

3.4.3 Other therapeutic uses of monoclonal antibodies

Monoclonal antibodies against T-cell surface antigens are used as immunosuppressive agents. The first antibody which has gained the status of an approved "drug" in the treatment of rejection episodes after organ transplantation is OKT3. Since this antibody is today used like an immunosuppressive drug, it will be discussed in Chapter 4.

4. Immunosuppression

4.1. What is an immunosuppressive?

The question as to which substances should be classified as immunosuppressives does not have a straightforward answer. Both antigens and antibodies may have an immunosuppressive effect under certain conditions. Even chemical substances such as alkylating agents or antimetabolites may, depending on the circumstances of their administration, promote or – more probably – inhibit the response to an antigenic stimulus. As we shall see, azathioprine, a drug frequently administered for suppressing rejection or "graft-versus-host" reactions, can exert an immunostimulatory effect if its antiproliferative properties can be channelled to act on the development of T-suppressor cells. Antiinflammatory substances can help attenuate the results of a cell-mediated immune reaction to an organ graft or to endogenous structures. This is also true of anticoagulants in certain situations. Compounding these difficulties is the fact that the biochemical and molecular mechanisms that lead to immunosuppression are not yet fully understood. Classification of substances according to their molecular mechanism is therefore still some way off.

In view of the complexity of the situation, it is more practical to approach the question "What is an immunosuppressive?" from the clinical-therapeutic angle. We know that the host's immunological reaction to a grafted organ can be understood basically as a manifestation of a delayed-type hypersensitivity reaction. In autoimmune diseases both humoral and cell-mediated immune reactions to endogenous structures play an essential pathogenetic role. Type-II, type-III and type-IV hypersensitivity reactions are observed, depending on the condition involved. Type-II reactions are antibody-dependent cytotoxic reactions and are seen in idiopathic thrombocytopenic purpura in neonates, occasionally in the host reaction to an organ transplant, and in autoimmune reactions to formed elements of the blood (autoimmune hemolytic anemia) and the basement membrane of glomeruli in glomerulonephritis. Type-III hypersensitivity reactions are also antibody-mediated. They depend on the formation of immune complexes which activate complement and attract neutrophilic and eosinophilic granulocytes chemotactically, thereby causing local lesions. Manifestations of these local processes are found in pulmonary aspergillosis and after rapid lysis of the pathogens of syphilis, leprosy and typhoid during chemotherapy, as well as in farmer's lung and pigeon fancier's disease. In relative antigen excess, soluble antigen-antibody complexes enter the bloodstream and form deposits in the joints, kidneys, skin and choroid plexus, where they cause inflammatory reactions. Clinical manifestations of generalized type-III hypersensitivity reactions include serum sickness, polyarthritis associated with hepatitis B, hemorrhagic shock associated with Dengue fever and, of course, glomerulonephritis after streptococcal infection.

Type-IV hypersensitivity is the classic cell-mediated reaction already mentioned several times. Its morphological substrate in the presence of persistent antigen is the granuloma.

Thus, in the clinical situations with which we are concerned, a cell-mediated or humoral response to structures that are foreign or recognized as foreign is the "primum movens". Substances which suppress such reactions and thereby allow an organ transplant to take and to function or which reduce the symptoms of an autoimmune disease can, in operative terms, be described as immunosuppressive agents, even if a cast-iron classification based on their mechanism of action is not yet possible.

In the search for immunosuppressive agents or treatment modalities we can follow two different strategies. In the first place, we can look for agents which interfere with one or several steps of the immune response. Such agents, if used properly, should be able to prevent an unwanted immune response against a transplanted organ or against self antigens. They would, however, also be capable of suppressing physiological immune responses against infectious organisms. Their "therapeutic" specificity would, therefore, depend largely on the correct timing of their application. Secondly, we can try to imitate those mechanisms by which self-tolerance is induced during fetal development and maintained throughout adult life.

4.1.1 Blocking the immune response

For an antigen to trigger an immune response, it has to be engulfed by macrophages or dendritic cells and then presented in association with a histocompatibility antigen. Specific inhibitors of antigen uptake and processing are not yet known. Chloroquine, an antimalarial agent, has been reported as inhibiting the breakdown of proteins into small "presentable" pieces in the lysosomes. Apparently, this inhibition is due to a rise in lysosomal pH brought about by the alkalinity of chloroquine. It is possible but by no means certain that this property of chloroquine relates to its well-known antiinflammatory effects. In a more general way cyclophosphamide and azathioprine interfere with the immune response at an early stage. Both compounds reduce the antigen content in lymphatic organs – cyclophosphamide predominantly in spleen follicles and azathioprine more particularly in the lymph nodes. This effect may originate from reduced production of monocytes from promonocytes in the presence of azathioprine, or possibly from direct damage by the two substances to the antigen-containing dendritic cell.

So far, it has not been possible to interfere pharmacologically with the presentation of an antigenic peptide by a histocompatibility molecule. The recent elucidation of the structure of these molecules and of the way in which they bind and present antigen seems to open conceptual possibilities for the design of peptides for molecules which could occupy or inactivate class-I or class-II molecules and perhaps even subsets of these structures which are involved in the presentation of antigens. It is conceivable that certain histocompatibility molecules are specifically involved in the presentation of "self" antigens. The high incidence of certain histocompatibility alleles in autoimmune diseases could be interpreted in this way.

Recognition of the presented antigen by lymphocytes triggers activation of an antigen-specific lymphocyte by means of a direct signal emanating from a T- or B-cell receptor and a second, humoral stimulus from interleukin 1 (Il-1) and other lymphokines. Low-molecular-weight substances which interfere with the process of antigen recognition are not known, and are difficult to conceive because they would not only have to block the specific T- and B-cell receptors but would also have to possess structural features of the antigen to be recognized. More likely such effects could be achieved by monoclonal antibodies with a high affinity for T-cell receptors or for histocompatibility antigens, capable of masking structures on the surface of the antigen-presenting cell or lymphocyte that are essential to recognition.

The CD4 and CD8 antigens play a crucial role in the interaction of T-cells with antigen-presenting cells and in the subsequent activation of T-cells. For some time, these antigens were envisaged as having merely a "stabilizing" function. Consequently, they were termed "associative antigens". It has, however, become quite clear that these proteins play a more important role in T-cell activation. Monoclonal antibodies against certain CD4 epitopes were shown to prevent T-cell activation by mitogens or antigens, and in mixed lymphocyte cultures. Compounds which "inactivate" CD4 and perhaps also CD8 could, therefore, be expected to be immunosuppressive.

Lymphocyte activation which is initiated by the recognition of an antigen presented on a histocompatibility molecule by a T-cell receptor can be interrupted by cyclosporin A. The mechanism of this event is not completely understood. Obviously, however, cyclosporin prevents the transcription of the Il-2 gene and of other lymphokine genes, thereby aborting the clonal expansion following T-cell activation.

The expansion of antigen-specific cell clones that follows T-cell activation is also inhibited by antiproliferative substances such as antimetabolites, cyclophosphamide and probably also glucocorticoids.

Il-2 receptors are expressed in the presence of concentrations of cyclosporin A which are immunosuppressive, and exogenous supply of Il-2, even in the presence of cyclosporin A, results in expansion of already activated T-cell clones. Monoclonal antibodies against the p55 subunit of the Il-2 receptor (tac antibodies) stop Il-2 from occupying these receptors, thereby preventing proliferation of activated T-cells. A monoclonal antibody (OKT 3) directed against the CD3 complex which is responsible for signal transduction after antigen recognition blocks the function of this protein complex and prevents T-cell activation. This antibody has found clinical application in the treatment of rejection episodes after kidney transplantation.

Inhibiting induction of cytotoxic T-cells or blocking the function of these cells could be useful, particularly in certain autoimmune diseases, i.e. in situations in which the primary immune response has long since taken place and in which therapy can be directed only at the secondary reactions. Ideally, blocking the function of cytotoxic lymphocytes should affect only those cell clones whose specific reaction to endogenous structures renders them pathogenic. However, this level of specificity is most likely to be achieved with monoclonal antibodies which "neutralize" certain clones by way of antiidiotype interactions without impairing cell-mediated immune defences as a whole.

Pharmacological inhibition of the recruiting and activation of other effector cells such as macrophages, neutrophilic granulocytes or NK-cells has less to do with specific immunosuppression than with pharmacological inhibition of inflammation. The role of glucocorticoids in this context will be described when this class of substance is discussed.

Table 4.1 gives an overview of the most important approaches to immunosuppression.

Table 4.1. Immunosuppressive modalities in descending order of specificity

Specificity	Typical protocols
Nonspecific	Cytotoxic agents, steroids, total body irradiation
Lymphocyte-specific	ALS, thoracic duct drainage, local allograft or total lymphoid irradiation
T-cell	Monoclonal antibodies (e.g. orthoclone OKT_3)
T-subsets	Cyclosporin A, anti-tac monoclonal antibody, FK 506
MHC (HLA) specific	Blockers of MHC alleles associated with autoimmune disease (see Chapter 7)
Antigen-specific	To be defined

The majority of agents which are available today belong to the first two levels, they are either non-specific or predominantly directed at lymphocytes. Cyclosporin A anmd OKT_3 can be classified as T-cell specific agents. A therapeutically defined approach towards certain lymphocyte subsets may just be emerging: monoclonal antibodies against CD4, CD8 or CD2 represent this class of compounds. The ideal, a donor-antigen specific agent is at present not even conceivable. There are, however, experimental models in which tolerance to a specific donor can be induced. The most encouraging of these models will be briefly discussed at the end of this chapter.

4.1.2 Strategies leading to the induction of tolerance

It is now well established that self-tolerance is the result of two basic mechanisms: clonal deletion and induction of T-suppressor cells. A third mechanism called "clonal anergy" has recently been discovered. This phenomenon is observed when T-cells encounter their antigen and are inactivated instead of activated. This can happen if the antigen is presented by B-cells without a co-stimulatory signal from a bystander macrophage or dendritic cell. The extent to which this mechanism of tolerance induction can be explained pharmacologically is still unclear.

During ontogenesis T-precursor cells migrate into the thymus. There they rearrange their γ- and δ- and subsequently their α- and β-genes and in doing so develop their individual antigen specificity. The antigenic repertoire expressed at this level contains a wealth of specific structures, directed against "self" as well as against "non-self". Most of these young cells are subsequently killed by a mechanism not yet understood. Only those cells that display an affinity for class-I or class-II histocompatibility antigens expressed on the thymic epithelium avoid destruction. Again it is not clear by what mechanism T-cells which bind to epithelium are rescued. Possibly a cytokine acting at short range is involved.

It is perhaps at this stage that immature $CD4^+/CD8^+$ cells are programmed to become either T-helper cells ($CD4^+/CD8^-$) or T-killer (suppressor) cells ($CD8^+/CD4^-$). In any case, only T-cells which can recognize "self" class-I or class-II molecules survive this first selection step. In a second selection, these surviving T-cells then interact with so-called accessory cells (macrophages and dendritic cells) which present self antigens in conjunction with class-I and class-II receptors *(Fig. 4.1)*. This time the interaction is negative: T-cells which react with accessory cells are killed. Since the T-cells are already biased towards recognizing self MHC molecules by the first selection step, a large proportion of T-cells – if not all cells – would be killed during this second encounter. This is probably avoided by selection on the basis of avidity. Only cells that bind to "self" antigens presented on class-I or class-II molecules with high avidity are eliminated. The result of this double selection is a T-cell population which is MHC restricted but does not react against self in association with histocompatibility molecules *(Fig. 4.2)*. The antigen repertoire of T-cells now contains a window which corresponds to all the presented self antigens. If this mechanism

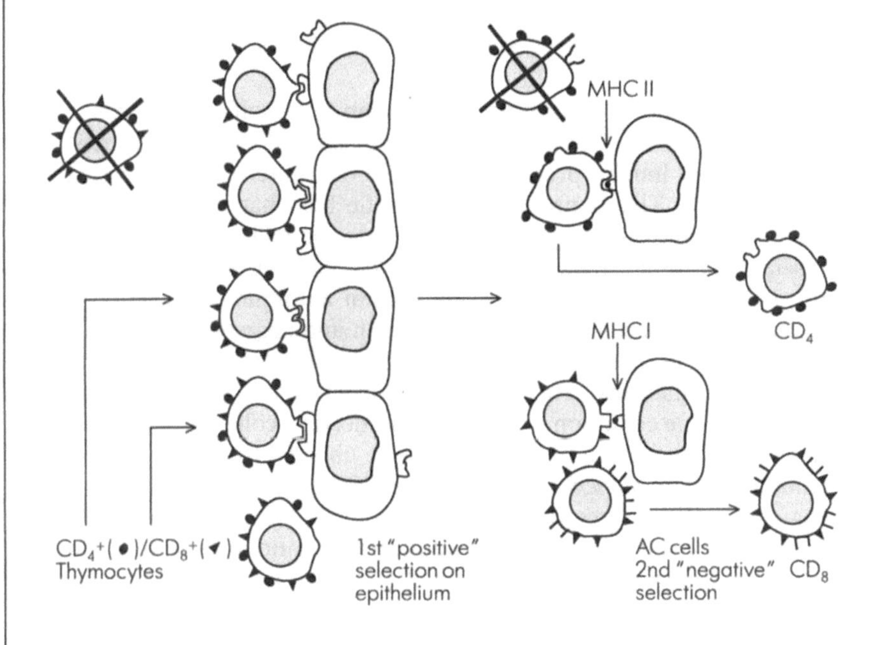

Figure 4.1. Positive and negative selection of T-cells in the thymus.
Double positive immature T-cells enter the thymus and interact with class-I and class-II MHC molecules on the thymus epithelium. Only cells with a T-cell receptor that recognizes MHC will be rescued from destruction (positive selection). Depending on the class of MHC which a T-cell can recognize it will develop into a CD_4^+/CD_8^- (T helper) cell or into a CD_8^+/CD_4^- (cytotoxic/suppressor) T-cell. In the second step accessory cells (dendritic cells, macrophages) present "self-antigens" to the T-cells which have passed the first selection. During the second negative selection those cells which react to "self-antigen" in the MHC environment strongly, are eliminated. Those that bind only weakly or not at all, can pass (see text).

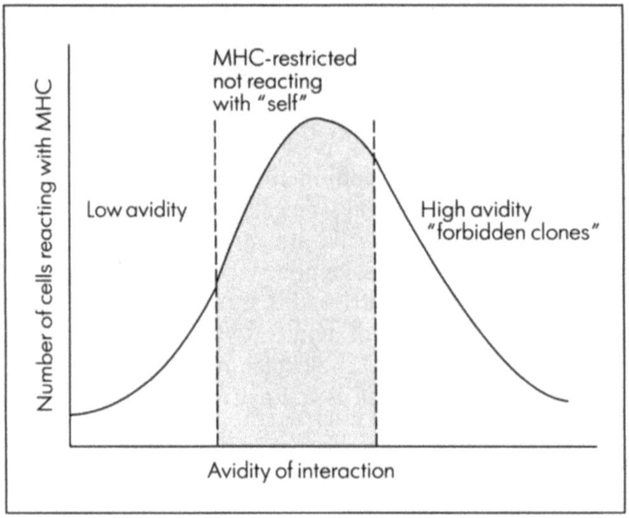

Figure 4.2. Distribution of T-cells before the second negative selection step. It is indicated that strong interaction of T-cell receptors with "self" is an exclusion criterion. Below a certain cut-off point, cells are MHC restricted but do not react with "self". Therefore, they can be regarded as useful in recognizing "non-self" in association with MHC.

were exhaustive it should lead to the elimination of all self-reactive cells. That, obviously, is not the case: in autoimmune diseases and even in "normal" individuals receiving a human protein like insulin or α-interferon, autoreactive T-cells are observed. This is probably due to the fact that not all self antigens are presented during ontogeny, because they may be relatively inaccessible and are consequently never "seen" by T-cells. If the deletion of "forbidden" clones does not suffice to protect any individual from autoimmune reactions, there must be additional mechanisms to prevent such autoaggression. The induction of T-suppressor cells directed against autoreactive T-helper cells may represent one of these mechanisms. There are many experimental examples indicating that an autoimmune condition like arthritis induced by collagen or experimental allergic encephalitis induced by myelin can be aborted by $CD8^+$ T-cells which are antiidiotypic with respect to autoreactive CD4-cells. However, these mechanisms have never been directly observed in humans. We have a reasonable idea of how to delete T-cell clones that are implicated in autoimmune reactions, but a therapeutic strategy based on the induction of T-suppressor cells cannot yet be envisaged.

We will therefore restrict ourselves to the description of fusion proteins that bind to activated T-cells only. This relative specificity is obtained by fusing or linking Il-2 with toxins like diphtheria toxin or ricin which can kill cells that carry a high-affinity Il-2 receptor and to which they are specifically addressed through the Il-2 moiety.

4.2 Azathioprine

4.2.1 Chemistry, history

Apart from the steroids and cyclosporin A, azathioprine is the most frequently used immunosuppressive. It was originally not conceived as an immunosuppressive agent but as a variant of the standard cytostatic 6-mercaptopurine. Azathioprine is methyl-nitroimidazolyl-6-mercaptopurine *(Fig. 4.3)*. By protecting the 6-mercapto group against methylation, it was hoped that the molecule would have a longer duration of action than unprotected 6-mercaptopurine. Though this was not the case, azathioprine has proved its worth in the context of cytostatic immunosuppressives.

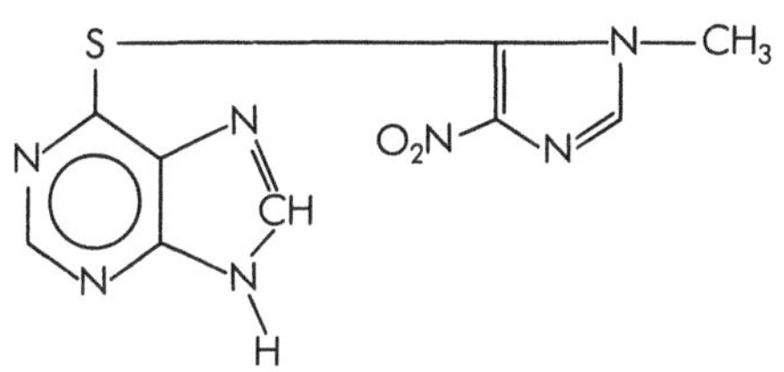

Figure 4.3. Molecular structure of azathioprine

4.2.2 Pharmacokinetics

Absorption of azathioprine after oral administration is 88%, and hence higher than that of 6-mercaptopurine (78%). Fifteen minutes after i.v. injections and an hour after oral administration of azathioprine, about 70% of the dose is available as 6-mercaptopurine and methylnitroimidazole. The half-lives of azathioprine and 6-mercaptopurine are relatively short: after i.v. injection that of azathioprine is 10 to 20 minutes and that of 6-mercaptopurine about 90 minutes. After oral administration the the plasma half-life of 6-mercaptopurine is between two and four hours. 6-Mercaptopurine, the active principle of azathioprine, has two metabolic pathways: one involves 6-methylation and subsequent oxidation, while the other consists of conversion of 6-mercaptopurine by xanthine oxidase into the cytostatically inactive 6-thiouric acid. 6-Methylmercaptopurine, like the non-methylated original compound, is phosphorylated within the cells to the corresponding mono-, di- and triphosphates. Azathioprine and 6-mercaptopurine are distributed evenly in the body without any tendency to accumulate in any specific organ. Only very small amounts of the two substances reach the central nervous system.

4.2.3 Mechanism of action

The cytotoxic mechanism of action of azathioprine is identical with that of 6-mercaptopurine. Whether this is a plausible explanation for all the immunopharmacological effects of the substance is an open question.

6-Mercaptopurine is phosphorylated intracellularly to thioinosine monophosphate (T-IMP). The responsible enzyme is hypoxanthine-guanine phosphoribosyltransferase. T-IMP then acts as a "bridgehead" in the biosynthesis of purine. It inhibits the conversion of inosine monophosphate (IMP) into adenylosuccinate, thereby blocking the release of adenosine phosphates. In addition, T-IMP inhibits IMP dehydrogenase, i.e. the enzyme that catalyzes the conversion of IMP to xanthine monophosphate. Suspension of this biosynthesis step also puts an end to the production of guanosine monophosphate in the cell *(Fig. 4.4)*. Moreover, by a feedback mechanism T-IMP can inhibit the first step in purine biosynthesis, the reaction of glutamine with phosphoribosylpyrophosphate, thereby putting a brake on purine biosynthesis.

We shall see that, compared with other antimetabolites and probably with 6-mercaptopurine, azathioprine is characterized by a certain selectivity for lymphocytes, particularly T-lymphocytes which mediate the delayed-type hypersensitivity reaction. This property conceivably derives from the nitroimidazole, a possibility that has been virtually ignored up to the present. However, imidazole is known to increase the cGMP concentration in lymphocytes, thereby also increasing the reactivity of such cells to mitogens and foreign antigens. It is perfectly possible that lymphocytes that have been "sensitized" by nitroimidazole constitute particularly sensitive targets for the activity of 6-mercaptopurine. In this connection, however, it should be borne in mind that a related molecule, nitrothiazolyl-2-imidazolidinone or niridazole, exerts an inhibitory action that is directed particularly at cell-mediated immunity. Reduced convertibility of lymphocytes by mitogens or antigens has been found three months after withdrawal of therapy in patients given this anthelmintic over a prolonged period. Cutaneous delayed-type hypersensitivity was also reduced for about the same time in these patients. It may not be the entire molecule that is responsible for the effect. The urine of patients given niridazole has been found to contain a metabolite, possibly the imidazolidinone, which does not have an anthelmintic effect but does have stronger immunosuppressive properties than niridazole itself. Niridazole potentiates the effects of azathioprine and steroids in preventing rejection of kidney grafts in dogs. It is still difficult to arrange these rather

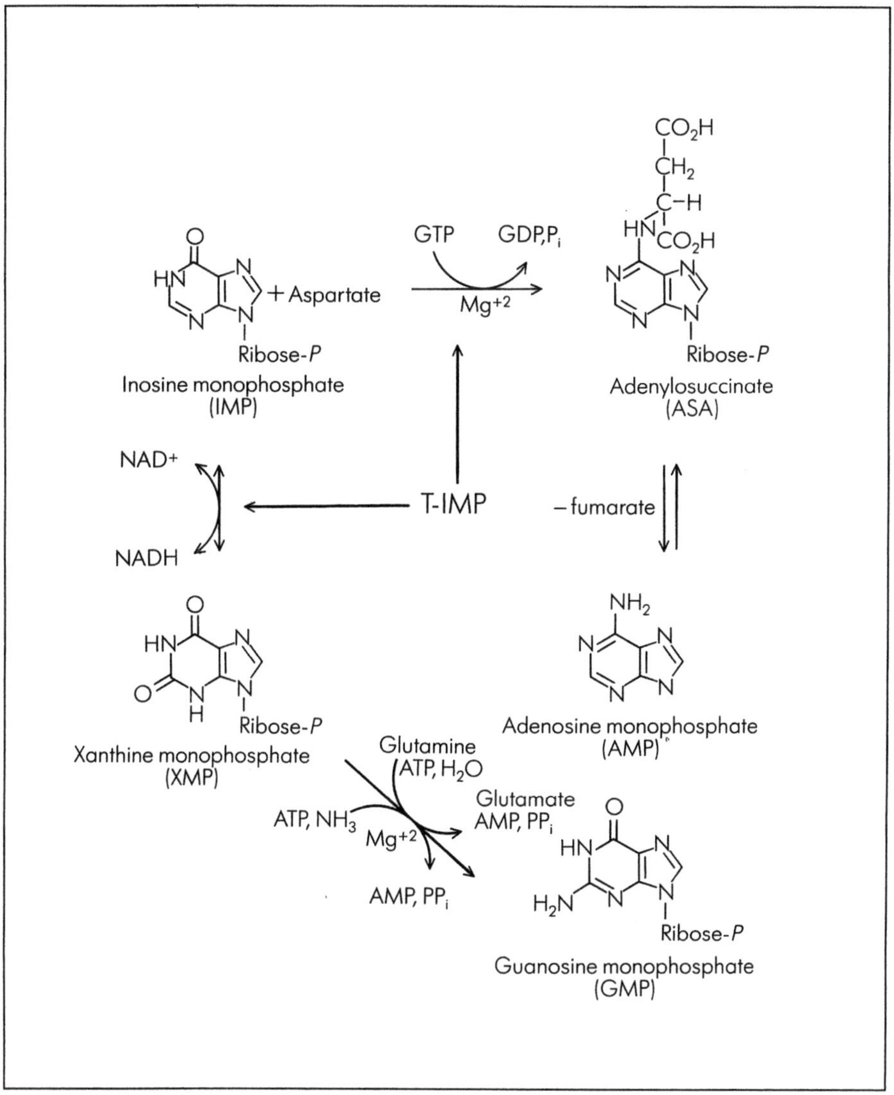

Figure 4.4. Diagram of the effect of thioinosine monophosphate (T-IMP) on the conversion of IMP to adenosine monophosphate and guanosine monophosphate. See text for further details.

heterogenous findings into a logical pattern. Obviously, however, the nitroimidazole group in azathioprine contributes to the overall effect of the drug.

4.2.4 Immunopharmacological effect of azathioprine

Azathioprine has distinct antiinflammatory properties. Compared with other antiinflammatory substances like aspirin or indomethacin, the onset of the antiinflammatory effect is slow. It is probably associated with inhibition of promonocyte maturation. The maturation of these cells is slowed down by azathioprine in the S- and G2-phase, consequently the number of mature monocytes leaving the bone marrow per unit of time is reduced. The release of neutrophilic granulocytes is also slowed down by azathioprine.

Under certain circumstances azathioprine inhibits humoral immunity, the synthesis of IgG antibodies being more significantly affected than the formation of IgM antibodies. The intensity of this effect depends on a number of parameters, e.g. the amount of antigen present. It is, however, especially dependent on the time of administration. In the classic model in which the primary immune response of the mouse to erythrocytes from another species is observed, azathioprine has a clear effect only if it is administered within 48 hours after immunization. This finding is consistent with the mechanism of cytostatic action of azathioprine and 6-mercaptopurine: resting cells are scarcely affected, while cells already involved in the mitotic cycle are very sensitive. For man, hardly any reliable data exist on the effect of azathioprine on humoral immunity.

Azathioprine lowers the number of lymphocytes in the bone marrow of rodents after only a short period of administration. Cell counts in the thymus are also reduced, with the cortisone-sensitive cortical cells being more significantly affected than the steroid-resistant lymphocytes in the thymus medulla. Peripheral lymphocytes and those located in the lymph nodes are relatively insensitive to azathioprine. In patients with rheumatoid arthritis the number of peripheral lymphocytes is reduced by an average of 40% after a six-month course of treatment with azathioprine, with T- and B-lymphocytes being more or less equally affected.

Patients treated for one to five months with prednisolone and azathioprine following a kidney transplant exhibited a substantial reduction in in-vitro NK-cell activity. A comparable reduction was found in ADCC. The same changes in even more pronounced form were seen in a group of patients treated for an even longer period with these substances. Control studies with prednisolone alone showed that azathioprine was probably responsible for the changes. Regression of such changes following withdrawal of the medication seems to take several months.

Azathioprine seems to have a stronger effect on T-lymphocytes than on B-cells. The concentrations of active substance needed to inhibit in-vitro induction of cytotoxic T-cells are in the 0.1–1.0 μg/ml range. In contrast, the concentrations required for inhibition of the humoral immune response to T-cell-independent antigens are about 300 times as high. In both cases azathioprine works only if it is added to the cell cultures with, or shortly after, the antigen. Pre-sensitized cells are largely insensitive to azathioprine. This suggests that it might have a stronger inhibitory effect on the activation phase following antigen recognition than on the formation or activity of effector cells. An interesting parallel to cyclosporin A!

Together with neuraminidase-treated sheep erythrocytes, T-cells spontaneously form rosettes. The receptor responsible for this phenomenon is acquired during maturation of the T-lymphocytes in the thymus. Very low concentrations of azathioprine (< 1.0 μg/ml) are needed to lower the proportion of rosette-forming lymphocytes. The effect is not seen immediately but requires one hour of incubation. It is reversible within 60 minutes on withdrawal of azathioprine. This indicates a rapid turnover of receptor protein in the membranes of T-lymphocytes. The effect is not obtained with 6-mercaptopurine alone, and therefore is evidence of the particular properties of azathioprine, vis-à-vis mercaptopurine. Similar conclusions may be drawn from the extraordinary efficacy of azathioprine in the mixed lymphocyte reaction. This reaction, a simple *in vitro* model for immunological incompatibility between two individuals, is completely inhibited by concentrations ranging between 0.1 and 1.0 μg azathioprine per ml. Here too, however, the substance is fully effective only if it is present in the incubation mixture from the outset, i.e. before DNA synthesis has begun.

Azathioprine lowers the antigen concentration in the spleen and lymphocytes. This effect is attributed to the fact that the substance reduces the density of antigen-presenting cells (macrophages and dendritic cells) in these organs. It also makes macrophages less susceptible to activation and impairs production of MIF (migration inhibitory factor), a lymphokine that inhibits migration of macrophages while activating them. In addition, azathioprine reduces the activity of NK-cells. In certain experimental conditions (particularly in the presence of large amounts of antigen) azathioprine interferes with induction of T-suppressor lymphocytes. The substance that has to be administered in such studies within the stringent limits of a "time window" can, under these circumstances, enhance a humoral immune response.

4.2.5 Clinical use

Azathioprine is usually administered together with steroids in organ and bone marrow transplantation. In the first few weeks following the graft, daily doses of 3–5 mg per kg bodyweight are given, followed by maintenance doses of 1–2 mg per kg bodyweight daily. The use of this substance in autoimmune diseases is being investigated in clinical studies. Accumulation of azathioprine may occur in patients with renal failure; the dosage should be reduced in such cases. Moreover, the daily dosage may be reduced by about 25% when azathioprine is administered together with the xanthine oxidase inhibitor allopurinol. Inhibition of this enzyme also blocks one of the two metabolic pathways of azathioprine.

Azathioprine causes the same side effects as those known to occur under 6-mercaptopurine. First in importance is bone-marrow depression, initially presenting as granulocytopenia. The substance is also potentially hepatotoxic: biliary stasis and cell death due to the direct effect of azathioprine predominate (toxic hepatitis!). As with other immunosuppression methods, infections occur during treatment with azathioprine. The fact that infections with CMV and other viruses of the herpes group are more likely to occur than bacterial infections is an indirect confirmation that azathioprine impairs cell-mediated immunity in particular.

4.3 Glucocorticoids

The glucocorticoids play an important role in endocrine regulation of virtually all functional systems of the body. We will not discuss here the metabolic functions (antianabolic-gluconeogenic) to which these steroid hormones owe their name. Hydrocortisone or cortisol (in man) and corticosterone (in rodents) also influence a large number of cell and tissue regulation processes central to the function of the immune system. This is as true of the relatively nonspecific defence reactions carried out by macrophages, neutrophils, basophils, eosinophils and mast cells as it is of the functioning of T- and B-lymphocytes, i.e. immune cells in the narrow sense. On the molecular level the manifold actions of the glucocorticoids are not fully elucidated. In particular, we do not understand the complex changes produced by the glucocorticoids in the distribution and redistribution of blood and immune cells in the macroorganism. Accordingly, the clinical use of glucocorticoids and of their synthetic analogs is resting to a large extent on empirical criteria. While knowledge of the underlying mechanisms is essential for understanding therapy with glucocorticoids, there is only at present a loose connection between this knowledge and the clinical use of glucocorticoids.

4.3.1 Cellular mechanism of action

The cytoplasm of many cells contains receptors which have a high affinity for glucocorticoids: lymphocytes, connective tissue cells, monocytes and macrophages all contain such receptors. These target cells have about $6-7 \times 10^3$ receptors per cell. There are two types of glucocorticoid receptor. Both bind cortisone, and one has a high affinity for dexamethasone, the other one for aldosterone. The latter is therefore called the mineralo-corticoid receptor. These receptors belong to a receptor family which is characterized by a ligand binding site, a so-called hinge region and a DNA binding sequence. Other members of this family are the receptors for thyroid hormone, sex steroids and retinoic acid. The dissociation constant for receptor and steroid is about 10^{-8} M. After binding of the ligand, the conformation of the receptor molecule in the cytoplasm is modified so that its affinity for interphase chromosomes in the cell nucleus increases. The "activated" steroid-receptor complex accumulates in the nucleus, where it is bound to chromosomal DNA. Within 30 minutes of this event, synthesis and accumulation of specific messenger RNA precursor molecules is observed in the nucleus. These molecules contain "introns" as well as "exons" the nucleotide sequences destined for expression. Introns are sequences which will not undergo translation. By a process known as "splicing", they will be excised from the mRNA molecules, and the free cut ends are rejoined. The processed mRNA, now "mature", is transported into the cytoplasm, where it is translated into protein. Subsequently this protein brings about the hormonally induced phenotype. There is strong evidence that the actual mechanism by which the steroid hormones act consists in turning "on and off" specific genes. Genes whose functional status is regulated by steroid hormones bear nucleotide sequences at their 5'-end which have a particularly marked affinity for steroid-receptor complexes. These sequences are 20 nucleotides long. If they are removed, the gene can no longer be regulated by steroid hormones. But which are the proteins whose synthesis is induced by glucocorticoids? The question cannot be answered in full. This group doubtless includes proteins which inhibit phospholipase A_2. In certain cell types (e.g. thymocytes), glucocorticoids can also induce proteins which regulate calcium and magnesium transport. It has never been proven, however, that all glucocorticoid effects conform to this basic pattern. For instance, is inhibition of histamine release from basophils or mast cells (a typical effect of glucocorticoids) brought about by induced synthesis of a specific protein?

4.3.2 Pharmacological effects

Synthetic glucocorticoids such as dexamethasone, triamcinolone and prednisone are used therapeutically in four indication fields related to the immune system: as immunosuppressants, as antiinflamatory agents, as antilymphocytic cytostatics in oncology and in the management of allergic diseases. The pharmacological effects described below do not fit exactly into these categories, but to some extent they all contribute to the therapeutic applications mentioned above.

4.3.2.1 Effect on the distribution of blood cells

Four to six hours after a single therapeutic dose of a glucocorticoid, a marked increase in the number of neutrophil leucocytes in peripheral blood is observed. This effect is due to the mobilization of neutrophils from bone marrow. All other white blood cells tend to decrease under the influence of glucocorticoids. This decline is most pronounced in monocytes and in B- and T-lymphocytes four to six hours after administration of the glucocorticoid and in basophils and eosinophils four to eight hours afterwards.

The lymphopenia observed after administration of glucocorticoids is, at least in man, not the result of increased lysis of lymphocytes but primarily of redistribution. Under the influence of glucocorticoids, lymphocytes and, in particular, T-lymphocytes migrate into the bone marrow and, to a lesser extent, into lymph nodes. This migration predominantly affects lymphocytes with the phenotype of T-helper cells ($CD4^+$). As with the eosinophilic and basophilic lymphocytes, the redistribution within the pool of circulating lymphocytes can be attributed to changes in the cell membrane, which, by increased affinity for the walls of small vessels, in particular small veins, prolong the sojourn in the "periphery". In addition, glucocorticoids also act on the vascular endothelium itself, thereby intensifying the effect on the blood cells. One effect which the change in lymphocyte circulation may have on immunological parameters is that lymphocytes and basophilic and eosinophilic leucocytes, which would normally be available for a cell-mediated immune response and for collateral inflammatory reactions, are temporarily prevented from coming into contact with the antigen.

Even at concentrations which are readily reached in therapy, monocytes and their differentiation products seem to be very sensitive to glucocorticoids. This is true with respect both to their redistribution and chemotactic reactivity and to their antigen-presenting and secretory functions. An important fact to note about the function of monocytes is that the secretion of soluble mediators, particularly of interleukin 1, is inhibited by glucocorticoids. Higher concentrations (10^{-3}–10^{-4} M) also impair the function of C3b and IgG Fc-receptors on the surface of monocytes.

4.3.2.2 Inhibition of lymphocyte activation

At a very early stage it was noticed that lymphocyte transformation brought about by concanavalin A or phytohemagglutinin can be inhibited by glucocorticoids in both *in vitro* experiments and in *ex vivo* studies in which animals or human volunteers are treated with glucocorticoids and their lymphocytes subsequently stimulated in vitro with mitogens. Both autologous and allogeneic mixed lymphocyte reactions were inhibited by corticosteroids, and a decline in Il-2 production was found. Addition of exogenous Il-2 is not able to reverse the inhibition in mixed lymphocyte reactions, suggesting that in the presence of 20 μg hydrocortisone per ml lymphocytes become insensitive to interleukin 1. According to recent research, interleukin-1 plays a central role not only in leukocyte activation but also in the development of fever, the release of prostaglandins and collagenase and other reactions. Glucocorticoid-induced inhibition of Il-1 secretion in activated monocytes and macrophages and the "desensitization" of lymphocytes to Il-1 might therefore be of decisive importance for the immunosuppressive and antiinflammatory effects of glucocorticoids.

Single doses of glucocorticoids scarcely have any effect on B-lymphocytes. If treatment lasts for several (3–10) days, a slight decline in IgG, IgA and IgM antibodies and, in many cases, an increase in specific IgE antibodies and the IgE fraction is seen. These changes are presumably caused by the inhibition of IgE-specific T-suppressor cells and set in about two weeks after treatment begins. The inhibition of IgG secretion, brought about by suppressor cells, can be reversed with corticosteroids. This phenomenon is observed in the treatment of common variable hypogammaglobinemia and in patients with active sarcoidosis, who are immunologically compromised because of a specific T-suppressor cell activity. This is another example of a predominantly immunosuppressive agent which in certain circumstances can induce the stimulation of an immune response.

4.3.2.3 Lytic effects on lymphocytes

Compared with the lymph cells of rodents, human lymphocytes are very insensitive to corticosteroids. Murine thymocytes are lysed after only six hours of incubation with 10^{-6} M dexamethasone, whereas human lymphocytes are scarcely affected by even longer incubation periods. If a more sensitive method of assessing cytotoxicity caused by steroids is employed, i.e. incorporation of nucleotides into the nucleic acids of cells, human thymocytes are found to be relatively insensitive in comparison with peripheral lymphocytes. Despite this relative lack of sensitivity of human lymphocytes to corticosteroids, the effect of glucocorticoids on lymphatic cells and organs in man has been known for a long time. The clinical entities of Cushing's syndrome (with atrophy of lymphatic tissue) and Addison's disease (with hyperplasia of lymphatic tissue) vividly illustrate the role played by the glucocorticoids in the lymphatic system. It was on the basis of this phenomenology that the treatment of immunological and inflammatory diseases and of neoplastic diseases involving the lymphatic organs with cortisone or synthetic glucocorticoids was introduced.

Clinical scientists are aware that certain forms of leukemia and lymphatic neoplasms respond to glucocorticoids, while others do not. Attempts have been made to correlate the responsiveness of lymphocytes with the quantity of glucocorticoid receptors they possess. A possible correlation seemed to be suggested by the positive relation between the presence of estrogen and progesterone receptors on the one hand and the response shown by certain forms of mammary carcinoma to hormonal treatment on the other. To date, however, no comparable correlation has been found between the number of glucocorticoid receptors and the *in vitro* sensitivity of normal and neoplastic lymphocytes in man. The reason may have been the heterogenous nature of the cell populations studied. If cells taken from patients with acute lymphocytic leukemia are characterized by means of monoclonal antibodies and their sensitivity to glucocorticoids examined on immunological criteria, differences are found which are reproducible: cells from patients with pre-B-cell leukemia or with "early" T-cell leukemia are highly sensitive *in vitro* to glucocorticoids, whereas cells which exhibit a more mature T-cell phenotype are insensitive. The number of glucocorticoid receptors is, at the very least therefore, not the sole decisive factor for corticosteroid sensitivity of a lymph cell. The developmental stage of the cell and their growth pattern also play a prominent part. Lymphocyte populations with a large portion of cells in the S-phase are, generally speaking, more sensitive than cell populations with a smaller proportion of S-phases.

The biochemical mechanism in corticosteroid-sensitive cells which leads to cell death has not been completely elucidated. Glucocorticoid-induced membrane changes apparently play a role by allowing an increased influx of calcium into the cell. Recently a calcium- and magnesium-dependent endonuclease was found in mouse thymocytes which is activated in the presence of pharmacologically and physiologically attainable concentrations of dexamethasone (10^{-7} M) or corticosterone (10^{-6} M) and within 90 minutes fractionates the DNA in thymus cell nuclei. Investigators showed that this activation requires *de novo* RNA and protein synthesis: actinomycin D (5 μg per ml) and cycloheximide (5 μg per ml) prevent the activation of this enzyme by glucocorticoids. In the presence of these inhibitors of RNA and protein biosynthesis, DNA is also not fractionated. The enzyme only works in the presence of 5 mM Ca^{++} and 10 mM Mg^{++} and it can be inhibited by zinc sulfate. The endonuclease cuts the DNA between the nucleosomes, thus giving rise to "oligonucleosomal" fragments. Lymphocytes from lymph nodes have the same number of glucocorticoid receptors as thymocytes and also contain the endonuclease. However, these cells are insensitive to dexamethasone at the selected concentration of 10^{-7} M, and DNA-fractionation does not take place. Glucocorticoids are obviously unable to activate the enzyme in these cells.

4.3.2.4 Phospholipase A_2 inhibitors

In addition to inhibition of Il-1 secretion and inhibition of the secretion of mediators by basophilic granulocytes and mast cells, one mechanism in particular is responsible for the antiinflammatory and antiallergic activity of the glucocorticoids: the inhibition of phospholipase A_2 by steroid-induced proteins. As long ago as the 1970s, investigators had found that glucocorticoids inhibit prostaglandin synthesis not, as with aspirin and other antiinflammatories, by inhibition of cyclooxygenase but by preventing the release of arachidonic acid from phospholipids. Not long afterwards it was found that this effect is caused by a non-dialysable second messenger molecule. As with other steroid effects, the inhibition of phospholipase A_2 depends on occupancy of specific receptors and intact RNA and protein biosynthesis. Inhibitors of RNA and protein synthesis can block the inhibitory action of glucocorticoids on prostaglandin synthesis in macrophages and leucocytes. In 1980 it was reported that the second messenger, which causes the inhibition of phospholipase A_2 and thus blocks the prostaglandin cascade, is a protein with a molecular weight of 15,000 daltons. It was shown that this protein, designated macrocortin, specifically inhibits phospholipase A_2, the key enzyme in prostaglandin and leucotriene synthesis, thereby interrupting the release of arachidonic acid. The substrate supply of cyclooxygenase and lipoxygenase is reduced, and subsequently prostaglandin and leukotriene synthesis declines. Following the discovery of macrocortin, other corticosteroid-inducible proteins were found which inhibit phospholipases. Lipomodulin was isolated from the leucocytes of rabbits (MW 40,000) and renocortin from the cells of the medullary interstitium of rat kidney (MW 15,000 and 30,000). These proteins all have the same mechanism of action. There is strong evidence that macrocortin is a phosphorylated fragment of lipomodulin, which must first be dephosphorylated by a phosphatase before it is effective.

Today these proteins are all encompassed by the term lipocortins. The lipocortins are related to a family of calcium and phospholipid-binding proteins called calpactins, which are components of the cytoskeleton and of membranes. The exact mechanism by which these proteins inhibit phospholipase A_2 is not known. However, it has been shown that the inhibitory effect of lipocortin on phospholipase A_2 is dependent on the substrate concentration. This finding has been interpreted to indicate that lipocortin does not directly interfere with phospholipase A_2 but rather acts by sequestering the phospholipid substrate, thus making it unavailable for the enzyme.

Recent studies have shown that peritoneal cells of rats possess two types of phospholipase A_2 activity. One type (optimum at pH 4.5) is released during phagocytosis into the surroundings of the cells; the other (optimum at pH 8.5) exhibits the same activity in phagocytosing cells and control cells. Acidic phospholipase is a component of the lysosomes and independent of calcium ions. The alkaline enzyme, in contrast, is a component of the cell membrane and requires calcium for its function. Glucocorticoid-induced proteins with a molecular weight of 200,000 dalton selectively inhibit membrane-bound phospholipase A_2, while another fraction, also steroid-induced, with a molecular weight of 40,000 daltons, just as selectively inhibits the lysosomal, phagocytosis-induced enzyme. If leucocytes are incubated with the first of these two fractions, only membrane-bound phospholipase A_2 is inhibited; if incubation takes place only with the protein having a molecular weight of 40,000 daltons (lipomodulin?), only the lysosomal enzyme is inhibited. The latter inhibition is particularly pronounced during phagocytosis, i.e. during activation and elimination of the lysosomal enzyme. It is still uncertain how the phospholipase A_2-inhibiting protein can enter the cell. The process may be pinocytosis or a carrier-mediated mechanism.

Whatever the case, the induction of specific proteins which selectively inhibit phospholipases appears to be the central mechanism responsible for the antiinflammatory and some of the antiallergic effects of the glucocorticoids *(Fig. 4.5)*.

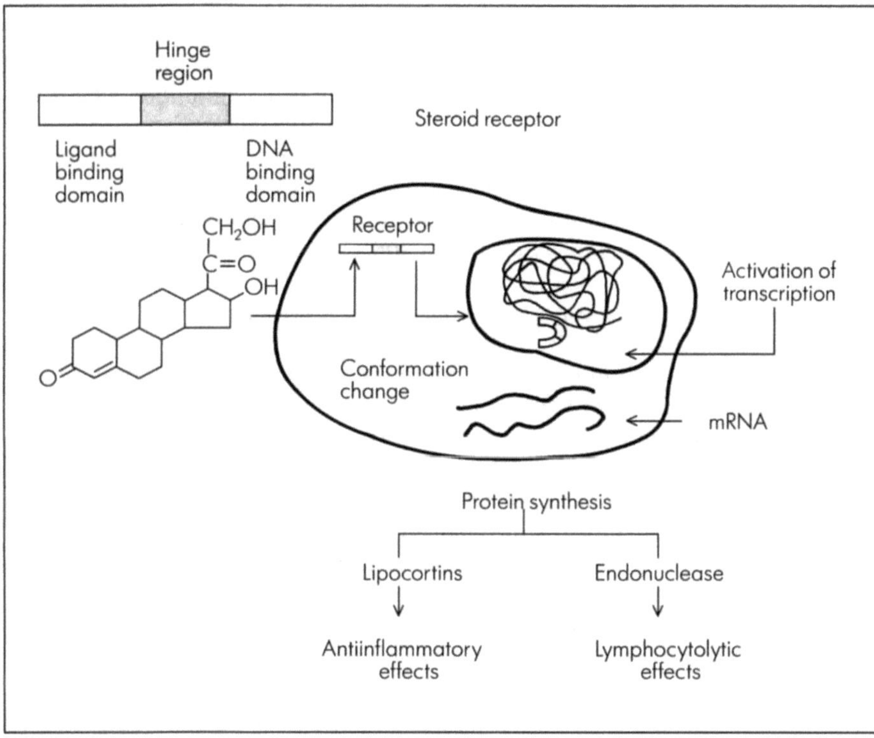

Figure 4.5. The antiinflammatory and lymphocytotoxic effects of glucocorticoids as a consequence of "activation" of specific genes and of de novo protein synthesis. Details in the text.

4.4 Cyclosporin A

Transplant surgery, which came into existence in the 1950s, was the driving force behind the development of an effective and safe immunosuppressive drug. At first, cytostatics, originally developed to combat tumours, were employed in immunosuppression. This method was very nonspecific; all proliferating cells, and not just those involved in an immune reaction of the immune system, were damaged. A second stage of drug-induced immunosuppression saw more selective activity with azathioprine and, in particular steroids. Among their many effects, steroids have marked lymphocytotoxic activity, which may be manifested as immunosuppression (see above). In addition, they are antiinflammatory. The two decades in which prednisone and azathioprine dominated the choice of immunosuppressive medication coincided with the development of other immunosuppressants, which aimed at reducing the number of lymphocytes or at damaging lymphocytes. These measures include antilymphocyte and antithymocyte serums and drainage of the thoracic duct in transplant recipients. The recent introduction of cyclosporin A is a further step along the road to a more selective form of immunosuppression. Cyclosporin A is active only against lymphocytes which are about to react to an antigenic stimulus. This substance can thus be employed to suppress a specific, i.e. temporally and qualitatively delimited, immune response, without suppressing other immunological functions. Cyclosporin A is evidence of the fact that the immune system can be selectively manipulated and that the development of the science of immunopharmacology is a practical task and not just wishful thinking.

Cyclosporin A was discovered in 1970 as the metabolic product of two imperfect fungi, *Tolypocladium inflatum* Gams and *Cylindrocarpon lucidum* Booth. The substance mixture in which cyclosporin A was found first attracted attention because of its antifungal properties, which were, however, too weak to warrant further development.

From earlier research into ovalicin, an immunosuppressant exhibiting prohibitive toxicity, it was known that microbial metabolites exist which have only weak antimicrobial activities but possess rather pronounced cytostatic and immunosuppressive properties. In this context, the neutral peptides from the above-mentioned imperfect fungi which had shown some antifungal activity were tested in a mouse model which permitted measurement of their cytostatic effect and of the formation of hemagglutinating antibodies to sheep erythrocytes. This model provided the first evidence of a pronounced immunosuppressive effect and the absence of any cytostatic properties. The substance suppressed the immune response, but did not prolong the survival of animals which had been inoculated with L1210 mice leukemia cells. Similar findings were reported in other models and in comparative experiments with spleen cells of mice and mastocytoma cells in vitro. These results prompted researchers to isolate the active ingredient, clarify its structure and improve fermentation yields.

Cyclosporin A was later found to be a highly potent immunosuppressive compound, which, in contrast to all hitherto known cytostatics or immunosuppressants like azathioprine, produced no bone marrow toxicity. It was shown that cyclosporin A is not lymphocytotoxic, that the immunosuppression which it produces is reversible and that it elicits similar effects in all animal species investigated.

4.4.1 Chemistry

Cyclosporin A is a neutral cyclic undecapeptide which contains a hitherto unknown nine-carbon amino acid. The molecule is highly lipophilic *(Fig. 4.6)*. Total synthesis of the molecule and a number of analogues has now been achieved. Biological investigation of these substances has yielded a fairly accurate picture of the relationship between their structure and effects. The amino acids 1, 2, 3 and 11 apparently are decisive for the immunosuppressive activity of cyclosporin A. An essential element is the carbon chain of the C_9 amino acid in position 1 and the methylvalin in position 11.

Some changes can be made to the amino acid in position 2. Alkyl residues of 2–3 carbon atoms in this position display good biological activity. Threonine^2-cyclosporin A possesses potent immunosuppressive properties. The introduction of a serine in position 2, however, weakens the effect of the compound. It can be seen that hydrophobic interactions play an important role in the interaction of the aliphatic chain in position 2 with the cyclosporin receptor. In contrast, the hydroxyl group in (threo^2) cyclosporin A does not seem to have any binding function.

4.4.2 Immunosuppressive properties

Cyclosporin A suppresses cell-mediated and humoral immune responses, although its activity against cell-mediated reactions predominates. The mixed lymphocyte reaction is suppressed as is the transformation of lymphocytes by phytohemagglutinin or concanavalin A. The maximum effect can be obtained with concentrations ranging from 40 to 200 ng per ml. The substance inhibits delayed hypersensitivity reactions in various species and experimental models. The dose necessary for this effect ranges, depending on the species or the model, from 20 to 150 mg per kg by mouth. The reactions were inhibited both by early treatment during the sensitization phase and by administration of cyclosporin A immediately or a few days after the dose of the precipitating antigen. At an early stage cyclosporin A was tested in a number of animal models for its effect on cell-mediated immune reactions. The results were convincing: inhibition of rejection reactions following organ transplants and of "graft-versus-host" reactions after bone marrow transplants. Cyclosporin A also proved to be effective in experimentally induced autoimmune disease (e.g. allergic encephalitis of the rat, guinea pig and rhesus monkey). The dosage required during the sensitization phase was 25 mg per kg. Therapeutic activity to prevent paralysis required somewhat higher doses. The prophylactic effectiveness of cyclosporin A in adjuvant arthritis of the rat was found to be markedly greater on a mg/kg basis than azathioprine or phenylbutazone. In this model,

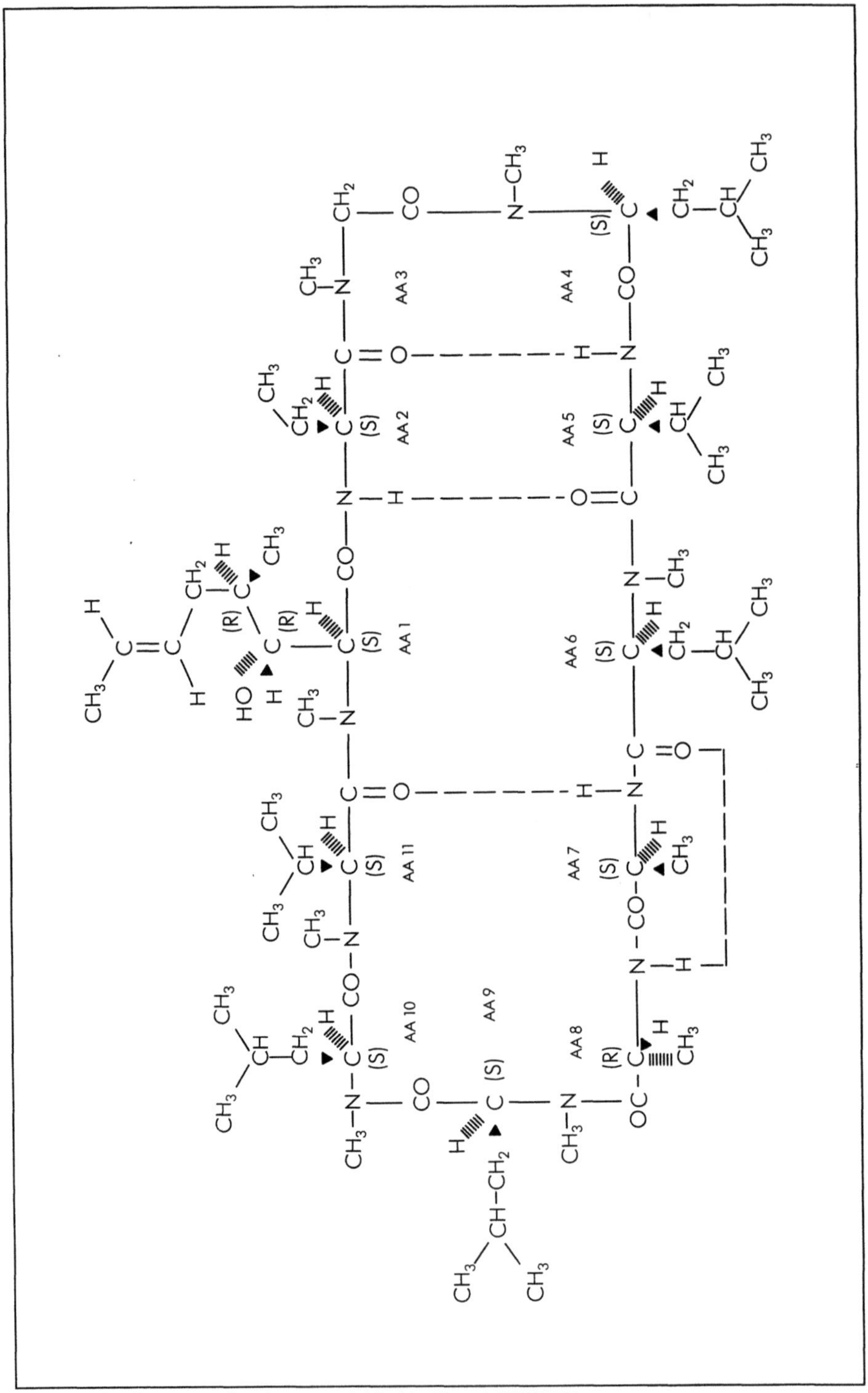

Figure 4.6. Structure of cyclosporin A ($C_{62}H_{111}O_{112}$; MW 1202).

cyclosporin A is just as effective as phenylbutazone. In contrast, cyclosporin A was found to be ineffective in treatment of experimentally induced inflammatory models such as cheek pouch granuloma in the hamster or carrageenan edema of the rat paw. Cyclosporin A also has no effect on experimentally induced fever. However, a dosage of only 10 mg cyclosporin A per kg can completely prevent allergic uveitis induced in the rat by injection of a glycoprotein obtained from the mammalian retina. Doses of up to 50 mg per kg are needed to prevent a lupus erythematosus-like syndrome in female (NZB/NZW) F_1 mice. At the age of 5–6 months, these animals are found to have high titres of anti-DNA antibodies. Four to six weeks later they develop glomerulonephritis with proteinuria, azotemia and, ultimately, fatal renal failure. Administered at a daily dose of 60 mg per kg from the fifth month of life, cyclosporin A can largely prevent proteinuria. Higher prophylactic doses (100 mg per kg daily) ensure survival of 60% of all animals after the 64th week, in contrast to 0% of the control animals.

Transplant experiments in a number of animal species provided specific evidence for the most important therapeutic applications in man. In most of these experiments, cyclosporin A prolonged survival of the transplant. An important finding was that in many cases cyclosporin A only had to be administered for a short time to achieve long-term and even permanent acceptance of the transplant. This is the situation, for instance, with respect to heart, kidney or liver transplants in rats. There are other situations in which the substance protects the transplant only as long as it is administered: skin transplants in mice, rats and rabbits, pancreas transplants in rats and kidney transplants in dogs. In all studies, cyclosporin A protects allogeneic organ transplants for as long as it is administered. When the drug is withdrawn, a phase of relatively weak immune reactivity follows. During this phase, the "defences" against a number of unrelated transplants or antigens are still subnormal. However, the body is increasingly inclined to reject transplanted organs or tissues during this period. In the third phase, some transplant recipients may become specifically tolerant to the tissue antigens of a particular donor. This phase is frequently characterized by poor specific reactivity of the peripheral lymphocytes, while the alloreactive repertoire of the lymphocytes in the lymph nodes is completely unaffected. It has been postulated that this therapeutically desirable state of specific hyporeactivity can be attributed to macrophages which phagocytose and destroy complexes of antigen and lymphocytes reacting specifically to this antigen. Another explanation, supported by experimental results, is the induction of specific T-suppressor cells, which suppress activity directed against the transplant at the level of the T-helper cells. The ability to accept a transplanted organ permanently can be transmitted by lymphocytes of tolerant rats to irradiated rats of the same strain. This finding might also be explained by induction of T-suppressor lymphocytes.

The transplant of bone marrow cells from one animal to another of the same species which has been irradiated or immunosuppressed with cyclophosphamide or other cytostatics usually results in graft-versus-host disease or reaction (GVHD). This disease is caused by the induction of cytotoxic lymphocytes from the transplanted bone marrow, which are directed against the host tissues.

Cyclosporin A inhibits this reaction in mice only at relatively high doses of several hundred mg per kg. Rats and rabbits are far more sensitive to cyclosporin A. The lowest dose in rats which can completely suppress GVHD is 30 mg per kg orally for a three-week period. In rabbits, a 28-day course of 10 mg cyclosporin A per kg i.m. reduced GVHD to below 25%, compared with more than 80% in untreated animals.

4.4.3 Mechanism of action

On the cellular level the mechanism of action of cyclosporin A is fairly well understood. Elucidation is more difficult at the subcellular or molecular level. Cyclosporin A inhibits the activation of resting T-cells. This reaction requires two signals: firstly, recognition of the "right" antigen in connection with class I and II MHC antigens and, secondly, stimulation of lymphocytes by interleukin-1, i.e. a humoral signal emanating from the antigen-presenting cell.

$$T \xrightarrow[(2)]{(1)} T'$$

In the notation proposed by K.J. Lafferty, (1) refers to the signal represented by antigen-recognition and (2) to stimulation by Il-1. Activated T-cells are marked by expression of the receptor for interleukin-2. If interleukin-2 is brought into contact with such cells *in vitro,* clonal expansion of these cells can be observed. This reaction is not inhibited by cyclosporin A at concentrations up to 1 μg per ml. Inhibitory effects, which occur at a dosage of several mg per ml are in all likelihood an expression of cytotoxicity, which is observable at these concentrations. Activated T-cells produce interleukin-2 only after renewed contact with antigen or mitogens. This reaction is suppressed by cyclosporin A at concentrations ranging from 10 to 1000 ng per ml. The reaction can thus be inhibited as shown in Lafferty's notation:

$$T' \xrightarrow{(1)} 1 \text{ (=lymphokine)}$$

There is evidence, however, that lymphokine production becomes insensitive to cyclosporin A about eight hours after it is triggered by an antigen. This finding can be interpreted to mean that cyclosporin A interrupts transmission to the cell nucleus of the stimulus which emanates from antigen recognition. What is clear is that cyclosporin A impairs neither antigen-binding by T-cell receptors nor the interaction of Il-2 with its receptor. In a recent publication it was shown that cyclosporin A selectively inhibits the transcription of the gene for interleukin-2 in a transformed human permanent T-cell, a "Jurkat cell". First it was shown with authentic Il-2 DNA that phorbolmyristine acetate (PMA) and phytohemagglutinin trigger the synthesis of Il-2 messenger RNA in Jurkat cells. The intracellular concentrations of this mRNA peak six hours after induction by the above-mentioned mitogens and then decline until they are no longer detectable at 24 hours. Non-induced cells do not contain any Il-2 mRNA and also do not synthesize interleukin 2. When cyclosporin A was added to the cell cultures at the time of induction, no mRNA synthesis took place or, if it did, it was at least markedly inhibited.

Specific mRNA synthesis was completely suppressed at concentrations of 100 ng per ml of the active substance. 30 ng per ml produced almost total inhibition and 10 ng per ml still detectable inhibition of the synthesis of Il-2mRNA. Under the same experimental conditions, the expression of two other inducible genes was not inhibited. It is particularly noteworthy that the Il-2 receptor was normally expressed even in the presence of cyclosporin A. These experiments would seem to indicate that cyclosporin A inhibits the transcription of the Il-2 gene rather selectively and without any evidence of general cell toxicity or general impairment of transcription. *Since the synthesis and secretion of gamma interferon, MIF and interleukin 3 are also impaired by cyclosporin A, it can be assumed that cyclosporin A selectively inhibits the transcription of a limited number of inducible genes of T-lymphocytes and that this effect explains all or most of its other immunological actions.*

It has been demonstrated that cyclosporin A binds with a dissociation constant of about 2×10^{-7} M to the calcium-complexing protein calmodulin, thereby inhibiting calmodulin-dependent phosphodiesterase. More recent experiments, however, have led to the identification of a cytoplasmic protein which binds cyclosporin A with an even lower dissociation constant (10^{-8} M) than calmodulin. More importantly, this protein, which is called cyclophilin, binds derivatives and analogues of cyclosporin A in precise correspondence with the immunosuppressive activities of these agents: highly active compounds are tightly bound by cyclophilin while less active agents or inactive ones show only weak attachment or no affinity at all. The relationship of cyclophilin to the overall mechanism of cyclosporin action, especially to the temporary "shut-down" of lymphokine genes, however, is not yet completely understood (see Chapter 7).

4.4.4 Absorption, pharmacokinetics

As already mentioned, cyclosporin A is a highly lipophilic molecule. In order to be absorbed it must be taken in dissolved form. Solutions in olive oil have proved useful in experiments and also in initial clinical investigations. An oral solution is available today for use in man: absorption after oral ingestion is about 37%. The first-pass effect, i.e. degradation of the substance on first passing through the liver, is 27% and absolute bioavailability is barely 30%. The principal data on pharmacokinetics, distribution and elimination of cyclosporin A are shown in *Table 4.2.* It should, however, be borne in mind that absorption of cyclosporin A is subject to intra- and interindividual fluctuations: a given dose will not result in the same blood levels when applied to different individuals. Even in a single individual, absorption rates may vary from dose to dose. Regular monitoring of the blood level of cyclosporin A is therefore recommended. Sensitive and accurate procedures such as radioimmunoassay or high-performance liquid chromatography are available for this purpose. It

Table 4.2. Pharmacokinetics of cyclosporin A

Absorption		
Oral absorption	37%	
First-pass effect	27%	
Absolute oral bioavailability	27%	
Time to peak blood concentration	2–4 hr	
Steady-state blood concentration (12 mg/kg/day)	100– 200 ng per ml (min.)	
	500–1000 ng per ml	
	Distribution	
Binding to plasma protein	90%	
Distribution volume	800 l/60 kg bodyweight	
	Metabolism	
Extent of metabolism	99%	
Number of metabolites	about 10	
Elimination half-life	2 hr (alpha-phase)	
	24 hr (beta-phase)	
Total blood clearance	400 ml/min	60 kg bodyweight
Renal clearance	0.4 ml/min	

is, however, important that the analyses should be performed in whole blood since almost 50% or even 60% of cyclosporin A, depending on its plasma concentration, accumulates in the erythrocytes. Although a population of high-affinity binding sites on T-lymphocytes should already be saturated at 50–100 ng cyclosporin A per ml blood, it is recommended in transplant patients that the cyclosporin A level be kept between 200 ng and 700 ng per ml.

4.4.5 Side effects

Cyclosporin A causes a number of side effects, most of which are of little importance for therapy. The drug's toxicity mainly affects the kidneys. In dogs, chronic toxicity studies failed to reveal any particular signs of nephrotoxicity, even after doses of 45 mg per kg. Rats, however, reacted more sensitively: in subacute investigations this animal species showed vacuolar degeneration of the proximal tubule and even tubular necrosis at doses as low as 36 mg per kg. Damage to the pars convoluta of the tubule is also observed in man. The development of these lesions depends on the concentrations of active substance and the extent and duration of the ischemia to which an organ is exposed. Since the transplanted kidney is exposed to ischemia until incorporated into the recipient's arterial blood supply and is susceptible to damage, particularly if warmed, the lesions are, understandably enough, mostly observed in the *transplanted organ*. Nephrotoxicity is therefore first and foremost a complication of kidney transplantation. In other indications nephrotoxicity is also a concern but it is easier to recognize and does not occur as regularly. The particular sensitivity of transplanted kidneys to cyclosporin is corroborated by experimental findings in rats. In these animals, cyclosporin given in the equivalent of therapeutic doses is only nephrotoxic if other predisposing factors are present at the time of cyclosporin application. These factors include heminephrectomy, hypertension, ischemia or the application of additional nephrotoxic agents. A number of criteria exist for differentiating between a rejection reaction and toxic renal damage due to cyclosporin A; though they do not provide absolute certainty, they should nevertheless be observed. Typical of the rejection reaction is onset within the first thirty days after the transplant procedure, and a rise of over 25% in baseline serum creatinine values within 3–4 days, given a cyclosporin A concentration in the blood of about 200 ng or less per ml. If, however, the disorder sets in more than 30 days after transplantation and if serum creatinine rises by 25% within one week given cyclosporin A levels in excess of 200 ng per ml, a toxic functional disorder is more likely. The differential diagnosis often necessitates biopsy, though this does not always provide a clear answer. The existence of a dense, cellular infiltrate unequivocally points to a rejection reaction, as does a reduction of 25% or more in renal volume.

Following cyclosporin A treatment in bone marrow grafts, carefully monitored dosage was associated with only low-grade nephrotoxicity which was reversible under continued therapy. More serious disturbances were found only in connection with blood levels which were still in excess of 500 ng per ml between the doses, i.e. at the lowest levels on the blood level curve. The spontaneously hypertensive rat provides the most sensitive model for producing, quantifying and explaining cyclosporin A-induced renal damage. In addition to tubular lesions one also observes in this model foci of arteriolar damage which can either be characterized by fibrinoid necrosis of the media or by endothelial proliferations which often obliterate the vessel. In these animals, intensive stimulation of the renin-angiotensin-aldosterone system is observed under cyclosporin A. In the light of the data thus obtained, it may be concluded that raised sympathetic tone, inhibition of renal prostaglandin synthesis, particularly of PGI_2 and PGE, and heart failure with reduced renal blood flow all contribute to the renal damage caused by cyclosporin A.

Distinct impairment of renal function was observed in 17 heart transplant recipients treated with cyclosporin A for one year or longer, in contrast to 15 comparable heart transplant recipients given azathioprine. All the parameters monitored (plasma flow, glomerular filtration rate, renal blood flow) deteriorated during long-term therapy with cyclosporin A, despite careful maintenance of active substance concentrations below 200 ng per ml between doses. In addition, tubulointerstitial and glomerular changes correlating in severity with the observed impairment of glomerular filtration were seen in biopsies from 5 of the patients treated with cyclosporin A.

Hepatotoxicity associated with cyclosporin A is characterized by hyperbilirubinemia (conjugated bilirubin), moderate elevation of aminotransaminases and a slight rise in alkaline phosphatase. Hepatotoxicity depends greatly on the levels of cyclosporin A in the blood. Histologically, cyclosporin A does not cause very typical hepatic changes, apart from centrilobular fatty degeneration. Following bone marrow transplants, cyclosporin A-induced liver damage must be distinguished from the graft-versus-host reaction (GVHR). The following criteria are generally applied: in the GVHR not only the liver but also the skin and the intestinal tract are usually involved; alkaline serum phosphatase is always *markedly* increased in any GVHR affecting the liver; and it is characteristic of cyclosporin A-induced liver toxicity that elevated bilirubin levels are rapidly normalized following withdrawal of the medication.

Other toxic effects of the drug are overshadowed by the renal and hepatic toxicity of cyclosporin A. The drug may occasionally cause focal or generalized convulsions, particularly in the presence of existing brain damage and at high blood concentrations.

Hirsutism may occur during treatment with cyclosporin A – a finding that is perhaps underpinned by the fact that cyclosporin A produces an almost "normal" coat in the nude (nu/nu) mouse. Gingival hyperplasia is often observed. This clinical finding can be reproduced experimentally. In man, adequate dental and mouth hygiene seems largely to counteract this effect.

A considerable number of the clinical and experimental side effects are a direct consequence of immunosuppression. Chronic cyclosporin A treatment in dogs often gives rise to cutaneous papillomatosis which might be of viral origin. Under cyclosporin A there is a particular risk of infection from microorganisms that can be eliminated only if T-cell function is intact. They include herpesviruses and, more particularly, cytomegalovirus, as well as a number of pathogenic fungi. The severity and incidence of infectious complications occurring under cyclosporin A depend to a large extent on the organ transplanted. Almost all patients suffer from CMV infection, which becomes symptomatic in 18–30% in the first year after the transplant and the immunosuppressive therapy. These acute episodes are always associated with viremia. Severe fungal infections have been found only in patients with a liver transplant. Patients treated with cyclosporin A do not exhibit particular sensitivity to the majority of extracellular or facultative intracellular bacterial infections. This tallies with the findings of animal studies. Protection against such infections is mediated by circulating antibodies, complement, neutrophils and occasionally macrophages as well. These mechanisms are not impaired by cyclosporin A. Animal studies show, however, that cyclosporin A increases sensitivity to herpes viruses. Massive immunosuppression with cyclosporin A may occasionally cause infections similar to those occurring in patients with AIDS (acquired immune deficiency syndrome). For instance, *Pneumocystis carinii* pneumonia occurs more frequently in renal-transplant patients receiving cyclosporin A therapy than in those given azathioprine and prednisone.

Lymphomas are a chapter in themselves. Organ-transplant patients taking immunosuppressive medication are at much (up to 50 times) greater risk of developing certain tumours, particularly lymphomas, than a control population of comparable age. Up to May 1983, the Cincinnati Transplantation Tumor Registry (CTTR) had recorded 314 lymphomas among 1,767 malignant tumours observed in 1,661 organ recipients: this amounts to 18%. Unlike other tumours, which often have a latency of many years, lymphomas develop relatively soon (1–153.5 months, or 29 months on average) after the transplant procedure. 10% of these tumours occur within four months of the transplant. In the same period, only 3% of the non-lymphocytic tumours are observed. The most common lymphomas were reticulum cell sarcoma (155 cases), Kaposi's sarcoma

(60), unclassifiable lymphomas (42), B-cell lymphomas (26) and Hodgkin's disease (10).

Any comparison of these data with those obtained in organ-transplant patients treated with cyclosporin A is complicated by the disparity in the size of the population groups treated. By the spring of 1983, 2,000–2,500 patients had been treated with cyclosporin A in connection with an organ transplant. Up to that time, the CTTR had registered 23 patients with malignant tumours, 17 of them lymphomas. The proportion accounted for by lymphomas was therefore substantially higher than in the population that had been treated with other immunosuppressive agents. It was also notable that the lymphomas occurred very soon (i.e. 1–17 months or six months on average) after the transplant. Unlike lymphomas occurring under "conventional" therapy and frequently exhibiting CNS involvement, none of the patients on cyclosporin A showed any signs of CNS involvement. Interesting though these differences are, it should be borne in mind that only one of the 17 patients with a lymphoma had been given cyclosporin A as the sole immunosuppressive medication. *A recent overall assessment of the lymphoma incidence in cyclosporin-treated patients after several years of drug usage does not confirm the higher frequency of lymphoma observed in earlier studies.*

It remains to be seen whether these results imply a particular risk of lymphoma in patients treated with cyclosporin A. The short induction time after transplantation is consistent with a tumour of viral origin. There are two possible etiologies in this connection. On the one hand, latent infections involving oncogenic viruses might be activated by an immunological reaction such as rejection of a transplanted organ. On the other, immunosuppressed patients might be particularly at risk of de novo infections with tumour viruses such as the Epstein-Barr virus. According to more recent results this latter mechanism seems to occur more frequently than the former one. Several authors claim that lymphomas induced by EBV infection disappear spontaneously upon discontinuation of the immunosuppression. Finally, lymphomas might also be the result of a reaction between antigenically altered lymphocytes and normal lymphocytes.

In the course of a local GVHR, secretion of an angiogenesis factor could result in intensive proliferation of mesenchymal and endothelial cells. This mechanism would explain the development of Kaposi's sarcoma in particular.

4.4.6 Clinical use

Cyclosporin A has very quickly established itself in immunosuppressive treatment following organ transplants, particularly kidney or bone-marrow transplants. Most authors concur in the view that the use of cyclosporin A with or without adjunctive prednisolone in the first year following kidney transplantation results in a higher survival rate for both transplant and patient than any other therapy can produce. This statement requires qualification, however: besides the choice of immunosuppressive, the outcome of a kidney transplant depends on a number of other factors which can have a telling effect on the overall picture. These include treatment of the organ to be transplanted, particularly its re-warming time and perfusion time prior to grafting. Long perfusion times are associated with a higher rate of initial functional defects. Further important factors that play a – usually positive – role in the outcome of a transplant procedure are matching of donor and host HLA antigens, and performance of blood transfusions before the graft. It should, however, be pointed out that kidney transplant centres that have already optimized their methods seem to have less to gain from the adjunctive use of cyclosporin A than centres whose results, whilst retaining the existing treatment methods, could still be further improved. In Minnesota, J. S. Najarian and his group did not perceive any advantages for kidney-transplant patients taking cyclosporin A over a group of comparable patients who had been given azathioprine, prednisone and a total of 14 doses of antilymphocyte globulin (30 mg per kg per day). Two years after the transplant, the survival rate in patients treated with azathioprine, ALG and prednisone was 91%, as against 88% in the cyclosporin A group. The two-year survival rate for transplanted organs was 82% in the cyclosporin A group, compared with 77% in the azathioprine group. Within 600 days of the transplant, 58% of the patients treated with azathioprine, ALG and prednisolone had to be treated on account of a rejection reaction, as against 31% in the cyclosporin A group. The number of intercurrent bacterial, viral and mycoplasma infections in kidney transplant patients was much higher in the azathioprine group than in the patients receiving cyclosporin A. Only fungal infections were observed somewhat more often in the cyclosporin A group than in the conventionally treated group. The data published by Najarian are, however, the exception. The *overall impression* gained from the available studies is more accurately represented by data derived from a European multicentre study involving eight transplant units. In this study, functioning transplants were observed after one year in 72% of patients treated with cyclosporin A, as against 52% in the control group given only azathioprine and prednisone in a not quite standardized dosage. This difference of 10–20% in favour of cyclosporin A patients seems – at least for one-year survival – to be readily reproducible. However, how these findings are going to look after two or, for that matter, five years is an open question. In the Canadian multicentre study, it looks as if differences between the two groups might level out in the long run. The ultimate value of cyclosporin A in kidney-transplant patients has therefore still to be proved. *To summarize the results so far available: Compared with other forms of immunosuppression, cyclosporin A offers advantages that become evident at least one year after the transplant in the form of a 10–20% improvement in transplant survival and a reduction of about 50% in rejection reactions and intercurrent infections. The most important side effect is nephrotoxicity: even today, it is sometimes difficult to differentiate correctly between a rejection reaction and toxic renal failure.* In the hands of particularly experienced specialists, other methods of immunosuppression can produce results that are not far behind those of cyclosporin A.

According to Thomas Starzl, probably the most experienced surgeon in this field, the use of cyclosporin A has transformed liver transplantation from a difficult experiment of unpredictable outcome to a therapeutic modality that, in the right indication, can be readily recommended. The long-term success rates achieved with this measure cannot yet be compared with those of kidney transplantation. There are various reasons for this: the indication for transplanting a liver is more difficult to define; malignant liver tumours are sometimes the cause of the transplantation, and these may have already metastasized at the time of surgery, thereby rendering even a successful transplantation meaningless in the long term. One problem has since been probably overcome: absorption of cyclosporin A is poorer and more variable in liver-transplant patients than in healthy subjects, and grafts may be rejected. This outcome can be prevented by administering cyclosporin A i.v. for 28 days. The 30-month survival rate for liver-transplant patients taking cyclosporin A in one of the large American centres was almost 60%, as against only 24% after treatment with azathioprine and prednisone.

Cyclosporin A has also improved the results in transplantations of heart, lung and pancreas. If the indication is stringently defined, a 9[illegible]% recovery rate of patients with heart transplants can be achieved with cyclosporin A, compared with only a 70% rehabilitation rate using "conventional" therapy. Organ rejection and infections under cyclosporin A are reduced by about half the rate observed under conventional immunosuppressive therapy.

In bone marrow transplantation cyclosporin A has rapidly become a standard therapeutic agent. Survival rates depend naturally not only on the bone marrow transplant and concomitant therapy but also on the underlying disease. Furthermore, the closer the match between donor and recipient HLA loci, the better are the results. In aplastic anemia, an 80% survival rate was obtained after four and a half years in patients with bone marrow transplants. The survival rate in the same period was only 30–40% for patients treated with methotrexate.

Although cyclosporin A first made its mark in the field of organ transplantation, the greater benefit of this new immunological agent (in quantitative terms) may lie in the field of autoimmune diseases. The effect of cyclosporin A on experimentally induced autoimmune diseases has already been mentioned. In 1983 the findings of a Canadian research team startled the scientific world by showing that cyclosporin A can prevent congenital diabetes mellitus in Brattleborough (BB) rats. BB rats are inbred animals which become manifestly diabetic in adolescence. The predisposition to this disease is genetically dominant and linked to the histocompatibility complex. Although antibodies to islet cells are observed in the course of this form of diabetes, the primary mechanism leading to destruction of the islet cells seems to be cell-mediated. The assumption that human type-I diabetes mellitus is also an autoimmune disease is based on the histological appearance of the islet cells, the presence of islet cell antibodies and the frequent association of type-I diabetes with other autoimmune diseases such as hyperthyroidism, Hashimoto's thyroiditis, myasthenia gravis, Addison's disease and pernicious anemia. Lastly, there is a strong overrepresentation of the HLA allele DQ 3.2 in cases of juvenile insulin-dependent diabetes. In a clinical pilot trial which was conducted on the hypothesis that type-I diabetes mellitus is in fact an autoimmune disease, 41 patients were treated with cyclosporin A for periods ranging from two to twelve months. Patients were not admitted to this study unless, when fasting, they had normal concentrations of the immunoreactive C-peptide, a part of proinsulin, and had been treated for own blood sugar and to administer insulin as needed and also to adhere to an individually designed diet. In addition, they received 10 mg cyclosporin A per kg daily at the beginning of the study. Care was taken to maintain cyclosporin A blood levels between 100 and 200 ng per ml.

Sixteen of the 30 patients admitted to the trial within six weeks of the onset of diabetes became insulin-independent. Their C-peptide plasma concentrations were within the normal range, while antibodies to islet cells declined. Only 2 of 8 patients admitted to the trial 8–44 weeks after onset of diabetes attained the same result. That means that under therapy with cyclosporin A far more patients became insulin-independent than would be expected from the natural course (48% as opposed to 3%). Astonishingly, normalization of glucagon-stimulated C-peptide concentrations paralleled the decline in insulin dependence. These results are encouraging and warrant a controlled multicentre trial to explain the findings. A central point is the duration of therapy. Does immunosuppression have to be continued for a whole lifetime or can the therapy be reduced or even terminated after some months or years? BB rats in which cyclosporin was withdrawn at the age of 120 days have a lower than 25% recurrence rate for diabetes.

Cyclosporin A has already been tested in a number of other autoimmune diseases. Reliable positive findings on the effectiveness or ineffectiveness of the substance can only be obtained for a few diseases. Uveitis, which is caused by autoimmune mechanisms and is a feature of Behçet's syndrome, responds very well to therapy with cyclosporin A. However, as soon as cyclosporin A is withdrawn, the illness recurs. Controlled trials are now being conducted to quantify the effectiveness of cyclosporin A in primary rheumatoid arthritis, lupus erythematosus, multiple sclerosis, myasthenia gravis, thyroiditis, psoriasis and many other autoimmune diseases. Even if not all these investigations produce positive results, we can expect cyclosporin A to occupy an important place in the management of some of these diseases.

How is cyclosporin A tolerated in long-term, perhaps even lifelong, or intermittent therapy? Will there be irreversible renal toxicity, not to mention other side effects? The very fact that these questions must be asked proves that cyclosporin A does not yet completely satisfy the demand for a selective, efficacious and safe immunosuppressive drug. The development of other cyclosporin agents such as cyclosporin G or dehydro-cyclosporin C is therefore awaited with some impatience.

4.5. FK 506

FK 506 is a new immunosuppressive agent which was isolated from a strain of *Streptomyces (S. tsukubanensis* in 1984). Structurally, FK 506 is a macrolide. Its molecular weight is 822. FK 506 is insoluble in water but can be dissolved in ethanol, methanol or acetone. The drug was found during a screening programme designed to identify agents which inhibit Il-2 secretion *(Fig. 4.7)*.

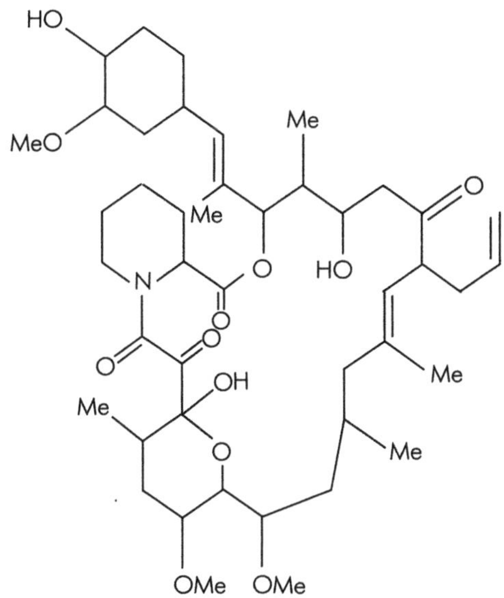

Figure 4.7. Chemical structure of FK 506.

4.5.1 Pharmacology

FK 506 suppresses phenomena related to T-cell activation such as lymphoblast formation in mixed lymphocyte cultures or in response to antigens, generation of cytotoxic T-cells, production of Il-2 and γ-interferon and expression of the Il-2 receptor. All of these effects can be observed at subnanomolar concentrations, which means that the compound is about 100-fold more potent *in vitro* than cyclosporin A.

FK 506 has also been shown to be extremely active in prolonging allograft survival after experimental organ transplantation, though in this situation the compound is only 10 to 30 times more active than cyclosporin A. Furthermore, the compound is effective in certain experimental autoimmune diseases. At doses between 1 and 10 mg/kg orally it completely suppresses the symptoms of an experimental uveoretinitis which can be induced in rats by injection of retinal proteins in complete Freund's adjuvant. Good efficacy was achieved even when the compound was given on day 7 to 12 after immunization. Cyclosporin A produced similar effects at doses between 10 and 30 mg/kg.

In a carefully conducted experimental study by the group of T. Starzl in Pittsburgh it was shown that FK 506 at doses >1.5. mg/kg is effective in maintaining allogcncic rcnal grafts in dogs for up to 90 days. Similar rcsults wcrc obtaincd with liver transplants in dogs and with renal transplants in cynomolgus monkeys and in baboons. Upon discontinuation of FK 506 therapy, most animals rejected their transplants but in some cases very prolonged maintenance of grafts occurred, indicating tolerance induction. Short courses of i.m. drug administration resulted in an unexpectedly long survival of grafts after cessation of therapy. Comparable results were obtained in dogs after segmental pancreas transplantation.

Although there is some phenomenological resemblance between the activities of cyclosporin A and FK 506 the two drugs seem to complement each other. Clearly synergistic effects could be obtained in unidirectional mixed lymphocyte reactions with concentrations at which neither of the two compounds shows any activity when tested alone. A similar synergism can also be observed with FK 506 and azathioprine. At least some of these synergistic effects appear also *in vivo:* in the study on renal allograft survival in dogs mentioned above, a dosage regimen of 0.5 mg FK 506, 5 mg cyclosporin A and 5 mg prednisone (per kg/day) proved to be the most effective modality in comparison with FK 506 given alone or in a combination of only two drugs. The blood levels necessary for clinically relevant immunosuppressive effects appear to be in the range of 1–10 ng/ml. In dogs the biological half-life of FK 506 was found to be 6.3 hours compared with 6.1 hours in baboons.

Like cyclosporin A, FK 506 binds to a cytoplasmic protein which displays *cis-trans* prolyl-peptidyl isomerase activity, but is distinct from cyclophilin.

4.5.2 Toxicity

FK 506 has been claimed to induce severe vasculitis in dogs at doses which were only weakly immunosuppressive. In baboons the compound was found to cause hyperglycemia and severe elevation of liver transaminases at therapeutic doses. Not all of these findings, however, have been confirmed. Arteriitis of the type seen after treatment with FK 506 is a common finding in beagle dogs and not clearly attributable to drug treatment. Some studies indicate that at immunosuppressive doses, FK 506 may exert in dogs only mild liver changes, which are reminiscent of erythromycin toxicity in humans. In baboons, only minor elevation of liver transaminases was observed.

A decisive assessment of the drug will not be possible until the results of systematic toxicity studies, including pharmacokinetic and metabolic parameters, become available. The apparent synergism of FK 506 with cyclosporin A and azathioprine leaves grounds for hope that this compound may show clinical usefulness, even if it is not used as a treatment modality in itself.

4.6 Orthoclone T3 (OKT3)

Orthoclone T3 is the first monoclonal antibody which gained the status of an accepted treatment of kidney transplant rejection episodes. This antibody originated from one of the first attempts to immunize mice against human T-cells and to obtain monoclonal antibodies specifically directed at T-cell antigens.

4.6.1 Physical properties

The OKT3 antibody is a mouse monoclonal IgG directed at the T3 (CD3) antigen which is present on all T-cells. This structure is closely associated with the T-cell receptor though not covalently linked to it. It is instrumental in transducing the signal generated by antigen recognition at the T-cell receptor to the cell nucleus. OKT 3 is provided today in > 95 % purity as a non-pyrogenic chemically homogeneous material that is free of mycoplasmas, viruses or other microorganisms. In view of these properties OKT3 can be classified as an immunosuppressive drug although it is a biological agent.

4.6.2 Immunological actions

OKT3 binds the CD3 complex and thereby interrupts the transmission of the specific signal generated at the T-cell receptor by antigen recognition to the cell nucleus. In mixed lymphocyte cultures OKT3 prevents the transformation of T-cells. More specifically, it strongly inhibits the reaction of cytotoxic T-cells against cells with a major histocompatibility difference. This effect occurs in the absence of complement. It is not due to killing of cytotoxic T-cells but rather to incapacitation of these cells. The inhibitory effect of OKT3 is clearly concentration-dependent. Almost complete suppression of T-cell killer function is observed at concentrations between 1 and 10 μg/ml, depending on the experimental conditions.

When applied *in vivo,* OKT3 antibodies display three immunological effects. The most important effect probably corresponds to the phenomenon observed also *in vitro:* the function of T-cells engaged in antigen recognition is immediately blocked. The immunosuppressive effects of OKT3 depend on this phenomenon more directly than on any other effect. Secondly, all mature T-cells, whether circulating or sessile, are opsonized. These opsonized cells are then rapidly taken up by the mononuclear-phagocytic system. Within the first 30 min after an i.v. dose of OKT3, T-cells virtually disappear from the circulation. The third phenomenon to be mentioned in this context is modulation of the T-cell surface. When T-cells begin to reappear in the circulation four to five days after a bolus injection of OKT3 they do not express the CD3 structure, although the presence of other T-cell markers clearly denotes their identity. The addition of OKT3 to T-cell cultures causes clumping, internalization and/or shedding of CD3 molecules. The result of this modulation of CD3 both *in vitro* and *in vivo* is a non-functional T-cell.

4.6.3 Therapeutic applications of OKT3

The standard dose for OKT3 is 5 mg per day intravenously. At this daily dose, plasma levels reach 1 μg/ml within three to four days and remain stable for the duration of the treatment. This concentration has been shown *in vitro* to completely block the killer function of cytotoxic T-cells.

OKT3 antibodies, if properly used, have been found to be both safe and effective in the treatment of rejection episodes after kidney transplantation. Other clinical uses are under investigation. In reversing rejection episodes after kidney transplantation, OKT3 has shown efficacy in more than 90% of all cases two to seven days after initiation of treatment.

In a randomized trial, OKT_3 reversed rejection in 94% of the cases, compared to a 75% reversal rate obtained with conventional therapy (steroids and azathioprine). In later studies, it was convincingly shown that OKT_3 could also reverse a large proportion of those rejection episodes which had failed to respond to prolonged courses of steroids in high doses. In a group of 80 patients falling into this category, 65% responded to 'rescue' treatment with OKT_3. In fact, 54% of these allografts which had been close to abandonment under steroid therapy remained functional for at least six months after the episode.

These figures are encouraging. There are, however, some serious limitations associated with OKT_3 therapy which became evident during the first clinical trials and which have only been partially overcome in subsequent trials. 45 to 60 minutes after the start of OKT_3 therapy almost all early patients experienced an acute toxic syndrome characterized by chills, fever, nausea and vomiting, wheezing and – sometimes – diarrhea. In patients with reduced left ventricular function, frank heart failure can be precipitated. This syndrome became so typical and occurred so regularly that it was termed 'first dose' syndrome. It appears to be due to the rapid lysis of T-cells and the subsequent liberation of large quantities of cytokines which, in turn, lead to the release of mediators from platelets, granulocytes and mast cells. The similarity of this reaction to symptoms induced by agents like thromboxane A_2 and serotonin has been explicitly mentioned by some authors. In more recent treatment protocols, the 'first dose' syndrome could be considerably mitigated by the application of high doses of steroids immediately before and after the first dose of OKT_3.

The second limitation of OKT_3 to be identified was the formation of antibodies against mouse monoclonal antibodies. It occurred in 86% of the patients receiving OKT_3 during the early trials. There are two types of antibody: an anti-mouse isotype directed against the Fc portion of the OKT_3 molecule and antiidiotype antibodies. The latter type, which occurs in the majority of patients, represents a serious impediment to the OKT_3 effect. Antibodies start to appear seven to ten days after the initiation of treatment. The application of steroids during the ten-day OKT_3 treatment and repeated on the first and on the fourth day after discontinuation of the antibody therapy can reduce the occurrence of anti-OKT_3 antibodies to about 38%.

Finally, patients whose first rejection episode was successfully managed with OKT_3 often developed further rejection episodes within one to eight weeks after cessation of OKT_3 therapy. This difficulty was also overcome, at least partially, by modifying the initial protocols: first, the duration of OKT_3 therapy was extended from ten to fourteen days with the option of continuing treatment in patients who did not show complete reversal of rejection symptoms even after two weeks. Second, the dosages of concomitant immunosuppressive therapy (azathioprine-prednisone) were markedly reduced during OKT_3 treatment. With these modifications one-year graft survival rates of patients with rejection episodes treated with OKT_3 amounted to 75%.

In summary, one may conclude that OKT_3 is the first monoclonal antibody preparation with a defined role in the treatment of rejection episodes after kidney transplantation. For this indication the preparation has obtained FDA approval. There is evidence that OKT_3 is also effective in aborting rejection episodes in liver transplantations. At present, the potential role of this 'drug' as a prophylactic immunosuppressive agent after organ transplantation is being investigated.

The advent of genetically engineered chimeric antibodies which contain human constant regions and restrict mouse sequences to the variable region or – even better – to the sequences which are needed to determine antigen complementarity is likely to make this modality more attractive than it is today.

4.7. Immunotoxins

As already mentioned, immunotoxins which comprise a carrier molecule and a toxic moiety have shown interesting immunosuppressive effects in animal experiments and are likely to be investigated in humans in the near future.

The most advanced concept is based on the fact that high-affinity Il-2 receptors are only expressed by activated T-cells but never by "resting" cells. After the transfer of an allogeneic organ, T-cells which recognize foreign MHC molecules will become activated. These cells then express high-affinity Il-2 receptors which bind Il-2 with a kd of almost 10^{-12} M! It has been possible to construct a gene which contains the complete nucleotide sequence of Il-2 at the 3' end fused to the translocation site and the catalytic site of diphtheria toxins at the 5' end. Another similar construct starts with Il-2 at the 5' end followed by the translocation sequence and the catalytic domain of *Pseudomonas* exotoxin at 3'. Such constructs, if expressed, will result in the formation of immunotoxins which carry Il-2 at one end and the catalytic moiety flanked by the translocation sequence of a toxin on the other side of the protein *(Fig. 4.8)*.

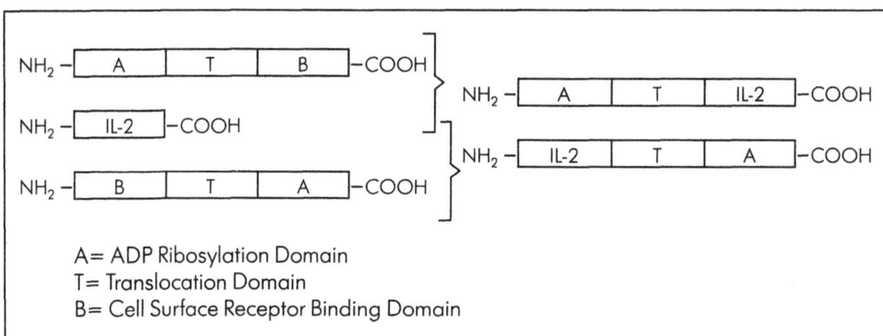

Figure 4.8. Recombination of Il-2 and diphtheria toxin (upper scheme) and pseudomonas (lower scheme) exotoxin. The constructs comprise IL-2, the catalytic domain of the toxins and the translocation domain. The receptor binding domain is exchanged for IL-2.

4.7.1 Mechanism of action

The activation of T-cells results in the expression of Il-2 receptors. These receptors comprise two subunits, the so-called "tac" antigen with a molecular weight of 55,000 daltons which by itself constitutes the "low affinity" receptor and a second subunit of 75,000 daltons. Together these two subunits form the complete receptor, which displays an extremely high affinity for Il-2 and therefore makes the activated cells vulnerable to the immunotoxin. After binding to the receptor the Il-2-toxin is internalized together with the p75 receptor subunit. The toxin moiety is then translocated into the cytoplasm across the phagosome membrane by virtue of the translocation sequence of the toxin. Finally the catalytic part of the toxin transfers ribosyl-ADP to elongation factor 2, interrupting cellular protein synthesis. Since the catalytic step can be repeated many times, a small number of toxin molecules will eventually inactivate all EF-2 molecules and kill the cell. The binding of Il-2-*Pseudomonas* exotoxin is followed by an analogous sequence of events.

The selectivity of this method rests on two circumstances: in the first place, on the low kd of the Il-2-receptor complex. Secondly, on the fact that the Il-2-toxin is internalized through the p75 subunit of the Il-2 receptor. The expression of the p55 subunit or tac subunit alone will afford Il-2 binding only with a kd of 10^{-8} M. The p75 subunit, which seems to be the only subunit expressed on NK-cells and macrophages, binds Il-2 with a kd $4{-}8 \times 10^{-10}$ M. It should therefore be possible to "titrate" the high-affinity receptor on activated T-cells without running the risk of poisoning NK-cells and macrophages.

Adult T-cell leukemia is a disease characterized by an uncontrolled proliferation of immature T-cells which carry the high-affinity form of the T-cell receptor represented by both subunits. It has been speculated that this disease would be amenable to treatment with Il-2-toxins. In view of the dissociation constants of the three forms of Il-2 receptors and Il-2, such treatment could indeed be designed to eliminate leukemic cells with a high degree of selectivity.

In animals, immunotoxins are potent immunosuppressive agents which can make the permanent engraftment of allogeneic organs possible. This efficacy is as yet unconfirmed in humans. Conceptually, Il-2-toxins are extremely attractive: if used properly, which means at the right time and in the correct dose, these agents should be able to destroy clones of T-lymphocytes which react against a set of transplantation antigens or against self antigens. Functionally, this relatively selective destruction of certain clones of T-lymphocytes would be comparable to the deletion of "forbidden clones" during ontogeny. The generation of such "windows" in the antigenic repertoire of T-cells should induce specific tolerance. Translated into a clinical context, this could mean that a transplanted organ is stably accepted or that an autoimmune process is abrogated while the ability of the immune system to react against all other antigens would remain unimpaired. Even if this goal were not attainable, the one-time elimination of autoreactive or alloreactive T-cell clones might still be expected to reduce the necessity for further conventional immunosuppressive treatment with respect to both time and dose.

5. Substances with an Antiallergic Effect

5.1 Immediate-type hypersensitivity reactions

Immediate-type hypersensitivity is the hallmark of any allergic reaction. It develops when contact with a specific antigen triggers the formation of IgE antibodies which bind to the Fc_ε receptors of mast cells or basophilic leucocytes. Renewed contact with the same antigen then leads to "bridging": adjacent antibodies on the cell surface are interconnected by antigen molecules through their antigen-binding portions. At the Fc receptor the antigen-antibody reaction gives rise to a signal that passes through a chain of biochemical reactions which will be described below in some detail. Eventually the signal leads to the release of mediators from the granules of mast cells and basophilic leucocytes.

The IgE-antibody-mediated reaction is not the only mechanism capable of bringing about degranulation of mast cells. Complement components such as C3a and, in particular, C5a can cause depletion of histamine stores by way of their own receptors. Ionophores such as the substance A 23187 can channel calcium into mast cells and basophils and bring about the release of mediators. f-Met tripeptides, i.e. substances of predominantly bacterial origin, induce the release of histamine by way of specific receptors located on basophilic leucocytes. Receptors for these tripeptides are also found on neutrophils and monocytes. This is possibly the mechanism involved in the bacterially induced release of histamine in bronchial asthma. Various neuropeptides including bradykinin, substance P, somatostatin, vasoactive intestinal peptide (VIP), neurotensin as well as endogenous opiates all have been reported as releasing histamine from rat mast cells, especially from peritoneal mast cells which correspond in type to human mast cells located in the dermis and in the intestinal submucosa. Lastly, some polycationic substances are also known to bring about degranulation by exerting a direct effect on the membrane of mast cells. These substances include 48/80, which is a polymerization product from methoxy-N-methylphenylamine and formaldehyde in a ratio of 1:1 and is used exclusively for experimental purposes. Further substances in this group are polymyxin B, an antibiotic with membrane activity, protamine, tubocurarine, dextrans with a molecular weight between 10^4 and 10^6 daltons, the bee poison mellitin, a peptide from snake venom, and a cationic protein from lysosomes.

The mediators that trigger an immediate-type hypersensitivity reaction vary from species to species. In man, guinea pigs and dogs, histamine is the most important initial triggering factor in hypersensitivity reactions, whereas in rats this role is taken by serotonin. The primary effector organs of a *generalized immediate-type hypersensitivity reaction* also vary according to the species involved. The lungs and larynx are the most important effector organs in man. In the guinea pig the lungs react most sensitively whereas the hepatic veins dilate in the dog, and in the rat the intestinal tract is the main effector organ.

Table 5.1. Anaphylactic reactions in different species

Species	Major pharmacological mediators	Effector organs	Clinical manifestations
Man	Histamine Leukotrienes Kinins	Lungs Larynx	Dyspnea Hypotension Urticaria Laryngeal edema
Guinea pig	Histamine Leukotrienes Kinins	Lungs	Respiratory distress Asphyxiation
Rat	Serotonin Kinins	Intestine Lungs	Circulatory collapse Hemorrhage
Dog	Histamine Kinins Serotonin	Hepatic veins	Blood congestion in hepatic veins, visceral hemorrhage

Accordingly, the primary symptoms of anaphylactic shock also vary from species to species *(Table 5.1)*.

However, hypersensitivity is influenced not only by preformed substances, but also by other mediators which are synthesized and released from cells following the mobilization of the preformed substances stored in the granules. In man, such substances include the arachidonic acid-derived products of lipoxygenases, i.e. the leukotrienes C, D and E, originally designated SRS-A or "slow-reacting substance of anaphylaxis", the hydroxyeicosatetraenoic (HETE) and hydroperoxyeicosatetraenoic (HPETE) acids (also steps of the lipoxygenase pathway), the prostaglandins (resulting from the action of cyclooxygenase) and platelet-activating factor (PAF) (1-O-alkyl-2-acetyl-sn-glyceryl-3-phosphoryl-choline).

5.1.1 Histamine

Histamine is synthesized from histidine by decarboxylation. L-histidine decarboxylase, the enzyme responsible for this reaction, is located in the cytoplasm of basophils and mast cells. Histamine, the product of this enzyme, is formed in the cytoplasm and bound to a low-molecular-weight protein in the granules. Binding and release are coupled with a cation exchange.

Histamine acts through two different receptors, which are designated H_1 and H_2 receptors. In man, the effects that characterize the development of a hypersensitivity reaction are concentrated in the vascular system: the smooth muscles of the smaller blood vessels relax under the action of histamine. Both H_1 and H_2 receptors are implicated in this reaction. Since histamine tends to constrict larger veins, increased blood flow through the dilated arterioles and reduction of venous return result in a rise in blood volume in the capillary bed. Vascular endothelial cells show constrictor responses to histamine. As a result, in the capillary and postcapillary small veins, gaps arise between the endothelial cells, thus exposing the basement membrane, which is freely permeable to fluid and plasma protein. Increased capillary pressure and greater permeability of the vascular wall cause edema. The vasoconstrictor effects are due largely to the H_1 receptors while the relaxing effects are mediated by the H_2 receptors.

Outside the cardiovascular system histamine usually causes contraction of smooth muscle. Here, too, activation of the H_1 receptors for the most part brings about contraction, and that of the H_2 receptors relaxation. The bronchial muscles of the guinea pig are particularly sensitive to histamine, of which even tiny concentrations give rise to extremely long lasting contraction of the smooth muscle of the bronchial tree, resulting in death. People with bronchial disease (chronic bronchitis, bronchial asthma) are also extremely sensitive to histamine, whereas healthy individuals are relatively insensitive. The reaction of certain animal species such as the cat or the sheep to histamine even takes the form of relaxation of the trachea or bronchi.

Histamine regulates its own release by means of a negative feedback mechanism involving H_2 receptors on basophils and mast cells. H_2 receptors which mediate inhibition of secretory functions are also found on other white blood cells. Histamine inhibits the release of lysosomal enzymes from neutrophils, and also has an inhibitory effect on secretion of antibodies by lymphocytes and on secretion of lymphokines by T-cells. It impairs the cytolysis of allogeneic tumour cells that are triggered by cytotoxic T-cells. T-suppressor cells also have H_2 receptors on their surfaces. Studies in guinea pigs have shown that, following immunization, T-suppressor cells synthesize a suppressor factor that is induced by histamine (histamine-induced suppressor factor or HSF). Synthesis of this factor can be suppressed by cimetidine, an H_2 antagonist (see Chapter 6). More recently, the effects of histamine on B-cells have also been studied. Mononuclear cells from healthy individuals were activated in vitro with pokeweed mitogen (PWM). In such cell cultures, chlorpheniramine (a H_1 receptor antagonist) in concentrations between 10^{-6} and 10^{-4}M but not cimetidine suppressed the synthesis of both IgE and IgG to values in the range of 10–20% of the controls. These findings may indicate that histamine influences B cells via its H_1 receptor.

5.1.2 Further primary and secondary mediators

Besides histamine, the "primary", i.e. preformed, factors include the following substances: eosinophilic chemotactic factors, a neutrophilic chemotactic factor, heparin, an α-chymotrypsin, N-acetyl-b-D-glucosaminidase, kallikrein and arylsulfatase A. The structure and function of these substances are summarized in *Table 5.2*.

The metabolic products of arachidonic acid and the platelet activating factor are substances which are only produced upon cell activation. Their effects are to some extent similar, and resemble those produced by histamine. On a molar basis the leukotrienes C, D, and E are at least one hundred times as effective as histamine, as judged by contraction of the guinea-pig intestine. Bronchial muscles in man also react very sensitively to the leukotrienes, which are formed not only by mast cells and basophils but also by neutrophils and macrophages in response to appropriate physiological stimuli.

Table 5.2. Properties of "primary" and "secondary" mediators of mast cells

Mediators	Physicochemical properties	Biological effects
"Primary" factors		
– Histamine	MW 111	Contracts smooth muscle. Increases vascular permeability. Modification of immune response.
– Eosinophilic chemotactic factors	Ala-Gly-Ser-Val-Gly-Ser-Glu	Recruitment of eosinophils and neutrophils to the site of the reaction.
– Neutrophilic chemotactic factor	Protein, MW 750,000	Attracts neurophilic granulocytes
– Heparin		Antiinflammatory properties
– Alpha-chymotrypsin	MW 29,000	
– N-acetyl-b-D glucosaminidase	MW 150,000	Breakdown of polysaccharides
– Kallikrein	MW 1,200,000	Releases kinin from plasmakininogen
– Arylsulfatase A	Arginine esterase	Inactivates leukotrienes C, D and E (SRS-A)
"Secondary" factors		
– Leukotrienes C, D and C (SRS-A)	MW 400	Contract smooth muscle, increase vascular permeability
– Prostaglandins	Arachidonic acid PGE_2, TXA_2, PGD_2, PGI_2	Contract and relax bronchial muscle. Platelet aggregation, vasodilatation, chemotaxis
– HHT, HETE	Eicosatetraenoic acids	Like prostaglandins
– Platelet-activating factor	1-O-alkyl-2 acetyl-sn-glyceryl-3 phosphoryl-choline	Platelet aggregation. Increases vascular permeability, causes shock. Releases vasoactive amines.

Platelet activating factor is a phospholipid which is released from platelets and, in turn, causes platelet aggregation and the release of vasoactive amines such as histamine and serotonin from the aggregated platelets. The factor is, however, also formed in mast cells and basophilic granulocytes. The molecule is broken down by phospholipases, especially phospholipase D. This enzyme is present in eosinophilic granulocytes. These cells are attracted to the site of the hypersensitivity reaction by chemotactic stimuli. Once on the scene, they exert a down-regulating influence on the entire process.

On the one hand, the clinical manifestations of an immediate-type hypersensitivity reaction are influenced by the pharmacological properties of the "primary" and "secondary" mediators that are released by mast cells and basophils. On the other hand, they also depend on the type of antigen and on the way in which an organism is exposed to antigen. Local skin manifestations consist of redness, edema and itching (histamine!). Entry of an allergen through the airways is followed by allergic rhinitis, i.e. hypersecretion, vasodilatation of the conjunctiva as well as the mucous membranes of nose and throat, sensitivity to light, and itching. A generalized hypersensitivity reaction occurs when a readily soluble and rapidly disseminating allergen affects the entire population of mast cells and basophils virtually simultaneously. Preformed and secondary mediators are released throughout the body and trigger a serious, often fatal, syndrome characterized by generalized edema, affecting the larynx and lungs in particular, and by severe cardiovascular collapse. Such reactions are observed in sensitized subjects, for instance after parenteral administration of penicillin.

5.1.3 IgE antibodies

Of the immunoglobulins present in the human body, IgE antibodies are quantitatively the least well represented:

They account for only 0.002% of the entire immunoglobulin in the body, and their concentration in normal serum ranges from 17 to 450 ng per ml. Physiologically, however, they are of great importance, since they are normally synthesized in the mucosa of the gastrointestinal tract and bronchial tree and their effect can be very considerably amplified by the mast cells also located in the mucosa. What is more, the antigens that trigger synthesis of IgE antibodies differ from those responsible for inducing synthesis of other antibody classes. The former are mostly substances that penetrate the body through mucoepithelial surfaces and then have to be eliminated again by local inflammatory processes, i.e. by formation of edema, diapedesis of phagocytic cells, phagocytosis and finally by intracellular degradation. The IgE system is extremely effective. Therefore, its effector mechanisms must be regulated within very narrow limits in order to protect the macroorganism against harmful elements and, at the same time, avoid damage from excessive reactions. The *fine regulation* of the IgE mast cell system is facilitated by the fact – already mentioned – that only very small amounts of IgE are required for the system to be fully effective, and by the very short biological half-life of the IgE antibody, which is only two and a half days, as compared with a mean half-life of 21 days for IgG antibodies!

IgE is regulated by systems that have been studied only in the last few years. Strictly speaking, the findings apply only to the animal models in which they have been elucidated, i.e. the mouse and the rat. Individual investigations have, however, shown that IgE regulation in man has a certain similarity to that in the mouse and the rat.

5.1.3.1 Regulation of IgE synthesis in rodents (according to K.Ishizaka)

The synthesis of IgE is regulated by isotype-specific mechanisms. This means that normal B-cells which have been activated by B-cell activators like pokeweed mitogen, EBV or *Staph. aureus* Cowan require additional stimuli in order to synthesize IgE. The most important of these stimuli appears to be represented by Il-4. This lymphokine causes an 'isotype switch' from IgM or IgD to the synthesis of IgE. The molecular mechanisms leading to this change in antibody production are not entirely clear. It has, however, been shown that activated

B-cells, which synthesize IgM and IgD produce 'sterile' transcripts of the $C\gamma 1$ and C_{ε} loci. Subsequently, switch recombinations bring these opened DNA loci into contiguity with the already rearranged VDJ region. It is not clear whether this occurs at the DNA level or at the level of RNA splicing. Some findings seem to indicate that additional stimuli represented by direct 'cognate' interaction with selected auto- or alloreactive T-cell clones strongly enhance IgE secretion after the isotype-switch has occurred. The T-lymphocytes responsible for the regulation of IgE secretion carry Fc_{ε} or Fc_{γ} receptors or both on their surface. They are of a Lyt^{+} (helper) phenotype. When stimulated by macrophages which present antigen and secrete type one interferon (α or β) these T-cells in turn secrete a 15,000 dalton protein which binds to the Fc portion of IgE molecules. This protein is called IgE-binding factor (IgE-BF). Proteins with a molecular weight of 60 or 30 kd are also secreted but the biological activity of these factors is less than that of the 15 kd protein.

Depending of its state of glycosylation, IgE-BF can either stimulate or inhibit the secretion of IgE in IgE producing B-cells. The IgE potentiating factor (IgE-PF) carries both N-linked, mannose-rich oligosaccharides and O-linked oligosaccharides with sialic acid residues in the terminal position of both types. In contrast the IgE-suppressive factor (IgE-SF) carries only O-linked oligosaccharides whose terminal residue is galactose – N-acetylgalactosamine. On account of these different glycosylation patterns, IgE-PF can bind to both concanavalin A and lentil lectin, while IgE-SF has no affinity for either substance but binds to peanut agglutinin.

A gene specifying the synthesis of IgE-binding factor has recently been isolated from a mouse T-cell hybridoma and cloned in COS 7 cells. The nucleotide sequence analysis of this gene revealed a coding region for 556 amino acids with two potential sites for N-glycosylation and several sites for posttranslational proteolytic cleavage. In COS 7 cells, this gene gives rise to a 60 kd and to an 11 kd protein both of which carry the N-glycosylation sites. Under normal conditions, COS 7 cells carrying the IgE-BF gene form IgE-potentiating factor. However, when incubation is carried out in the presence of tunicamycin, an inhibitor of N-glycosylation, the same cells give rise to synthesis of the non-glycosylated factor which suppresses IgE formation and secretion.

In summary: IgE-PF and IgE-SF share a common structural gene. The biological activity of the factors is decided by a post-translational glycosylation process (Fig. 5.1.).

In vivo, the amount of IgE antibody that is synthesized in response to a specific antigen depends on the ratio of the glycosylated (potentiating) factor to the non-glycosylated (suppressing) factor. The same Fc_{γ}- and/or Fc_{ε}-receptor-bearing T-helper cells which form the IgE-binding protein also synthesize and secrete a kallikrein-like enzyme, GEF (glycosylation-enhancing factor). This enzyme promotes glycosylation of the IgE-binding protein and thus the secretion and synthesis of IgE. GEF is a serine protease. It stimulates phospolipid methylation, Ca^{++} uptake and the formation of diacylglycerol through the activation of phospholipase C. It also activates other membrane-associated enzymes such as methyltransferases and phospholipase A_2. Consequently, it induces the release of arachidonic acid from phospholipids. Taken by themselves, these results

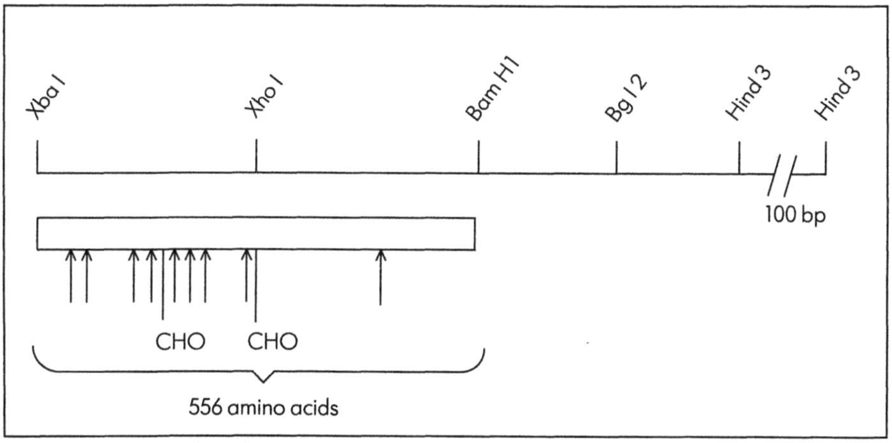

Figure 5.1. The nucleotide sequence of the cDNA clone reveals a putative protein-coding region of 556 amino acids. The peptide (bottom bar) contains two potential sites for N-linked glycosylation (CHO sites = Asn-x-Ser residues). The molecular weight of the peptide calculated from the predicted amino acid sequence is about 62 kd. Whether this factor induces or suppresses IgE synthesis depends entirely on the glycosylation in the N-linked glycosylation sites. Arrows: Sites for posttranslational proteolytic cleavage.

are not easily interpretable against the background of the stimulation of glycosylation which we have just discussed. However, they become more meaningful if we look at them in context with glycosylation-inhibiting factor (GIF) which is the other basic element in the regulatory cycle which determines IgE secretion. In rodents GIF is formed by a subset of T-suppressor cells (Lyt 2^+) as a response to antigens presented together with complete Freund's adjuvant. Under these conditions Lyt 1^+ helper cells produce γ interferon while Lyt 2^+ T-suppressor cells secrete GIF. Together, γ interferon and GIF inhibit the glycosylation of IgE-BF in specific T-helper cells. GIF has a molecular weight of 13,000. It reacts with antibodies directed against lipocortin, a cytoskeletal Ca^{++} binding protein which seems to be involved in the regulation of phospholipase A_2. For some time, GIF was considered to be a phosphorylated fragment of lipocortin: it acted on phospholipase only after treatment with alkaline phosphatase. Today, a direct precursor product relationship between lipocortin and GIF is considered unlikely. However, the two molecules appear to be related. As one might expect, glucocorticoids induce GIF formation in normal spleen lymphocytes.

GIF prevents glycosylation of the IgE-binding proteins and is instrumental in inhibiting IgE formation and secretion. The intensity of an IgE response is therefore determined by the ratio of GEF to GIF *(Fig. 5.2)*. Which of the two factors is predominant depends on the type of antigen involved and probably also on the form in which it penetrates the body. Spleen cells from rats which had been immunized with aluminium hydroxide-absorbed KLH (keyhole-limpet hemocyanin) formed IgE-potentiating factor on renewed contact with the antigen. When the same rats had been immunized primarily with KLH in Freund's complete adjuvant, the spleen lymphocytes formed IgE-inhibiting factor on renewed contact with the antigen. In the mouse, initial immunization with

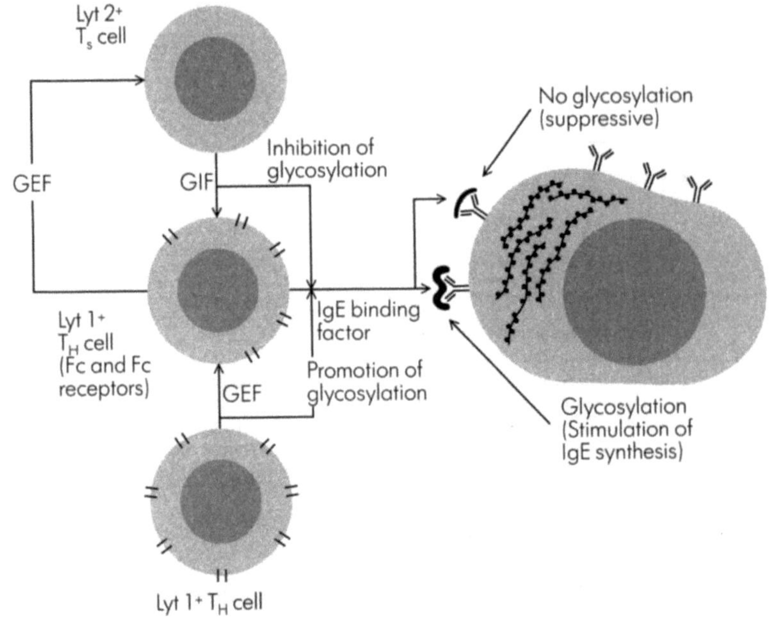

Figure 5.2. Regulation of IgE synthesis according to K. Ishizaka. GEF = glycosylation-enhancing factor. GIF = glycosylation-inhibiting factor. See text for explanation.

$Al(OH)_3$-absorbed antigens also seemed to intensify IgE synthesis, while the same antigens (e.g. ovalbumin), without adjuvant and administered i.v., brought about suppression of IgE synthesis.

The fact that the glycosylation-enhancing factor is a kallikrein-like enzyme is remarkable. It is thought that, by cleavage of a kininogen, this factor produces a kinin in lymphocytes which, in an as yet undetermined manner, brings about glycosylation of the IgE-binding protein by mechanisms which involve phospholipase activation but are otherwise not understood. Interestingly, other serine proteases like trypsin, plasmin, kallikrein and bradykinin, which of course is a cleavage product of kininogen formed by the action of kallikrein, all promote glycosylation of the IgE-binding protein to some extent.

Even more interesting than these findings is the fact that GIF, the glycosylation-inhibiting factor, appears to be similar to a phosphorylated fragment of lipocortin. After all, lipocortin, a membrane protein that can be induced with glucocorticosteroids, inhibits phospholipase A_2 and thus also the formation of leukotrienes and prostaglandins. The interconnections have not all been fully elucidated as yet. What is important, however, is the indication that glucocorticosteroids prevent glycosylation of IgE-binding protein, thus promoting the formation of an IgE-suppressing factor. It is not yet known whether GEF and GIF compete with each other directly in the sense that GEF activates phosphoolipases A_2 and C and GIF inhibits these enzymes by a mechanism reminiscent of lipocortin. An agonistic-antagonistic relationship between the two factors at the level of membrane associated enzymes is, however, a realistic possibility to explain a large number of regulatory phenomena involving IgE-binding factors, GEF and GIF.

Under certain conditions antigen-specific T-cells form GIF or GEF which are also antigen-specific. One such protocol runs as follows: BDF1 mice were primed with aluminium-absorbed ovalbumin. After two weeks, their spleen cells were taken and incubated in the presence of ovalbumin for three days in order to activate antigen-primed T-cells. The activated T-cells were then propagated either with Il-2 alone or with Il-2 and GIF. The cells grown with Il-2 alone formed IgE-BF and antigen-specific GEF, when they were incubated with syngeneic macrophages which had been pulsed with ovalbumin. In contrast the cells which had been grown in the presence of Il-2 and GIF formed IgE-suppressive factor and antigen-specific GIF upon stimulation with ovalbumin-primed macrophages.

T-helper cells forming antigen-specific GEF and T-suppressor cells secreting antigen-specific GIF were fused with suitable tumour cells. Some of the resulting T-cell hybridomas then formed the antigen-specific factors as a response to macrophages presenting ovalbumin. Antigen specificity in this context means that these factors confer glycosylation enhancement or inhibition to Lyt 2^+ T-cells only in response to one particular antigen, e.g. ovalbumin, but not to any other antigen.

Antigen-specific GIF appears to consist of two peptide chains, one of which recognizes the antigen and the MHC "environment" in which it is presented, the other mediating the lipocortin-like activity.

Unspecific GIF when injected into immunized mice suppresses a primary IgE and IgG immune response. The material can also suppress the ongoing antibody response when injections are started 2 weeks after immunization, at a time, when titers have already reached peak levels, though under these conditions, inhibition is not complete. While nonspecific GIF exerts a general immunosuppressive effect, antigen-specific factor reacts only to one particular antigen against which it is, however, much more active than nonspecific GIF. The induction of antigen-specific T-cells producing antigen-specific GIF may open an important possibility for the treatment of human atopic diseases.

Analogous to GIF, antigen-specific GEF also appears to have two chains, one carrying the serine protease activity and the other providing the antigen specificity. *In vitro* the antigen-specific enhancement of antibody responses has been demonstrated. It was also shown that this antigen-specific response, like the analogous effects of GIF are MHC restricted. *In vivo* activity for antigen-specific GEF has not yet been demonstrated.

All the results described above were obtained with rodents or with cells from these animals. We must therefore ask ourselves to what extent the conclusions drawn from Ishizaka's experiments also apply to man. If one analyses the evidence derived from experiments with human cells or from clinical observations one finds a general, but not always specific, correlation between the two sets of data.

In the first place, there is evidence that IgE secretion in humans is tightly controlled by T-cells. The socalled hyper-IgE syndrome is a condition characterized by elevated serum IgE, recurrent infections and chronic pruritic dermatitis. In this disease one finds a selective deficiency of $CD8^+$ T-suppressor cells. Also mononuclear peripheral blood cells from these patients cannot generate normal suppressor T-cell activity after incubation with concanavalin A. Similar observations were made in patients with atopic dermatitis. Secondly, T-cells from atopic patients, but not from normal individuals, were found to secrete soluble factors which induce the formation of IgE in normal B-cells. In contrast, when IgG secretion was taken as the end point, there appeared to be no difference between T-cells from normal and atopic individuals. If T-cells from atopic donors were incubated with tunicamycin, their capacity for secreting IgE inducing factors was abolished. This finding seems to indicate that the activity of the IgE inducing factors secreted by human T-cells is dependent on glycosylation similar to that observed in rodent systems. Most of the studies relating to human cells were performed with peripheral mononuclear cells or with unseparated T-cells. Recently it was shown that the numbers of cells which carry Fc_ε receptors are quite different in normal and in atopic individuals, the values fluctuating between 0–1% and 1–8.5% respectively.

By separating Fc_ε R positive cells from the receptor negative T-cells in atopic donors and cultivating the cells in the presence of Il-2 and irradiated autologous mononuclear cells from peripheral blood (PBMCs), long-term cell-lines were established. It could now be shown that the Fc_ε receptor-positive but not the negative cells secreted factors which bound to immobilized IgE (not to IgG) and stimulated IgE secretion. These factors lost their activity after treatment with neuraminidase or trypsin. It was also found that these factors did not act on B-cells to induce isotype-switching but rather as differentiation signals. The physico-chemical properties of these factors were comparable to those of the corresponding rat factors.

It has repeatedly been observed that B-cells from atopic patients will respond to IgE inducing factors while "normal" B-cells will not. However, B-cells from non-atopic "normal" individuals will respond to total, unfractionated supernatants from T-helper cells. These findings suggest that factors other than IgE-binding factors must be involved in IgE secretion. The pursuit of this question led to the following model: B-cells carrying IgE molecules on their surface must first be activated by a suitable antigen and by MHC restricted interaction with T-helper cells. Only "activated" B-cells will be able to respond to IgE-binding and potentiating factors. In short, two signals are needed for activation of IgE synthesis.

5.1.3.2 Regulation of IgE synthesis (according to D. Katz)

The findings reported by D. Katz and his team give a somewhat different picture of the regulation of IgE, while still remaining compatible with the situation just described. Katz and his colleagues investigated IgE regulation in SJL mice. These inbred mice form only a limited amount of antibody as a reaction to stimuli which trigger a very clear IgE immune response in other mouse strains. But if these animals are subjected to sublethal whole-body irradiation with 250 rad several days before immunization with $Al(OH)_3$-adsorbed KLH, they react by forming very high titres of specific IgE antibodies. If, at the time of, or just prior to, immunization, these mice are injected with serum or ascites fluid from SJL animals that have been treated with Freund's complete adjuvant, IgE synthesis will be restored to the low level typical of such strains. From the body fluids of mice treated with Freund's complete adjuvant Katz and his group isolated a factor that inhibited IgE formation. They designated this protein "suppressive factor of allergy" or SFA, determining a molecular weight of 30,000–50,000 daltons for it. They also found, both in the serum of irradiated SJL mice and in "IgE high responder" strains, a glycoprotein which had the opposite effect, i.e it caused IgE synthesis to rise to a level many times as high as the particular control values. The molecular weight of this "enhancing factor of allergy", or EFA, was found to be 10,000–15,000 daltons. The SFA described by Katz is apparently also synthesized by thymectomized mice. It suppressed *in vivo* IgE formation even when no, or very few, T-cells were present. The synthesis of EFA and SFA is subject to a complex regulatory system in which B-cells and T-helper (Lyt 1^+) and T-suppressor (Lyt 2^+) cells intervene by synthesizing "IgE-immune regulants". Supernatants from human mixed lymphocyte cultures have been shown to exert activity similar to that of murine SFA, a finding that may have some bearing on the development of new therapeutics. This factor is apparently capable of selective suppression of pokeweed mitogen-induced IgE synthesis of human lymphocytes, i.e. without impairing IgG synthesis.

In the meantime, a number of permanently growing human T-cells have been isolated which synthesize a factor that selectively suppresses IgE synthesis. This factor is presumably identical with that described by Katz. Work is at present in progress to produce this protein by genetic engineering and investigate its therapeutic value.

5.1.3.3. IgE regulation in human cell systems

A coherent, though by no means complete, picture of the regulation of IgE synthesis in human cells has emerged only recently. While it shows certain parallels to the findings made in rodent systems, especially those reported by the Ishizaka group, there are also apparent discrepancies with the earlier findings. At present, therefore, it seems difficult to incorporate these different lines of evidence into a comprehensive unifying concept. There are two important new elements emerging from studies with human cells: the first one is the occurrence of two receptors for IgE, one high affinity receptor occurring on mast cells and basophils and a second low affinity receptor called Fc_ε R type II which comes in two subtypes called a and b. (The low affinity R binds IgE with a dissociation constant of only 10^{-7} M as compared to 10^{-10} M for the high affinity receptor.) The a subtype of this receptor occurs only on B-cells while the b subtype which is generated by a different transcriptional initiation site and by different RNA splicing occurs also on eosinophils, macrophages and platelets. The second important element concerns the role of Il-4.

Structure of Fc_ε RII

This receptor was first discovered on a human lymphoblastoid cell line. It consists of a protein with 321 amino acids with one possible N-glycosylation site and a site for O-glycosylation. This protein had previously been detected on human B-lymphocytes with the so-called CD23 cluster of antibodies. It is now established that Fc_ε RII and CD23 are identical. The molecular weight of this receptor protein, which has a short NH_2 terminal portion pointing towards the cytoplasm, a transmembrane region of 48 amino acids and a large extracellular carboxy-terminal portion, is 45 kd. Fc_ε RII shows homology with a chicken sialo-glycoprotein receptor or hepatic lectin. The extracellular part of the molecule can undergo autoproteolytic cleavage. This leads to the formation of several soluble fragments (37, 33, 25 and 12 kd), of which the first three can all bind to IgE. In other words: these soluble peptides derived from Fc_ε RII are IgE-binding factors. They bear, however, no homology to rodent IgE-BF. Some observations seem to indicate that soluble CD23 or Fc_ε RII stimulate IgE synthesis in primed B-cells. However, since the respective experiments were done with rather crude preparations of Fc_ε RII fragments, the stimulation of IgE secretion might have been caused by other factors, possibly those that are similar to rodent IgE-BF. Interestingly these crude preparations, when obtained from cells which had been cultured with tunicamycin, a glycosylation inhibitor, suppressed IgE synthesis. This phenomenon, of course, is reminiscent of the action of glycosylation inhibiting factor (GIF) which imposes upon rodent IgE-BF an activity that suppresses IgE synthesis in primed B-cells.

Il-4

Il-4, which in mice and possibly also in humans is the product of a special subset of T helper cells, enhances the expression of Fc_ε RII. It also induces in B-cells a 'switch recombination' which results in the synthesis of IgE instead of IgD or IgM. The factor also stimulates IgE synthesis. This effect might be the consequence of the increase in the Fc_ε RII expression already mentioned. Alternatively, it might result from an induced formation of other IgE-BFs analogous to the ones found in rodents. γ-Interferon antagonizes all Il-4 effects on B-cells: it prevents the switch from IgM or IgD to IgE synthesis, it suppresses the expression of IFc_ε RII and IgE-BF and it inhibits IgE formation. α-interferon and PGE_2 (IC_{50} = 1nM) exert similar effects: both compounds inhibit Fc_ε RII expression at the transcriptional level, reduce the secretion of IgE-BF and inhibit IgE production. These relationships are illustrated in *Fig. 5.3.*

Other compounds which interfere with the Il-4 induced expression of Fc_ε RII are bromo-cAMP (10^{-3} M), forskolin (10^{-5} M) and cholera toxin. All of these compounds, including PGE_2, raise intracellular levels of cAMP when used at

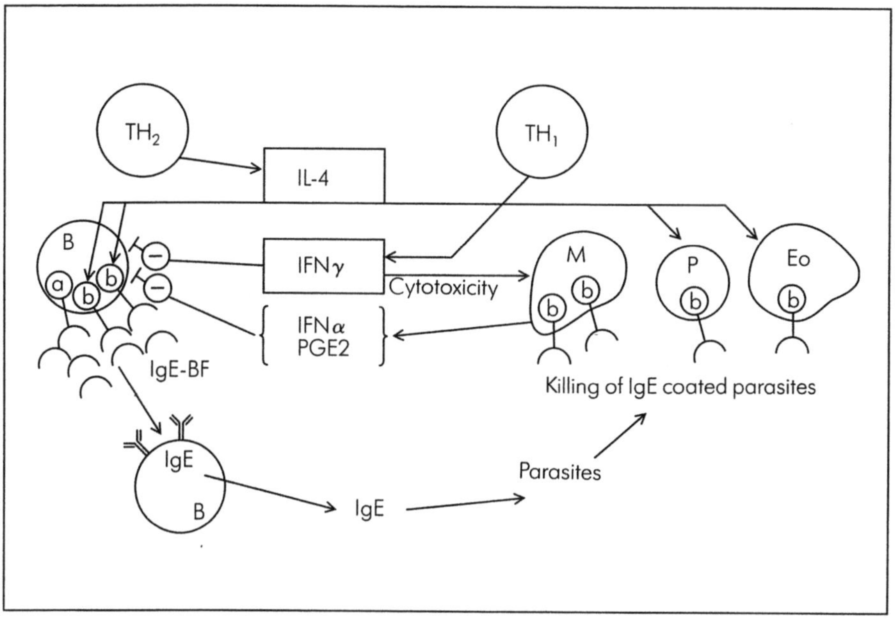

Figure 5.3. IL-4 and interferon-γ are generated by two different subsets of helper (CD4) cells. IL-4 increases the expression of Fc RII/CD23 type a and b, enhances the secretion of IgE-BF and stimulates IgE secretion. Interferon γ, interferon α and PGE2 antagonize all of these effects on B-cells. IL-4 also enhances the expression of Fc RII on monocytes (M), eosinophils (Eo) and platelets (P). The expression of the low affinity IgE receptors on the former two cell types leads to an increased killing of IgE-coated parasites.

the concentrations indicated. Thus it appears possible that these substances act by a common mechanism which must be different from that elicited by γ-interferon which, for its part, does not influence intracellular cAMP concentrations. None of the agents mentioned have any influence on the interaction of Il-4 with its receptor or the number of Il-4 receptor molecules per cell. Furthermore the internalization of Il-4 and the rate of its degradation are not affected by any of these agents.

5.1.3.4 Desensitization and IgE regulation

The isolation of factors that suppress IgE synthesis may eventually result in new approaches to the treatment of allergy. Until such factors become available, desensitization remains the standard method for the treatment of allergies. Desensitization can be achieved by the administration of the antigen to which hypersensitivity exists in low doses; these are increased in small increments over a long period of time. The form in which the antigen is administered is important: in man as in animal models, modification of the antigen can result in stimulation of IgG antibody synthesis and suppression of IgE antibody synthesis. In some cases this is achieved by aggregating low-molecular-weight antigens with glutaraldehyde or, as with pollen antigens, by coupling L-tyrosine to the antigen, which is also achieved through glutaraldehyde.

The effects of such "desensitizing" measures are well documented in many cases. The causes underlying the frequently observed clinical improvements have been less thoroughly investigated. In this connection the following mechanisms are under discussion:

1. Synthesis of "blocking" IgG antibodies. Such antibodies will limit the amount of antigen which is available for the stimulation of IgE formation. With fewer "allergizing" IgE antibodies present, the release of mediators from mast cells and basophils will also be reduced.
2. Induction of "tolerance" in IgE-producing B-cells.
3. Inhibition of T-helper cell function.
4. Induction of isotype-specific and/or antigen-specific T-suppressor cells and factors (this approach derives from the findings described above).
5. Regulation of IgE synthesis by antiidiotypic auto-antibodies.

The first of these mechanisms is considered the most plausible explanation for the phenomenon of desensitization since an increase in the IgG antibody concentration and a corresponding fall in the IgE titre are often associated with a clinical improvement.

5.1.4 Degranulation of mast cells

Degranulation of mast cells is the key event in all allergic reactions. Consequently, it is an important target of therapeutic strategies aiming at preventing or attenuating such reactions. The biochemical events which lead to the receptor-mediated release of *preformed mediators,* and the subsequent events that cause *secondary mediators* to be synthesized and released have been largely elucidated, even though the order in which they occur and their causal interconnections are not yet fully understood. The situation portrayed in *Fig. 5.4* should therefore

Figure 5.4. Survey of biochemical processes which bring about degranulation. See text for explanations.

Special abbreviations:

PI	Phosphoinositol
PI(4)P	Phosphoinositol-4-monophosphate
PI(4,5)P_2	Phosphoinositol-4,5-diphosphate
PE	Phosphatidylethanolamine
PMME	Phosphatidyl-N-monomethylethanolamine
PDME	Phosphatidyl-N,N-dimethylethanolamine
PLC	Phospholipase C
PC	Phosphatidylcholine
DAG	Diacylglycerol
IP_3	Inositoltriphosphate
Protein kinase Ci and a =	inactive and active
COG	Cyclooxygenase
LOG	Lipoxygenase
PLA_2	Phospholipase A_2
LPC	Lysophosphatidylcholine
PhD	Phosphodiesterase
MTase I and II	Methyltransferase I and II
R	Receptors

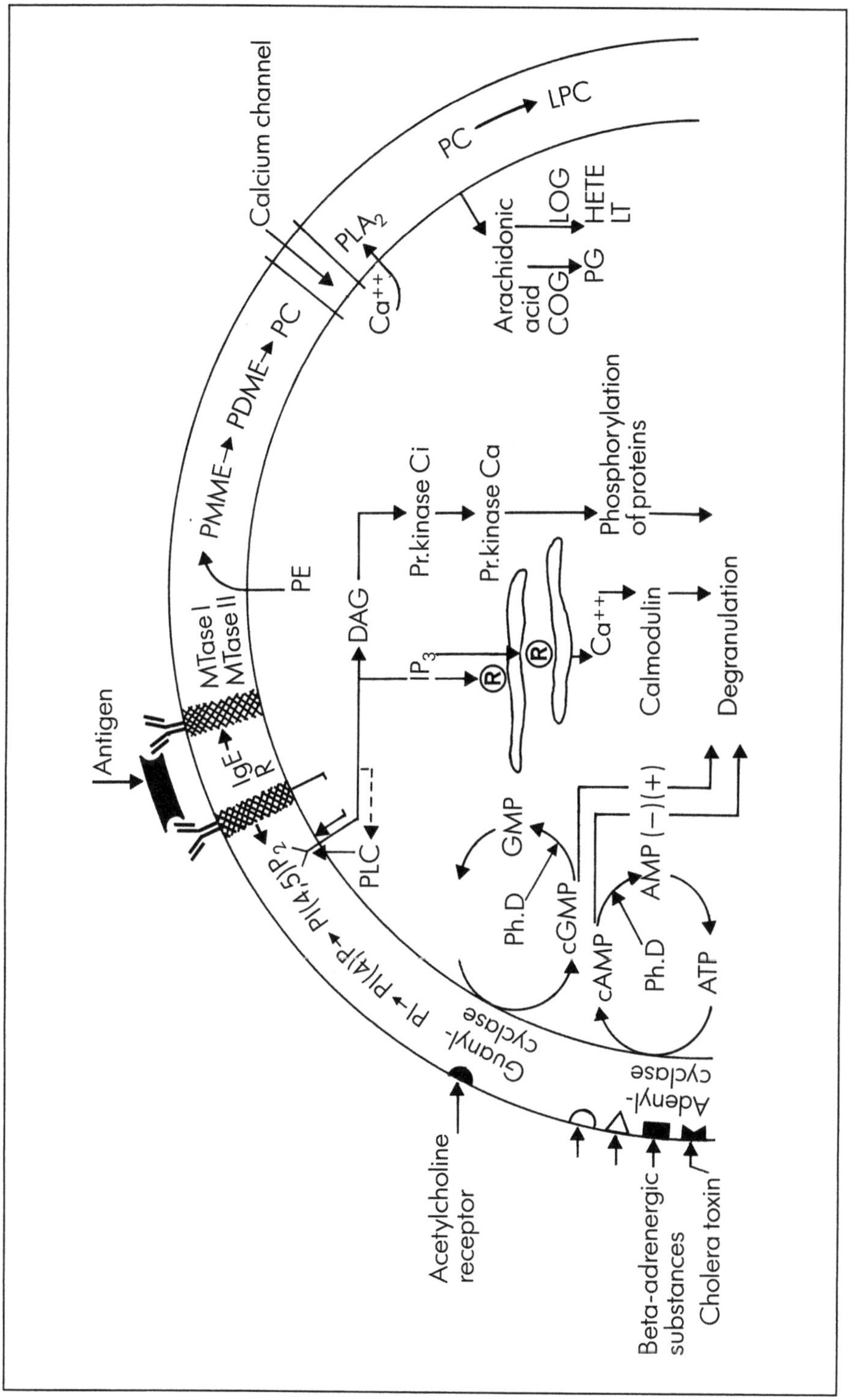
Antigen
IgE-R
MTase I
MTase II
PE
PMME
PDME
PC
Calcium channel
PLA$_2$
Ca^{++}
PC
LPC
Arachidonic acid
COG
LOG
PG
HETE
LT
DAG
Pr.kinase Ci
Pr.kinase Ca
Phosphorylation of proteins
IP$_3$
Ca^{++}
Calmodulin
Degranulation
PLC
PI
PI(4)P
PI(4,5)P$_2$
GMP
cGMP
Ph.D
AMP
cAMP
Ph.D
ATP
(−)(+)
Guanyl-cyclase
Adenyl-cyclase
Acetylcholine receptor
Beta-adrenergic substances
Cholera toxin

be taken with a grain of salt. "Bridging" of the antigen-forming arms of two adjacent cell-bound IgE molecules by an antigen causes a signal to develop which triggers a number of characteristic changes in the cell.

The early changes occurring within seconds of the antigen-antibody reaction include:

1. Hydrolysis of phosphoinositol-4,5-diphosphate to diacylglycerol and to inositol triphosphate.
2. Activation of a membrane-bound serine esterase, which activates methyltransferases directly or indirectly.
3. Sequential transmethylation of phosphatidylethanolamine in three steps to phosphatidyl-N-monomethyl-ethanolamine, phosphatidyl-N,N-dimethylethanolamine and finally phosphatidylcholine.

A result of these early events is the influx of Ca^{++} into the cell and – perhaps even more important – the mobilization of calcium from intracellular stores, in particular from the endoplasmic reticulum. The increase in the intracellular calcium concentration has three major consequences: together with the diacylglycerol released by cleavage of phosphoinositol calcium activates protein kinase C (PKC). In many tissues, the concentration of this enzyme greatly exceeds that of protein kinase A, the cAMP-dependent enzyme. PKC phosphorylates a large number of proteins at their serine and threonyl residues. It is not known what bearing the phosphorylation of cellular proteins has on degranulation of basophils and mast cells. This is also true of other physiological reactions which are triggered by protein kinase C. Secondly, the increase in intracellular calcium leads to an activation of calmodulin which in turn activates enzymes like Ca^{++}-dependent ATPase and phosphodiesterase which catalyses the breakdown of cAMP. In conjunction with the subsequent fall in cAMP levels, the calcium influx also activates microfilaments and microtubules which contract and thus bring the granules closer to the cellular membrane. Recent experimental evidence suggests that calmodulin antagonists are also invariably inhibitors of histamine and serotonin release from rat mast cells. In a study comparing the effects of a great number of calcium antagonists on protein kinase C and on calmodulin dependent enzymes (Ca^{++}-dependent ATPase and phosphodiesterase) it was shown that the degree of calmodulin antagonism paralleled the antisecretory effects of cloxacepride, oxatomide, picumast, prenylamine, thioridazine, fendiline and bepridile. The site of action of these substances was found to be distal to the calcium signal. Moreover, protein kinase C could be excluded as a target in these cases. The relationship between calmodulin antagonism and inhibition of histamine release did not depend on the signal which was used to trigger histamine release: substance 48/80, concanavalin A, antigen-IgE complexes and the calcium ionophore A 23187 all gave the same results. On the other hand, cromolyn sodium and ketotifen did not inhibit calmodulin-dependent enzymes. Their antisecretory activity, like that of terfenadine must, therefore, rely on alternative mechanisms.

A third important effect of the calcium ions concerns the activation of phospholipase A2, the enzyme that releases arachidonic acid from phosphatidylcho-

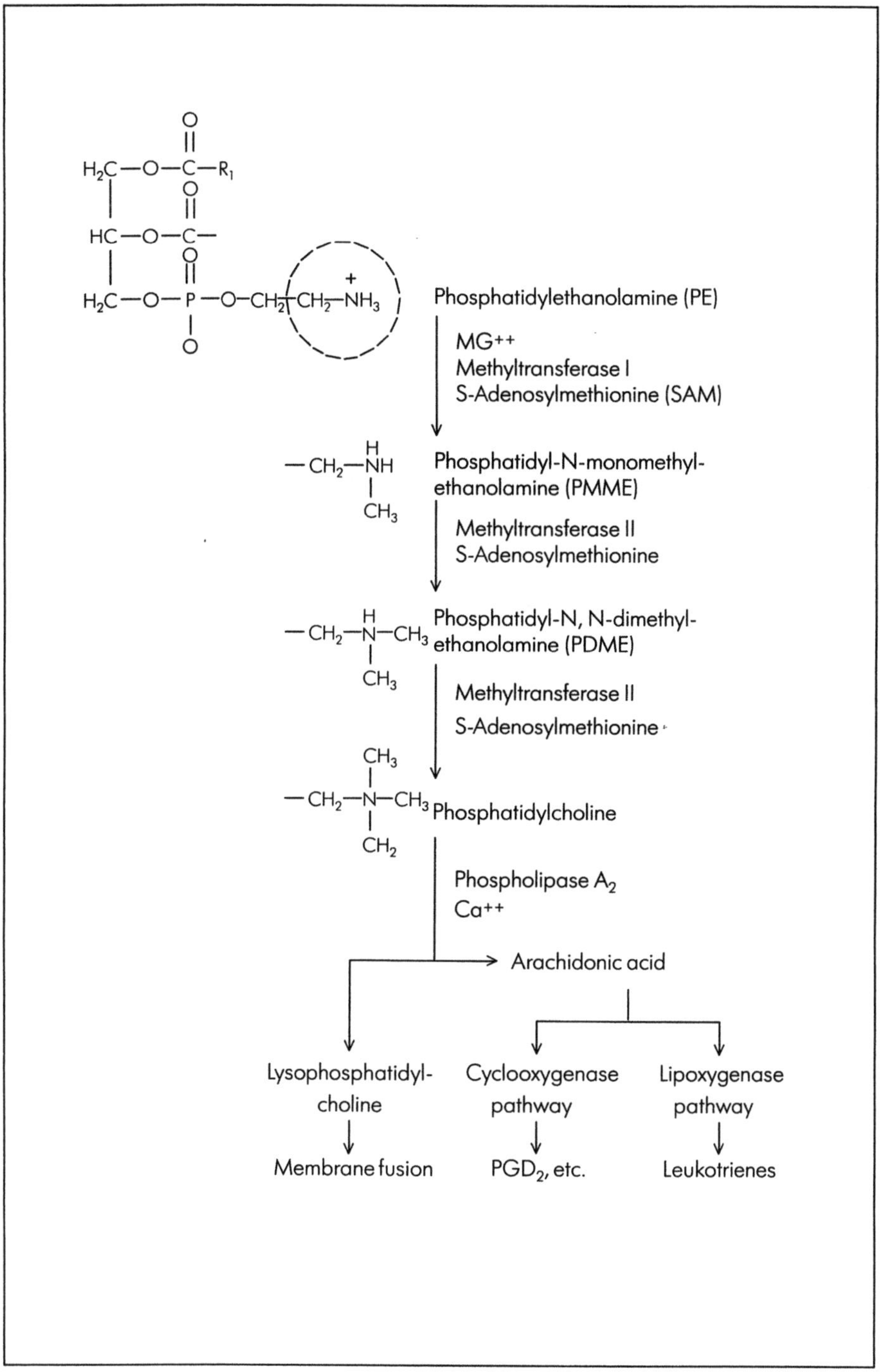

Figure 5.5. Diagram of the steps involved in methylation of phosphatidylethanolamine to phosphatidylcholine.

line and phosphatidylinositol, thereby providing the substrate used by cyclo-oxygenase to produce prostaglandins and thromboxane and by lipoxygenase to produce leukotrienes and hydroxy- and hydroperoxy-eicosatetraenoic acids. On the following pages, some of the elements of the reaction chain which are currently thought to have a particular bearing on degranulation are described in greater detail.

5.1.4.1 Phospholipid metabolism

It has long been accepted that changes in phospholipid metabolism are of decisive importance for the transduction of signals which are aimed at the cell membrane. Interest in this context was initially concentrated on methylation processes in which phosphatidylethanolamine is converted into phosphatidylcholine by the sequential transfer of three methyl groups originating from S-adenosylmethionine. Phosphatidylcholine is used as the substrate for the release of arachidonic acid by phospholipase A_2, which is activated by calcium ions. Also seen at this stage is lysophosphatidylcholine, which is responsible for membrane fusion and which may therefore play a role in the fusion of granular membranes with each other and of granular membranes with the cytoplasmic membrane *(Fig. 5.5)*.

In recent years, however, interest has shifted from this methylation sequence to the phosphatidylinositol metabolism, which is presumably directly receptor-dependent. Phosphatidylinositol is phosphorylated in the inner layer of the cell membrane to phosphatidylinositol-4-phosphate and in a further step to phosphatidylinositol-4,5-diphosphate (PIP_2). These reactions are catalysed by two specific kinases. Phosphoinositol-2,4-diphosphate is a compound that seems to be directly associated with various receptor functions, including those of the Fc receptors. Via a receptor-dependent phosphodiesterase, inositoltriphosphate and diacylglycerol are produced from PIP_2. These two products are *"second messenger"* molecules, i.e. substances which are formed as a response to external, receptor-mediated stimuli and which control cellular processes such as secretion, growth, contraction and other features *(Fig. 5.6)*.

The phosphodiesterase which is responsible for cleaving PIP_2 is presumably bound to the Fc receptor by way of a GTP-binding protein. The administration of non-hydrolysable analogues of GTP, e.g. $GDPCH_2P$ or GDPNHP, triggers activation of the phosphatidylinositol cycle, as does stimulation of the receptor via IgE antibody. Diacylglycerol activates protein kinase C, thereby inducing a number of phosphorylation reactions which, in association with elevation of intracellular calcium, give rise to a stimulus response characteristic of a specific cell. With mast cells the response is degranulation, i.e. release of preformed mediators. Inositol-1,4,5-triphosphate is apparently directly responsible for the release of calcium from intracellular stores, particularly from the endoplasmic reticulum. This process, too, is mediated by specific receptors which cannot be influenced by calcium antagonists such as verapamil or nifedipine. Although phosphatidylinositol accounts for only 6% of total phospholipids and PIP_2 in turn, makes up for only 5% of phosphatidylinositol, inositol triphosphate is

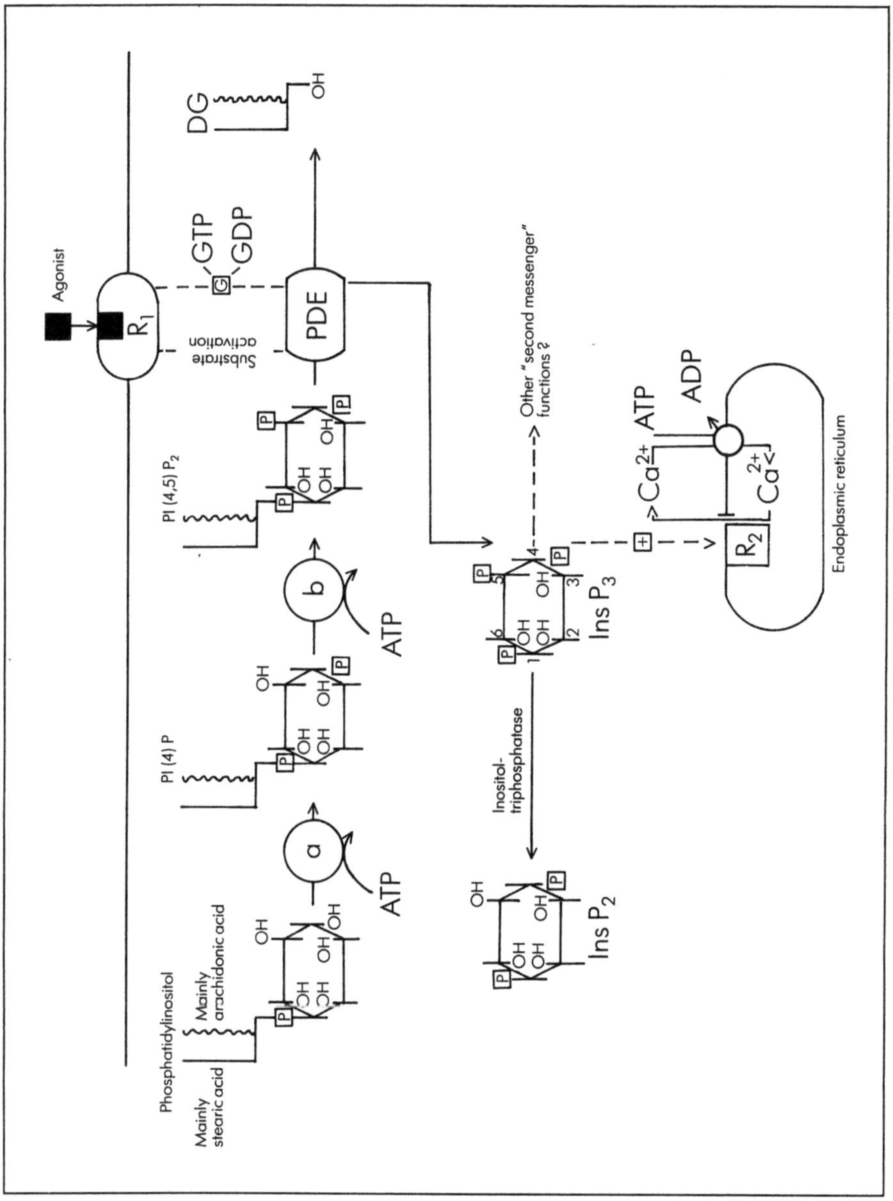

Figure 5.6. Hypothetical role of inosine triphosphate as intracellular second messenger. An agonist (antigen) binds to an external receptor and stimulates hydrolysis of IP (4,5)P_2 through a phosphodiesterase (PDE) to DAG and IP_3. DAG activates protein kinase C. IP_3 releases Ca^{++} from the endoplasmic reticulum via receptors on the reticulum. For further details see text (cf. Figs 5.5 and 5.7).

obviously formed sufficiently fast after receptor stimulation to be able to function as a second messenger. Since diacylglycerol and inositoltriphosphate exercise important functions as regulatory elements, mechanisms must exist which ensure not only the breakdown of these substances but also the constant availability of the precursor molecule PIP_2, without which the two internal messenger molecules cannot, of course, be generated. This is achieved by three cyclic processes which are mutually complementary: an inositol phosphate cycle, a lipid cycle and a cycle in which, at the expense of energy, PIP_2 is constantly synthesized and then reconverted to phosphatidylinositol. Through a number of sequential phosphatases, inosine triphosphate is converted again to inositol, which combines with CDP-diacylglycerol to form phosphatidylinositol. Diacylglycerol is either broken down to monoacylglycerol and arachidonic acid or – under energy utilization – converted into phosphatidic acid and then into CDP-DG, which in turn combines with inositol to form phosphatidic acid.

As a result of the interplay of the three cycles, the cell is in a constant state of reactivity. The price to be paid for this reactivity is energy in the form of a total of 2 mol ATP and 1 mol CTP. These building blocks are required for the fresh synthesis of one mol PIP_2. Thus the cell goes to considerable expenses in order to keep its functions regulable *(Fig. 5.7.)*.

5.1.4.2 Cyclic nucleotides

A direct connection between cyclic adenosine monophosphate (cAMP) and degranulation of mast cells has long been assumed. This assumption was based first on the fact that cAMP was the first molecule to be known as a "second messenger". In the absence of any other known intracellular signal molecules apart from the cyclic nucleotides, research was focused on the study of regulatory systems associated with these substances. The second reason for the assumption was the fact that a characteristic change takes place in intracellular cAMP concentrations immediately after crosslinking of the IgE molecules bound to Fc receptors. The antigen binding is followed five to fifteen seconds later by a short-lived, monophasic rise in cAMP concentrations. In cells that are stimulated by the substance 48/80 rather than by IgE, the early rise is followed by a monophasic fall in cAMP levels in the cell. These changes are, however, not directly tied up with the secretory process, as has been demonstrated only recently. They may be explained by the following sequence of events: adenyl cyclase, the enzyme that catalyses the conversion of ATP to cAMP, is stimulated by low concentrations of free calcium, and inhibited by the somewhat higher levels achieved within the first minute after activation of mast cells. Conversely, phosphodiesterase, the enzyme that cleaves cAMP to AMP, is activated only by high concentrations of calcium. Hence, as a result of the cAMP changes that occur within an antigen-stimulated mast cell, it is evident that, immediately after the stimulus, the formation of inositoltriphosphate (IP_3) causes calcium levels to rise in the cell. During the early stages of calcium influx or calcium mobilization, the ion forms a complex with calmodulin. This complex augments the activity of adenyl cyclase and thus also the concentration of intracellular

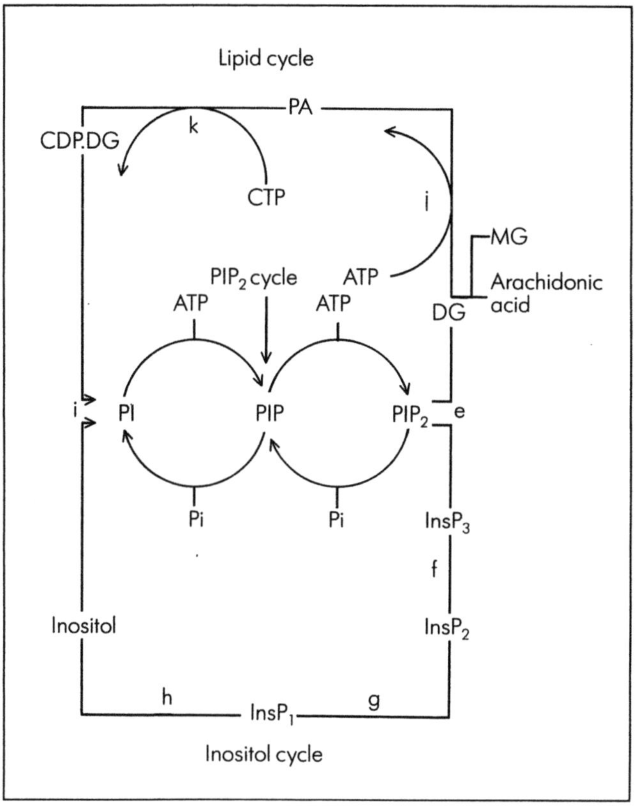

Figure 5.7. Inositol cycle. The phosphoinositol-diphosphate cycle constantly makes PI(4,5)P available for conversion of receptor-mediated signals. After activation of a receptor, $P(4,5)P_2$ is split into diaglycerol (DAG) and IP_3. A lipid cycle then transforms DAG into phosphatidic acid (PA) and CDP-diacylglycerol. In a parallel cycle IP_3 is dephosphorylated to inositol. Thus the building blocks required for the synthesis of $PI(4,5)P_2$ are again available for use.

Special abbreviations:

$InsP_1$, $InsP_2$, $InsP_3$	Inositol mono-, di- and triphosphate
MG	Monoacylglycerol
e	$PI(4,5)P_2$-phosphodiesterase
f	$InsP_3$-phosphatase
g	$InsP_2$-phosphatase
h	$InsP_1$-phosphatase
i	CDP-diacylglycerolinositol phosphatide transferase
j	Diacylglycerol lipase
k	CTP-phosphatidate cytidyl transferase
PA	Phosphatidic acid
PI	Phosphatidylinositol
PIP	Phosphatidylinositol-(4)-phosphate
PIP_2	Phosphatidylinositol-(4,5)-diphosphate

cAMP. The activity of adenyl cyclase declines in proportion to the rise in intracellular calcium levels. At the same time, however, the calcium-calmodulin complex, now present in higher concentrations, activates phosphodiesterase, thereby accelerating the breakdown of the available cAMP.

The initial rise in cAMP has little effect on the reactions leading to secretion. It is, however, certain that prolonged increases in the cAMP concentrations in the cell result in inhibition of secretion. Such cAMP increases may be caused by a number of antagonists, the receptors of which are coupled with adenyl cyclase. This group includes beta-adrenergic substances, histamine (H_2 receptors), prostaglandin E and cholera toxin. Phosphodiesterase inhibitors such as theophylline can increase intracellular cAMP concentrations, thereby exerting an inhibitory effect on secretory processes.

cAMP has an inhibitory effect on the breakdown of inositol phospholipids. Through this effect it also inhibits internal calcium mobilization and the development of DG, and, consequently, the activation of protein kinase C as well. Some findings suggest that both theophylline and cAMP can inhibit phospholipase, i.e. the enzyme that releases arachidonic acid from inositol phospholipids.

The formation of cGMP depends on other receptors, e.g. the acetylcholine receptor. The short-lived peroxides of arachidonic acid and prostaglandin endoperoxides can activate guanyl cyclase. The cGMP-dependent protein kinase G has a substrate spectrum similar to that of protein kinaseA, the cAMP-dependent enzyme. cGMP does not show antagonism to cAMP in all cells. In human lung fragments, however, histamine secretion is promoted by cGMP or a number of stable cGMP analogs. This does not apply to basophilic leucocytes.

5.1.4.3 Prostaglandins and leukotrienes

Among the secondary mediators that are formed by stimulated mast cells as well as by stimulated macrophages, neutrophils and other cells, the metabolic products of arachidonic acid are of particular significance, due to the chemical and biological diversity of the molecules that derive from arachidonic acid. As already mentioned, arachidonic acid is released from phosphatidyl ethanolamine by phospholipase A, and from inositol phospholipids by phospholipase C. This fatty acid is itself the substrate of two enzymes: cyclooxygenase, which generates the unstable endoperoxides PGG_2 and PGH_2 and then the prostaglandins, thromboxanes and prostacyclin; and lipoxygenase, which is responsible for the formation of the also highly unstable intermediate product LTA_4, from which the leukotrienes and the hydroxy- and hydroperoxy-eicosatetraenoic acids are derived.

The prostaglandins were originally investigated on account of their contracting effect on smooth muscle. Once pure prostaglandin preparations had been obtained, it became clear that these substances exerted a wide range of biological effects and that many of their precursors and metabolites were also biologically active.

All compounds deriving from arachidonic acid are 20-carbon compounds of prostanoic acid. The prostaglandins are designated alphabetically according to

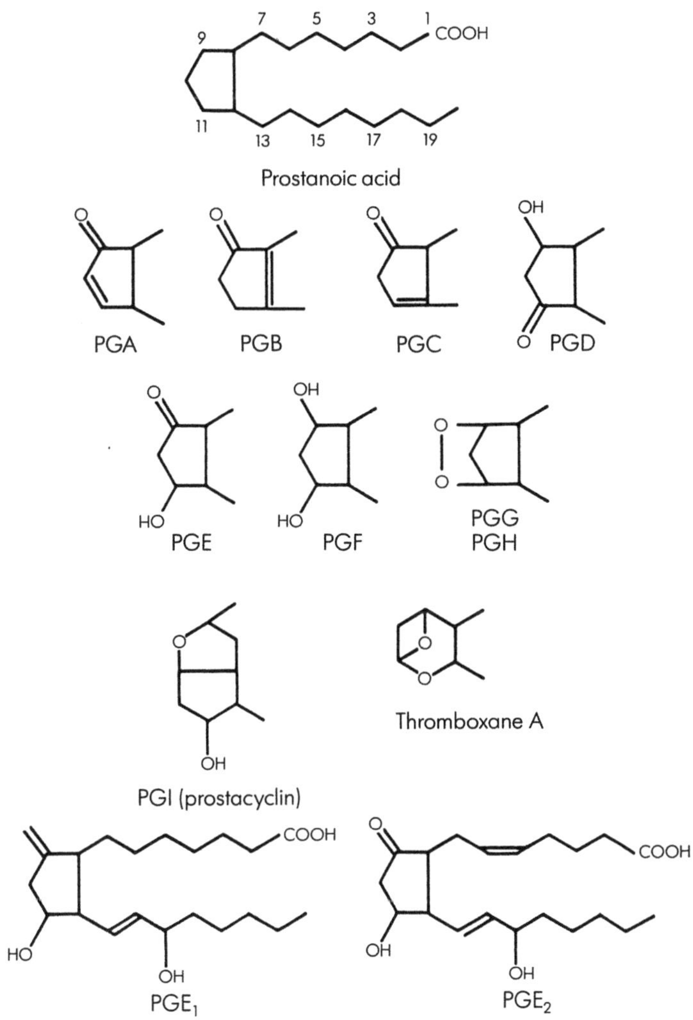

Figure 5.8. Structure and designation of the prostaglandins.

the oxidation pattern of the cyclopentane ring *(Fig. 5.8)*. The subscript numbers indicate the number of double bonds in the molecule. Prostaglandins and, in addition, products of the lipoxygenase pathway develop from arachidonic acid within a matter of seconds. Arachidonic acid itself is released from phosphatidylethanolamine or phosphatidylcholine by the action of phospholipase A_2.

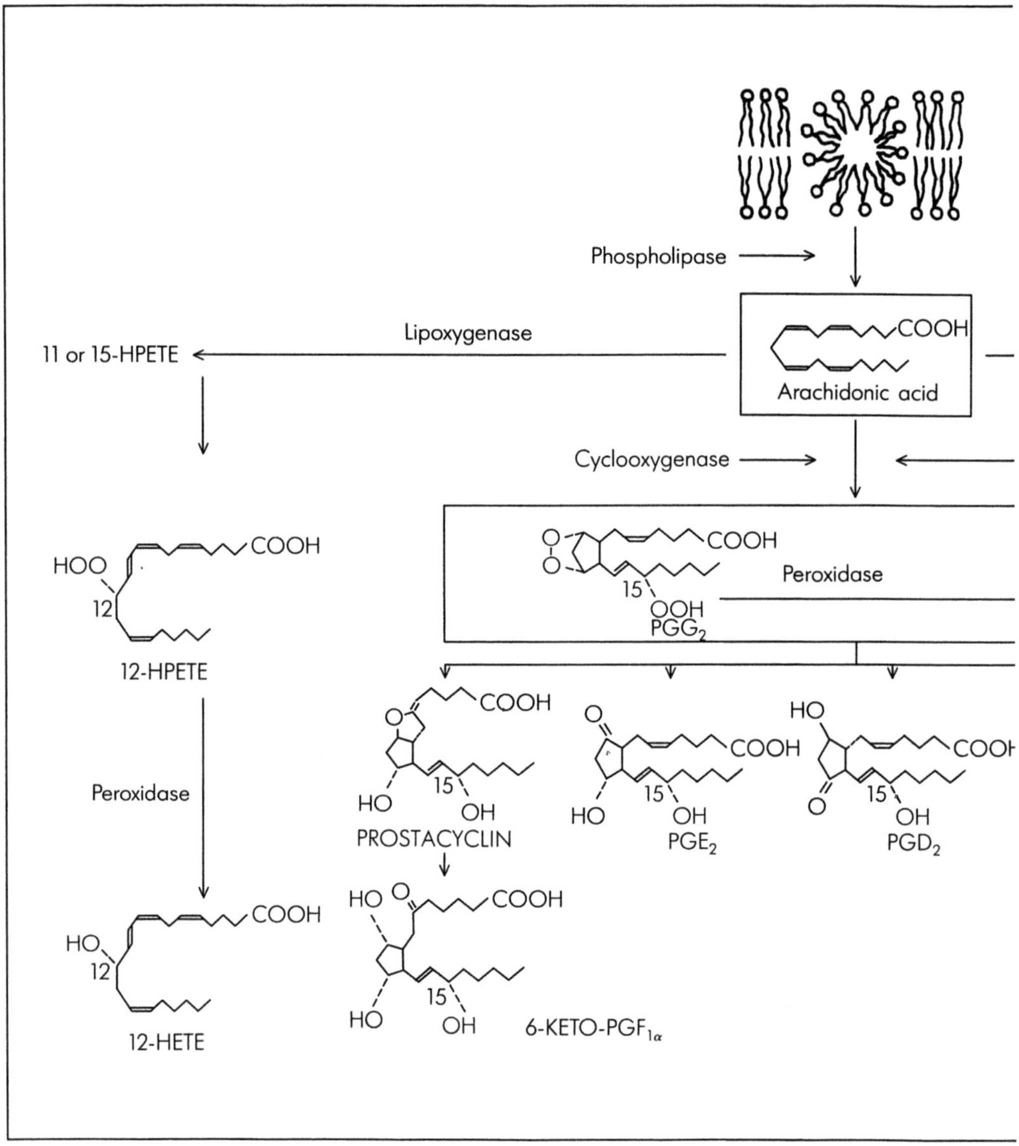

Cyclooxygenase, a membrane-bound enzyme that requires heme as a cofactor, initially converts arachidonic acid to PGG_2. A peroxidase transforms PGG_2 into PGH_2. Prostaglandin endoperoxide isomerase is responsible for conversion of the two very short-lived endoperoxides to prostaglandins E_2 or D_2. A 9-ketoreductase can convert PGE_2 to $PGF_{2\alpha}$. This latter can also develop directly from PGG_2. In many cases 9-ketoreductases are present in large concentrations, and can be activated by cGMP. A particularly important product of the cyclo-

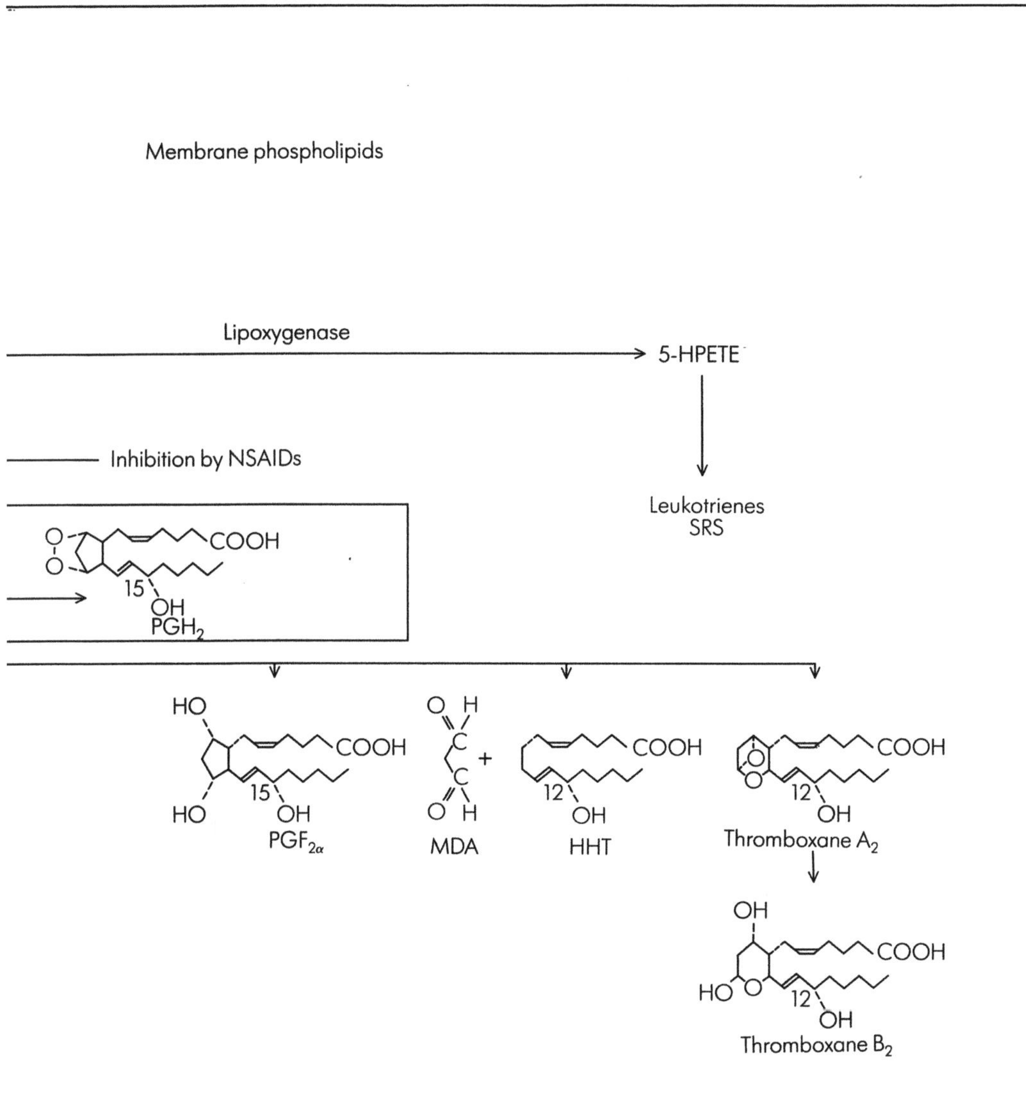

Figure 5.9. Arachidonic acid cascade. Biosynthesis pathway of prostaglandins, leukotrienes and hydroxyeicosatetraenoic acids. NSAID: nonsteroidal antiinflammatory drugs.

oxygenase pathway is thromboxane A_2. In aqueous solutions this substance has a half-life of only 36 seconds. Before being broken down into the more stable but inactive thromboxane B_2, it exerts a strong platelet-aggregating effect. PGI_2 or prostacyclin is a possible physiological antagonist of thromboxane A_2 in almost all cells except platelets. PGI_2 is also derived from the endoperoxides and is a powerful inhibitor of platelet aggregation. Its biological half-life is about ten minutes *(Fig. 5.9)*.

The leukotrienes are products of the lipoxygenase pathway. They owe their designation to having first been found in leucocytes and to the fact that their molecules all have three conjugated double bonds.

The leukotriene pathway involves transformation of the unstable LTA_4 to LTB_4. The action of a glutathione enzyme converts LTB_4 to the leukotriene LTC_4, which is itself converted by sequential cleavage to LTD_4 and LTE_4. *Non-enzymatic hydration* of LTA_4 results in 5,12-di-HETE and 5,6-di-HETE. Cellular cooperation between neutrophils and macrophages or platelets is obviously an important source for LTB_4 and other 5,12 HETE-isomers. The 5-HETE from leucocytes serves as the substrate for the 12-lipoxygenase from platelets; the reverse process also takes place. A 15-lipoxygenase which is found mainly in human eosinophils and in the bronchial epithelium is responsible for the formation of 14,15 and 8,15 di-HETE *(Fig. 5.10)*.

5.1.4.4. The biological role of prostaglandins and leukotrienes in immediate-type hypersensitivity

Many of the typical symptoms of allergic reactions are triggered or influenced by prostaglandins and leukotrienes at least to some extent. This is most clearly illustrated by comparing the manifestations of characteristic allergic conditions with the effects that can be induced with prostaglandins in humans. Allergic rhinitis, bronchial asthma and urticaria are typical allergic diseases. They are characterized by mucosal edema, capillary dilatation, hypersecretion, and infiltration of eosinophilic leucocytes. Furthermore, pruritus is a feature of urticaria and rhinitis and bronchial spasm of bronchial asthma. A comparison of these symptoms with the known effects of prostaglandin or leukotriene administration shows that PGE_2 and $PGF_{2\alpha}$ increase vascular permeability (formation of edema) and produce capillary dilatation; mucous secretion is promoted by $PGF_{2\alpha}$, PGA and PGB, while the hexaeicosatetraenoic acids are potent chemotactic agents for eosinophils. The leukotrienes C_4, D_4 and E_4, formerly designated "slow-reacting substance", and $PGF_{2\alpha}$ thromboxane, the endoperoxides and, according to recent investigations, PGD_2 in particular cause bronchoconstriction, an effect that is antagonized by prostacyclin (PGI_2).

Prostaglandins are typical tissue hormones. *On account of their local origin and short biological half-life they do not exert systemic hormonal activity.* By their action on the development of cyclic nucleotides the prostaglandins promote or inhibit the performance of cells involved in immediate-type hypersensitivity reactions. PGE_2 activates adenyl cyclase, elevates intracellular cAMP concentrations and thus inhibits release of histamine and other primary and secondary mediators from mast cells and basophils. This negative feedback effect of PGE_2 is not confined to mast cells and basophils but is also observed in macrophages, T-lymphocytes and, to a lesser extent, B-cells.

The bearing of PGE_2 on the formation of T-suppressor cells is, however, not quite clear. Some types of T-suppressor cell seem to need the presence of PGE_2 both for induction and maintenance of function. In such cases, inhibition of

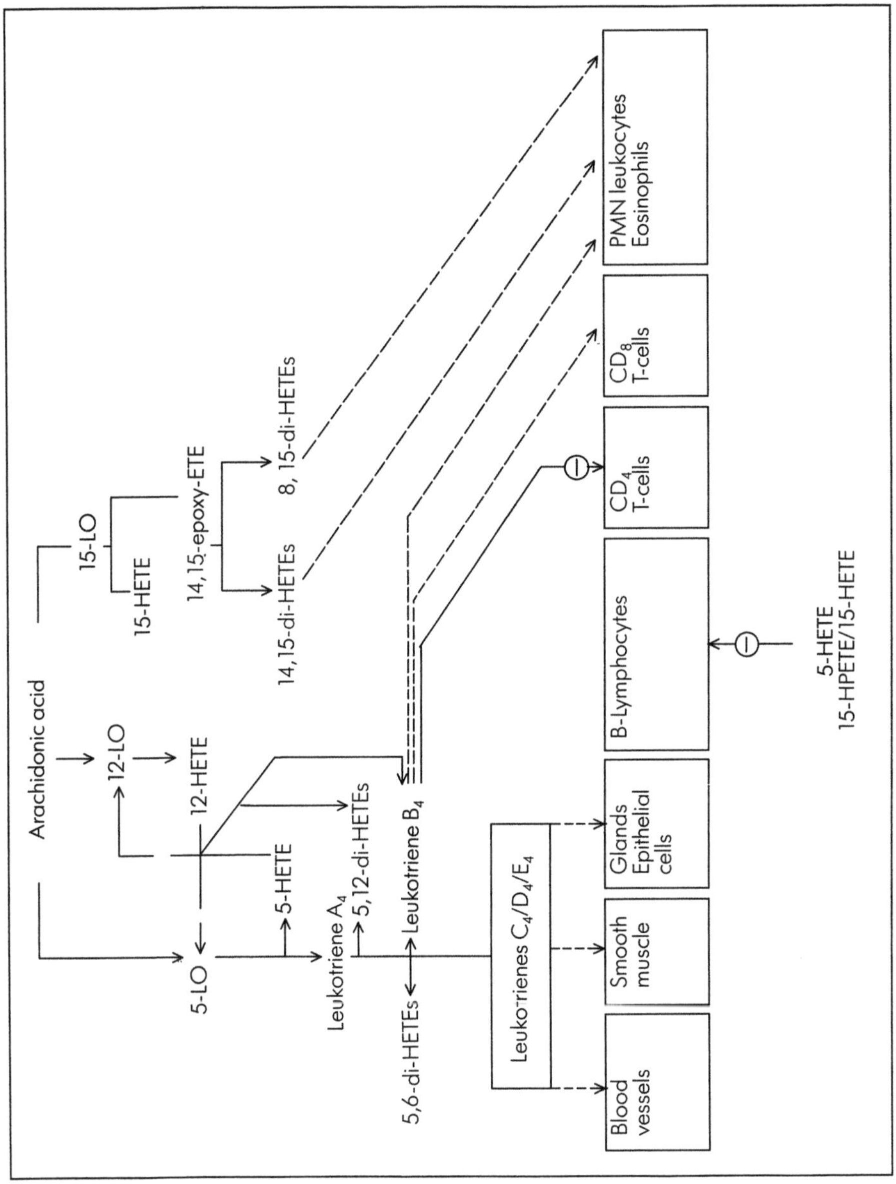

Figure 5.10. Products of the lipoxygenase pathway and their effects.

LO	Lipoxygenase
PMN	Polymorphonuclear
HPETE	Hydroxyperoxy-eicosatetraenoic acid
HETE	Hydroxy-eicosatetraenoic acid
Dotted lines	Stimulation, enhancement
	inhibition

PGE_2 synthesis by nonsteroidal antiinflammatory drugs results in disturbance of T-suppressor function and a more pronounced immune response.

Prostaglandins can also exert effects on certain organs by way of the autonomic nervous system. Histamine and possibly also prostaglandins stimulate afferent parasympathetic nerve endings in the bronchial mucosa. Like a reflex, these stimuli are conducted through afferent parasympathetic fibres back to the smooth muscle of the bronchial tree, where they bring about contraction of the smooth muscle and an increase in mucous secretion. Beta-adrenergic stimulation counteracts these effects. Alpha-adrenergic stimuli, e.g. noradrenalin, intensify contraction of the smooth muscle in the bronchial tree, promote release of further mediators and reduce pulmonary blood flow.

5.1.5 Antiallergic agents

This section is largely concerned with substances that can be designated antiallergic agents in the strict sense of the term. The drugs most frequently prescribed to combat allergic disease are the antihistamines, i.e. substances that block the H_1-receptors and thus all effects of histamine that are mediated by these receptors. Antihistamines therefore compensate for the effects of an immediate hypersensitivity reaction but do not interfere directly with the allergic process. They will therefore be discussed only in brief.

5.1.5.1 Antihistamines

The most prominent chemical representatives of the antihistamines are ethanolamines, ethylenediamines, alkylamines, piperazones and phenothiazines. More recent developments include a methoxyphenylethyl-piperinidyl-benzimidazolamine, astemizole, which differs from the conventional antihistamines in its almost complete lack of a centrally active sedative component.

Experimentally induced block of H_1-receptors by typical H_1-antagonists is effective in all smooth-muscle systems that are influenced by H_1-receptors, i.e. the gastrointestinal tract, bronchial tree and capillary and postcapillary blood vessels. Histamine plays an important, but not exclusive, role in the development of symptoms of an immediate-type hypersensitivity reaction. It is therefore hardly surprising that not all manifestations of an allergic reaction can be influenced by antihistamines with equal efficacy. In humans, edema formation and pruritus can be managed effectively with antihistamines. However, these drugs have no bronchodilating effect. In view of what we know today about the pathogenesis of bronchial asthma or bronchospastic reactions in man this is not surprising. Therefore the clinical value of H_1-blocking agents in allergic diseases resides predominantly in the ability of these agents to prevent and to antagonize histamine effects on the skin and on mucous membranes.

The CNS effects of antihistamines have already been mentioned. Some of these subjstances can prevent motion sickness and are therefore used accordingly. Presumably, this effect can be attributed to the antagonism of some H_1-blockers against acetylcholine.

Antihistamines are all readily absorbed from the gastrointestinal tract. Their clinical effects become manifest within 15–30 minutes after injection, and reach a maximum after two hours. Their duration of action varies from substance to substance. Sedation is the most frequent side effect. To some degree it is observed with most substances even when they are given in therapeutic doses. This effect is intensified by alcohol and can be neutralized by purines such as caffeine or theophylline.

In view of these facts the clinical use of antihistamines is necessarily restricted to mild, usually seasonal allergies, including pollen-induced rhinitis and conjunctivitis, some acute allergic dermatoses such as acute urticaria, and atopic and contact dermatitis. Antihistamines can also bring relief in insect bites. They are of very little value in bronchial asthma, and they have no place in the treatment of systemic anaphylaxis, which requires the administration of epinephrine and corticosteroids.

5.1.5.2 Cromolyn sodium

This substance owes its development to the systematic attempt to boost the bronchodilating effects of khellin, a mixture of chromones (benzopyrones) of plant origin, by producing large numbers of derivatives of the molecule. A bis-chromone was found which did not cause bronchodilatation but suppressed an allergen-induced asthma attack in a test subject when used prophylactically. Detailed pharmacological investigations later showed that cromolyn sodium suppressed passive cutaneous anaphylaxis in the rat and inhibited antigen-induced release of histamine in human lung tissue. These findings were interpreted to indicate that cromolyn sodium inhibits the release of histamine from mast cells and basophils. The substance not only suppresses IgE- and antigen-mediated mast cell degranulation but also prevents this reaction when it is triggered by other stimuli such as the calcium ionophore A 23178 or dextran. This was later directly demonstrated on rat peritoneal mast cells.

The exact chemical designation of cromolyn sodium is 1,3 bis (2-carboxychromone-5yl oxy)-2-hydroxypropane *(Fig. 5.11)*.

Since absorption following oral administration is very poor, *oral treatment with this substance is out of the question.* It is inhaled in fine-powder form for prophylaxis of asthma, with about 10% of the total dose being absorbed. The half-life of the substance in blood is approximately 80 minutes. Cromolyn sodium is not metabolized. About half the absorbed portion is excreted in unchanged form via the kidney, and the other half, also unchanged, with the bile.

Pharmacology: It has already been mentioned that the therapeutic action of cromolyn sodium was first discovered in man. Experiments on animal models and isolated cells and tissues were helpful in interpreting the prophylactic efficacy against allergen-induced asthma observed in man. Although we now have a fairly clear idea of the pharmacological properties of cromolyn sodium, the

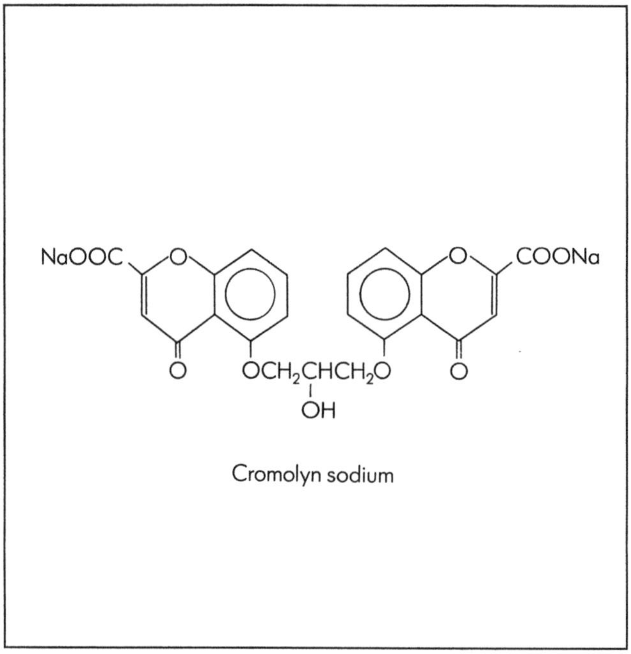

Figure 5.11. Structure of cromolyn sodium.

connection between the clinical efficacy of the substance and the "pharmacological profile" is rather questionable as will be clear from the following discussion of the pharmacological properties.

The prevention of cutaneous passive anaphylaxis in the rat has already been mentioned. This test involves sensitization of the dorsal skin of the rat by intradermal injection of IgE or IgG antibodies. Then cutaneous anaphylaxis is induced by intravenous injection of the allergen, mixed with a dye such as Evans' blue. As a result of the subsequent antigen-antibody reaction local mediators are released which increase vascular permeability. The extent of the reaction is evident from the passage of the dye into the surrounding tissue and can be quantified on the basis of the stained zones on the skin. Cromolyn sodium inhibits this reaction as a function of the dose administered, but is effective only if given in conjunction with the allergen. Administration of the substance *before* the antigen is applied will have no effect!

Cromolyn sodium also inhibits peritoneal anaphylaxis in which peritoneal mast cells are sensitized by intraperitoneal injection of IgE-containing plasma and the reaction is then induced by injection of antigen. "Self-tachyphylaxis" is typical of the effect of cromolyn sodium: if a large dose of the substance is injected 30–60 minutes before injection of the allergen together with an intrinsically active dose of cromolyn sodium the pharmacological efficacy of the second dose is abolished.

An attempt was made to use this effect to find other substances similar to cromolyn sodium by searching for compounds that exhibited "cross-tachyphylaxis" with cromolyn sodium.

Apart from the rat, the monkey is the only animal species in which cromolyn sodium suppressed immediate-type hypersensitivity reactions. Both passive cutaneous anaphylaxis and antigen-mediated release of mediators from monkey lungs were inhibited in a dose-dependent manner. Interestingly enough, cromolyn sodium is ineffective in guinea pigs. Despite the central role played by this animal species in the investigation of immediate hypersensitivity reactions, cromolyn sodium inhibits neither allergen-induced bronchoconstriction nor allergen-provoked release of histamine from mast cells or lung tissue. No antiallergic effects are exhibited by cromolyn sodium in the rabbit either. These as yet unexplained discrepancies between different animal models are indicative of the main difficulties with which one is confronted when extrapolating the results of animal experiments to man. An explanation for the difference in the behaviour of rats on the one hand and guinea pigs and rabbits on the other may reside in the fact that, in the rat as in man, IgE antibodies are the main vehicles of immediate-type hypersensitivity reactions, while this role is taken by IgG antibodies in the guinea pig and the rabbit.

Cromolyn sodium has recently been shown to inhibit certain allergic reactions which represent special forms of the Arthus phenomenon. In a rat foot-pad swelling model induced by rabbit anti-egg albumin antiserum, cromolyn sodium is very effective at doses between 10 and 100 mg bodyweight per kg. The model is characterized by late onset (maximum swelling 120 minutes after antigen challenge) and by massive neutrophil infiltration of the sensitized foot-pad. It is possible that this finding illustrates another facet of the compound's clinical profile without offering more than a partial explanation for the discrepancies between clinical efficacy and pharmacological profile.

Clinical findings: In man, cromolyn sodium inhibits the release of histamine from mast cells but not from basophils. Curiously enough, cutaneous passive anaphylaxis in man is not affected by cromolyn sodium. But the substance reliably prevents asthma, which is triggered by a number of different stimuli. This applies not only to induction by exposure to antigen, but also to asthma that has been induced by methacholine (a parasympathicomimetic) or histamine.

In predisposed subjects, physical effort, usually together with forced inspiration of cool air, triggers asthma. This reaction is inhibited by cromolyn sodium, although its association with the release of histamine is not readily apparent. The same is true for asthma induced by aspirin. Aspirin causes irreversible inhibition of cyclooxygenase, thereby blocking the biotransformation of arachidonic acid to prostaglandins. It is assumed that arachidonic acid not broken down on the cyclooxygenase pathway is metabolized through the lipoxygenase pathway, giving rise in turn to increased levels of leukotrienes C, D and E, which cause bronchoconstriction. Interestingly enough, cromolyn sodium inhibits this reaction as well.

Cromolyn sodium is of unquestionable value in the prophylaxis (or long-term treatment) of asthma. A striking feature of the studies performed with cromolyn sodium is the fact that subjective or symptomatic parameters tend to show an improvement under the therapy, in contrast to objective parameters such as pulmonary function. There is, however, evidence that pulmonary function, too, is improved by cromolyn sodium. It is difficult to predict the potential success of treatment with this substance. In view of the contradictory findings from animal experiments and human pharmacology it is scarcely surprising that the effect of cromolyn sodium is not confined to patients with asthma of unequivocally allergic origin. The following indicators show a positive correlation with therapeutic success: manifestation of asthma during adolescence; family history of allergic disease, positive skin tests for suspected allergens, FEV (forced expiratory volume) not less than 80% of normal for age, improvement of at least 20% in the FEV after inhalation of a bronchodilator, eosinophils in the sputum, rise of specific IgE serum antibodies and good response to oral administration of corticosteroids.

But even in patients falling into the category mentioned above cromolyn sodium may fail to act therapeutically. The main indication is bronchial asthma, but the substance is sometimes also prescribed in hay fever, conjunctivitis and food allergies.

Side effects: Cromolyn sodium is very well tolerated. Animal experiments have not revealed any systemic toxic effects. In asthma patients inhalation of cromolyn sodium occasionally causes local irritation of the bronchial mucosa, and bronchospasm, cough and nasal congestion. In addition to this local irritation, dizziness, painful swelling of the joints, nausea, headache and urticaria-type rash are sometimes observed. These symptoms are indicative of a hypersensitivity to the drug and can in extreme cases take the form of laryngeal edema and other typical manifestations of anaphylaxis.

Mechanism of action: Cromolyn sodium is a competitive inhibitor of phosphodiesterase, the enzyme that cleaves cyclic AMP. But the amount required for inhibition of this enzyme is two or three times as great as that required for inhibiting the release of histamine. As far as mast cell degranulation is concerned, a causal relationship between these two mechanisms is unlikely.

It is now evident that cromolyn sodium acts as a calcium channel blocker. It blocks the calcium channel associated with the IgE receptor, i.e. it inhibits the receptor-mediated influx of calcium into the cell. It has very recently been shown that the specific binding site for cromolyn sodium is on a protein that forms part of the calcium channel regulated by the IgE receptor.

It is not, however, clear whether this direct calcium-blocking action is responsible only for the stabilizing effect on mast cell granules or whether cromolyn sodium does not also inhibit the phosphoinositol cycle and thus the formation of diacylglycerol and inositol-triphosphate. In this context, too, reduction in calcium availability could be responsible for inhibiting the release of histamine. It should be borne in mind that phenothiazines and tricyclic antidepressants exert their inhibitory effect on mast cell degranulation by inhibiting calmodulin. Here, too, therefore, stabilization of mast cell granules involves a calcium-dependent process.

5.1.5.3 Ketotifen

Chemistry: Ketotifen is a benzocycloheptathiophene. The exact chemical name is 4,9-dihydro-4-(1-methyl-4-piperidylidene)-10H-benzo[4,5]-cyclohepta[1,2-b]thiophene-10-one *(Fig. 5.12)*. The substance was originally selected for clinical studies on account of its antihistamine properties. In addition to its properties as an H_2-histamine antagonist, the compound subsequently proved to exert other effects which make it suitable for treatment of allergy.

Pharmacokinetics: In contrast to cromolyn sodium, ketotifen is completely absorbed after oral administration. Peak concentrations of the parent substance are observed between two and three hours after ingestion, regardless of the dosage form employed. The plasma peaks following therapeutic doses show linear dose-dependence, also in long-term therapy. Ketotifen is characterized by a high first-pass effect (35%) in the liver. The unchanged substance is eliminated following biphasic kinetics: the half-life is 1.6 hours for the rapid phase and 20.4 hours for the slow phase. After a single oral dose, only 2% of the substance is excreted in the urine or feces. 70–75% of the metabolites are excreted with the urine and 20–25% with the feces. Of the 17 metabolites which are formed in different animal species, six are found in quantifiable amounts in human urine along with the parent compound. Only two metabolites, the N-glucuronide of ketotifen and the glucuronide of dihydroketotifen seem to occur in substantial amounts. Together they account for almost 80% of all the metabolites excreted in the urine. Within a wide concentration range of 1–200 μg per ml, at least 75% of ketotifen is bound to plasma proteins, though so weakly that the availability of the substance for interaction with cell receptors is not restricted.

Since children metabolize ketotifen more rapidly than adults, they require relatively high doses. On a milligram per kilogram basis, the required doses for children are about twice as high as those for adults.

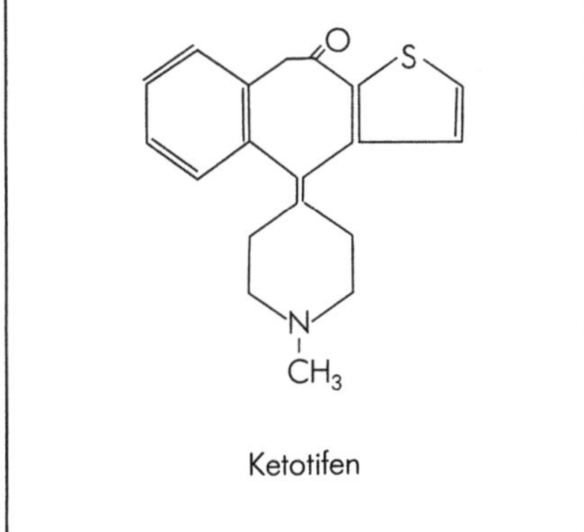

Figure 5.12. Structure of ketotifen.

Pharmacology: Ketotifen inhibits passive cutaneous anaphylaxis in the rat after both parenteral and oral administration. Given parenterally, ketotifen is about ten times as effective as cromolyn sodium in this test. Unlike the latter, ketotifen also inhibits anaphylactic reactions in the guinea pig. Ketotifen does not exhibit "self-tachyphylaxis", nor has cross-tachyphylaxis with cromolyn sodium been observed. On the other hand, ketotifen suppresses tachyphylaxis produced by isoprenalin and other beta-agonists. Since this effect is neutralized by beta-blockers such as propranolol, it can be assumed to be mediated by beta-receptors. These findings suggest a mechanism of action distinct from that of cromolyn sodium.

The antianaphylactic effect can be very easily distinguished from the antihistamine effect. The two activities are of varying duration, with the antihistamine effect lasting longer than the antiallergic effect. If ketotifen is administered together with an antihistamine such as clemastine or mepyramine, the antihistamine effect increases selectively, while the antianaphylactic effect, i.e. inhibition of passive cutaneous anaphylaxis, remains unchanged.

Ketotifen does not exert any appreciable anticholinergic or antiserotonergic effects, but in certain circumstances it inhibits the effects of leukotrienes C_4, D_4 and E_4, hitherto known by the collective designation "slow-reacting substance A". This effect does not seem to be based on direct antagonism: SRS-A-induced contractions of the guinea-pig ileum are inhibited by ketotifen in very high concentrations. If SRS-A is given to mechanically ventilated, anesthesized guinea pigs, the resulting bronchospasm can be appreciably reduced by pretreatment with low doses of ketotifen. This effect is attributed to inhibition by ketotifen of the influx of calcium into the smooth-muscle cells of the bronchial tree.

In isolated peritoneal mast cells, ketotifen inhibits the calcium influx induced by substance 40/80 and the subsequent release of histamine. Ketotifen also inhibits antigen-induced release of mediators from basophilic lymphocytes in atopic subjects. Ketotifen has an inhibitory effect on the release of leukotrienes from neutrophils. In view of the complementary role of neutrophils in hypersensitivity reactions, this effect may also have an important bearing on treatment of allergic reactions and of bronchial asthma.

Elevation of neutrophilic chemotactic factor in the serum of asthma patients after physical effort is suppressed by ketotifen. This effect does not occur after stimulation of the airways with an allergen, although even in these circumstances ketotifen inhibits the bronchospastic reaction. According to a very recent hypothesis the flare-up of asthmatic symptoms is due to increased formation and release of PAF in lung tissue. Ketotifen inhibits formation of this mediator and reduces its effects on the airways.

Ketotifen resensitizes the smooth muscle of the bronchial tree to beta-agonists. Neither cromolyn sodium nor antihistamines are known to have this effect.

Since ketotifen effectively inhibits immediate-type hypersensitivity reactions, the possibility that it also inhibits delayed-type cellular reactions or humoral immune reactions had to be excluded. The results of these investigations were basically negative. Ketotifen had no effect on *in vitro* mitogen-induced lymphocytic transformation, did not impair murine humoral immune reactions to sheep erythrocytes, and diminished the cutaneous reaction to tuberculin only very slightly and in very high doses (100 mg per kg). In the oxazolone skin test ketotifen clearly inhibited delayed-type hypersensitivity – although only when it was administered during the sensitization phase. Ketotifen had no effect at all on the secondary reaction to oxazolone.

Mechanism of action: Ketotifen exerts three main effects: *it is an H_1 histamine antagonist, it inhibits the release of mediators from mast cells and basophils, and it restores beta-adrenoceptor function in situations in which prolonged use of β-adrenergic bronchodilators has led to a loss of receptor function or to down-regulation of β-adrenoceptors.* The molecular mechanisms with which these effects, particularly the last two, are achieved have not been elucidated. Ketotifen exerts calcium-antagonist activity but differs appreciably from other calcium antagonists such as the dihydropyridines and verapamil. While these latter substances block the calcium channels which open on depolarization of the membrane in a "voltage-sensitive" way, ketotifen seems to act on other calcium channels. The calcium influx effected by depolarization is associated with an action potential. This process is influenced by nifedipine, verapamil and diltiazem. Ketotifen doses upwards of 10^{-6} M, on the other hand, inhibit the calcium influx which follows on sustained depolarization of the membrane of the smooth-muscle cell, as has been observed experimentally with high concentrations of potassium in the medium. Ketotifen has no effect on the cardiovascular system. Limitation of the intracellular calcium content – however this is achieved – should inhibit calcium-dependent processes such as degranulation of mast cells, hypersecretion of mucus (asthma, allergic rhinitis) and contraction of smooth-muscle cells. This would at least indicate the direction that any research should take in order to find a common biochemical denominator for the effect of ketotifen.

Clinical studies: Ketotifen inhibits antigen-induced bronchoconstriction in asthmatic patients. It also inhibits histamine-induced bronchoconstriction but not the analogous reaction brought about by acetylcholine. Asthmoid reactions following oral ingestion of aspirin or inhalation of benzoic acid or SO_2 are suppressed by ketotifen. Though the effect of the substance in asthma triggered by physical effort is at least questionable, ketotifen inhibits passive cutaneous anaphylaxis and other allergic hypersensitivity reactions in man as well. The therapeutic use of the drug has been concentrated on bronchial asthma: under long-term therapy with ketotifen there is a decrease in both the number and the duration of asthma attacks. The intrinsic or extrinsic nature of the asthma does not play a significant role.

The recommended dosage in long-term treatment is 1 mg twice daily by mouth. At this dosage the full effect is established within six to twelve weeks. The average response rate in all forms of bronchial asthma and in all age groups is 65–70%. Tolerance does not develop, and there have been no reports of any rebound effect after withdrawal of treatment.

Ketotifen can be readily combined with other standard antiasthmatic agents as well as glucocorticosteroids, theophylline, and with oral or local sympathicomimetics. Since ketotifen takes several weeks to become fully effective, withdrawal of concomitant therapy should begin only after several weeks of therapy with ketotifen. Since it has central sedative effects which become clinically evident in the first week or two of treatment, combination with theophylline is recommended since this substance also causes bronchodilatation but has an analeptic effect on the central nervous system.

In an open field study lasting one year and involving more than 8,000 patients, no serious side effects occurred under ketotifen. The most important adverse reaction was the above-mentioned sedation at the beginning of treatment.

5.1.5.4 Oxatomide

Although oxatomide belongs to a chemical group different from ketotifen, the two substances have much in common.

Oxatomide is 1-(3-4-diphenylmethyl-1-piperazinylpropyl)-1,3-dihydro-2-H-benzimidazole-2-one. It is readily absorbed after oral administration, and peak blood levels are reached after two hours. The distribution phase is a little over two hours. Oxatomide has a long elimination half-life of 18-19 hours. The substance is metabolized by oxidative N-dealkylation, and almost 75% is excreted with the bile and feces.

On account of its long half-life oxatomide only has to be taken in the mornings and evenings. Doses of 1–2 mg are given, depending on the indication. Treatment of bronchial asthma generally calls for daily dosages of 4 mg, while doses of 2 mg daily are usual in other allergic conditions.

Fewer data are available on oxatomide than on ketotifen. The literature shows that oxatomide exerts an H_1-antagonist effect and, over and above this, acts as a 5-HT antagonist. It is not known whether this effect is due to direct interaction of the active substance with a serotonin receptor or to another mechanism. The literature does not provide convincing support for a claimed effect directed against the action of leukotrienes C_4, D_4 and E_4.

Like ketotifen, oxatomide also exerts a direct antianaphylactic effect. At a concentration of 1 μg per ml, it reduces by 80% the IgE- and allergen-induced release of histamine from mast cells in human lung fragments. Half-maximal inhibition of histamine release (ED_{50}) was achieved in this particular trial protocol with concentrations between 10 and 20 ng per ml.

According to the data so far available, the main indication for oxatomide is chronic urticaria. With a course of treatment lasting between four and eight weeks good to very good results can be obtained in about 75 % of all cases of chronic urticaria. In allergic rhinitis, the effect of oxatomide is on a par with that of cromolyn sodium and distinctly inferior to the effect that can be achieved with steroids. Further indications for oxatomide are atopic dermatitis, food allergies and bronchial asthma. In the view of several authors, neither ketotifen nor the less thoroughly investigated oxatomide can be sufficiently distinguished from the more conventional H_1 blockers, which are to be considered a separate and distinct group of drugs. This view is perhaps too harsh. After all, the two substances can be distinguished pharmacologically from the antihistamines and from cromolyn sodium. There is, however, no evidence that the antianaphylactic components of the pharmacological profile play a clinically significant role. The clinical effects of both substances could easily be interpreted within the known range of antihistamine activity. The crucial experience still lies ahead. It would involve the development of substances similar to ketotifen or oxatomide, with no appreciable H_1-blocking properties but with clearly established antianaphylactic effects. If such substances were to prove effective in the above indications, then ketotifen and oxatomide could probably also be regarded as a distinct therapeutic category.

Neither subacute nor chronic toxicity studies of oxatomide have furnished any indications of specific toxicity. Only very high doses (40 mg per kg daily in the dog and 160 mg per 100 g of feed in the rat) produced abnormal findings suggestive of a poor general condition of the animals. This was obviously connected with a drug-related reduction in gastric acid secretion which was possibly due to a weak H_2 antihistamine effect.

No embryotoxic or teratogenic effects were found for oxatomide in the appropriate standard tests.

The substance is well tolerated clinically. Reports of side effects are confined to fatigue, which occurred in about 10% of patients treated with oxatomide. As with ketotifen and other antihistamines, this reaction is probably associated with a central anticholinergic effect of the substance.

6. Immunostimulation

6.1 Possible therapeutic strategies

The removal of a foreign antigen from a macroorganism requires a variety of reactions. Those that involve the recognition of the antigen by lymphocytes and a subsequent cellular or humoral immune response are classified as "specific". Others which entail the uptake and degradation of foreign materials by macrophages and related cells can be called "unspecific". Sometimes the events leading to the elimination of an antigen are quite simple. Certain antigens such as extracellular bacteria which have entered the host tissues are rapidly opsonized by pre-existing antibodies and then phagocytosed and killed by neutrophilic granulocytes or macrophages. This is the simplest case. Often, however, there are no opsonizing antibodies present, or – if there are – they have no bearing on the mechanism by which a particular antigen is eliminated from the body.

Macrophages and NK-cells possess an as yet poorly understood mechanism for distinguishing malignant from normal cells. This mechanism of recognition may in certain situations be sufficient to remove individual malignant or virally infected cells at the first encounter. More often, however, the immune response by which the "foreign" agent, live or non-live, is removed from the body has to be set up "from scratch". This necessitates several steps which involve not only components of the nonspecific immune system but also T-cells and B-lymphocytes. The complexity of the immune system allows for a large number of hypothetical points of attack and mechanisms which could be utilized to stimulate a particular immune response if this is therapeutically required *(Table 6.1)*. Whether or not all the forms of intervention listed in the table will become a permanent feature in the development of therapeutic strategies remains to be seen. Observations to date suggest that some of them may indeed result in the enhancement of biological defence mechanisms.

What should be the main strategies for the use of immunostimulatory agents? This question is best answered by considering the pathogenesis of the clinical conditions to be influenced. Acquired immune deficiencies stem from isolated disorders of certain cells or cell systems. Some of these conditions can be compensated by substitution of the deficient or defective element, e.g. gammaglobulins in congenital x-linked agammaglobulinemia. Other conditions can be managed by administration of thymic hormones, e.g. congenital thymic hypoplasia (Di George syndrome), mucocutaneous candidiasis in severe combined immunodeficiency, or the Wiskott-Aldrich syndrome. Strictly speaking, treatment of these conditions also involves substitution or partial substitution of hormones which assure the recruitment of functionally effective immune cells.

Therapeutic principles must be in line with the pathophysiology of acquired immune disorders as well. Transient granulocytopenia brought about by irradiation or cytostatic therapy can be experimentally influenced by agents which stimulate

Table 6.1. Facets of the immune response. Possible sites of action for immunostimulation

Site of action	Possible mechanism of action	Known substances
Antigen presentation	Absorption and processing of antigen. Expression of MHC antigens	Constituents of microbial cell walls. Interferons
Antigen recognition	Improvement of intracellular signal transmission by optimizing current reactions	
Lymphocyte activation	Expression of interleukin-2 receptors. Synthesis of interleukin 2 and other lymphokines	Gamma-interferon? Interleukin 1
Clonal expansion	Action of interleukin 2; amplification of T-helper functions	Interleukin 2
Recruitment of T-precursor cells	Thymus-dependent function Thymus hormones? Dendritic cells of thymus?	Thymosin fraction 5 Thymosin $alpha_1$
Induction of cytotoxic T-lymphocytes	Thymus-dependent Il-1 and Il-2-dependent	Isoprinosine (?) Thymosins THF, STF and other thymic hormones Interleukin 2
Enhancement of non-specific but specifically controllable effector mechanisms	Activation of macrophages (phagocytosis, Fc and C3b receptors, MHC complex, secretory functions) Recruitment of monocytes and macrophages	Microbial antigens Interferons (gamma-interferon, levamisole?, bestatin?) M-CSF GM-CSF
NK-cells	Recruitment and activation of NK-cells	Interferons (gamma-interferon) Interleukin 2
Granulocytes	Activation and recruitment	Neutrophil activation Inhibitory factor (NAF)? GM-CSF

macrophages; such agents enhance phagocytosis and reduce the number of circulating microorganisms. At the same time, they often stimulate the synthesis of colony-stimulating factors (CSFs) in a variety of mesenchymal cells which in turn speed up the production of new granulocytes from bone-marrow precursors. Substances that have this effect include glucans, peptidoglucans, muramyldipeptide and γ-interferon. The combined use of microbial immunostimulation and γ-interferon can activate macrophages to such an extent that they become cytotoxic for tumour cells. When used as an adjunct to more conventional methods this therapeutic approach may seem very promising. It does, however, have basic limitations: several macrophages are needed in order to kill one tumour cell. Because the number of macrophages that can be activated in the proximity of any one tumour cell is low, only a limited number of tumour cells can be dealt with by this mechanism.

Cytotoxic cells, NK-cells and LAK (lymphokine-activated killer)-cells as well as macrophages play an important role in the confrontation of the immune system with tumours. Gamma-interferon activates NK-cells and, in particular, speeds up differentiation of these cells from their precursors. Interleukin 2 is able to bring about not only clonal expansion of cytotoxic T-cells directed against tumour antigens but also the differentiation and proliferation of NK-cells directed primarily at tumour antigens. Il-3 and GM-CSF, probably also M-CSF, can augment the number of monocytes and macrophages. Consequently, these lymphokines should help to overcome the quantitative limitations of macrophage activation.

In the elderly, in patients with tumours, the chronically ill, or individuals with malnutrition, cell-mediated immunity is often impaired. Such individuals show an increased susceptibility to infectious agents against which T-cell-mediated reactions are required. The biochemical or molecular correlates of these immunological deficiencies are not known in detail. In phenomenological terms they are manifested as a reduction in the ability of T-cells to form rosettes with autologous or heterologous lymphocytes, and sometimes as an increase in T-suppressor lymphocytes in relation to T-helper cells. Thymic hormones, transfer factor, levamisole and purine derivatives such as isoprinosine have been reported to influence such functional disturbances of T-lymphocytes or individual T-cell subgroups to a certain extent. The sequential action of several colony stimulating factors such as Il-3 and GM-CSF leads to a substantial augmentation of lymphocytes in cynomolgus monkeys. If these findings can be transferred to humans, they would mark the beginning of a new therapeutic strategy which could effectively be applied to this problem. Cimetidine is known to reverse T-suppressor cell-induced suppression of cell-mediated immune reactions of the delayed type. This can be seen in the positive results obtained in skin reactions to typical allergens such as tuberculin, oxazolone or *Candida albicans*.

In many cases, however, an improvement is obtained only in the *in vitro* cell parameters and sometimes in the immunological parameters as determined in patients without a corresponding satisfactory improvement in the clinical course. Such discrepancies demonstrate that the connection between measurable immunological parameters such as rosette formation, mitogenic or antigenic transformation of peripheral lymphocytes, the behaviour of lymphocytes in mixed lymphocyte cultures, the T-helper/T-suppressor cell ratio and many other criteria, on the one hand, and the actual immunological competence of an individual, on the other, is not particularly well understood. These parameters provide, of course, only discrete items of information. What is more, the temporal relationship between objectifiable changes in immunological parameters and the clinical changes that might ensue is still unclear in many cases.

Therefore a great deal remains to be done before some of today's possible immunostimulatory strategies are fully understood immunopharmacologically and can be clinically implemented. In view of the successes already achieved in immunotherapy and of the urgent need for such therapeutic options, there can, however, be no doubt that this work will be done and that the targets set are basically within reach.

6.2 Endogenous substances

6.2.1 The role of gene cloning in the characterization and production of lymphokines and other endogenous proteins

Most of this section will be devoted to the interferons and the lymphokines, which are related substances in terms of origin and physiological importance. One of the interferons, gamma-interferon, is in fact a lymphokine. The major physiological role of these substances has already been discussed. The growing significance of these proteins for immunopharmacology and therapy is due to genetic engineering. Lymphokines and interferons occur in nature in very limited amounts. The production of sufficient quantities of alpha- and beta-interferons remained a problem even after the use of optimized cell cultures had become possible. Only genetic engineering can make sufficient amounts of these substances available under economically acceptable conditions.

The role of genetic engineering is, however, not confined to the production aspect. This technology has also been instrumental in putting order into the chaotic mass of factors that were postulated in immunology and cell biology on a largely descriptive basis prior to the advent of gene technology. Today the technology is instrumental in the identification of new factors and their receptors. By helping us to identify unambiguously the humoral and cellular components of the immune system gene cloning has become the methodological hallmark of immune pharmacology and immune therapy.

In view of the fundamental impact of gene cloning and gene expression for immunology and in particular for an understanding of lymphokines and their receptors a short description of the basic elements of this technology is called for. Research in the fields of immunology and cell biology has led to the establishment of many cell lines which, either physiologically or after induction with antigens, viruses or mitogens, produce lymphokines and release them into the medium in which they grow. Examples of induced lymphokine synthesis include the formation of gamma-interferon or interleukin 2 by the MO-cell or by Jurkat cells in the presence of concanavalin A. Since these cells synthesize certain lymphokines several hours after induction with an antigen or mitogen, they can also be assumed to contain the mRNA species which code for the proteins. Since the cell produces not only the desired protein but also thousands of others, the desired RNA is often present in a limited number of copies among 10,000 or more unrelated mRNA species in the cell. There are a number of ways in which the desired mRNA type can be enriched. Since mRNA carries polyadenylic acid sequences at its 3′-end, it can be separated from other cellular RNA species like rRNA and tRNA on chromatographic carrier materials which contain oligoxythymidylic acid. On account of the base complementarity between oligo dT and poly A, mRNA is retained on such columns and can be recovered by selective elution of the oligo dT column in pure form. Subsequently mRNA can be fractionated according to size by centrifugation in saccharose density gradients. Then, either in cell-free systems containing all the components required for protein synthesis or by injection into the eggs of the South African clawed toad *(Xenopus laevis)*, the individual fraction can be tested for the desired mRNA molecules: if the required mRNA is present it will be translated by the components of the cell-free system or by the protein synthesis machinery in the frog eggs. The desired protein will thus be synthesized, and can be demonstrated by means of a sensitive functional assay. Often, however, no such test is available, and if it is, it is not sufficiently sensitive to detect minute amounts of the newly formed lymphokine. In such cases, the mRNA has to be sought in other ways, for instance by first isolating and purifying a small amount of the desired protein. Then the amino acid sequence of a fragment of the protein is determined, if possible from the COOH or amino terminal. In experienced hands and with the right equipment this can be achieved with only a few micrograms of the pure protein. Given the amino acid sequence of a partial peptide, the rules of the genetic code will furnish the nucleotide sequence as well as the sequence of the complementary DNA strand. Thus, a DNA molecule can be synthesized that is complementary to part of the desired mRNA. In appropriate conditions hybrid double strands which can be separated from non-hybridized nucleic acids by absorption to nitrocellulose or other suitable material are formed between the desired mRNA and the "DNA probe".

Once the desired mRNA fraction has been enriched by one of these methods, it can be copied into a DNA strand by reverse transcriptase, an enzyme coded by RNA tumour viruses, thereby giving rise to mRNA-DNA hybrids. Hydrolysis in 0.1 M KOH breaks down the RNA strand, and the DNA strand can now be prolonged by DNA polymerase 1 to a double strand connected by a "hairpin loop". Treatment of the hairpin loop with S_1-nuclease results in a typical DNA double strand. Then the two ends of the cloned DNA and the sites on the plasmid or vector in which the new gene is to be inserted have to be modified in such a way that base complementarity will ensue at the ends of the molecules that are to be united. This can be done in several ways. For instance, residues of oligodeoxycytidylic acid are appended at the 3′-ends of this double strand with the help of terminal deoxynucleotidyl transferase. These "prepared" DNA fragments can then be incorporated into a plasmid in which treatment with a restriction enzyme and modification of the 3′-ends with oligodeoxyguanylic acid have created two ends which are complementary to the modified ends of the DNA fragment to be incorporated. The DNA strands can be joined again between the plasmid and the incorporated element by means of DNA ligase. The plasmid can now, by transformation, be incorporated into a microorganism or mammalian cell where it will multiply and be expressed.

A more global approach involves the use of gene banks. All mRNA from a cell which produces the lymphokine in question either constitutively or after induction is transcribed into cDNA. The cDNA molecules are then incorporated into a suitable plasmid of phage vector which is subsequently transformed into bacteria. In this way, a cDNA gene bank is obtained which should also contain the cDNA for the lymphokine which is to be isolated. Next, [^{32}P]-labelled mRNA from induced cells and non-labelled mRNA from non-induced cells is prepared. One now looks for labelled mRNA that binds to any of the cDNA clones in the presence of a large surplus of unlabelled mRNA from non-induced cells. Under these conditions, only mRNA species which are not present in non-induced cells should have a chance to bind to the complementary cDNA and in doing so identify a limited number of clones, each of which may contain the cDNA in question.

To have a better chance of obtaining a positive result with a reasonable number of individual specimens, the plasmid DNA from several colonies is combined in this test (*Figs 6.1* and *6.2*).

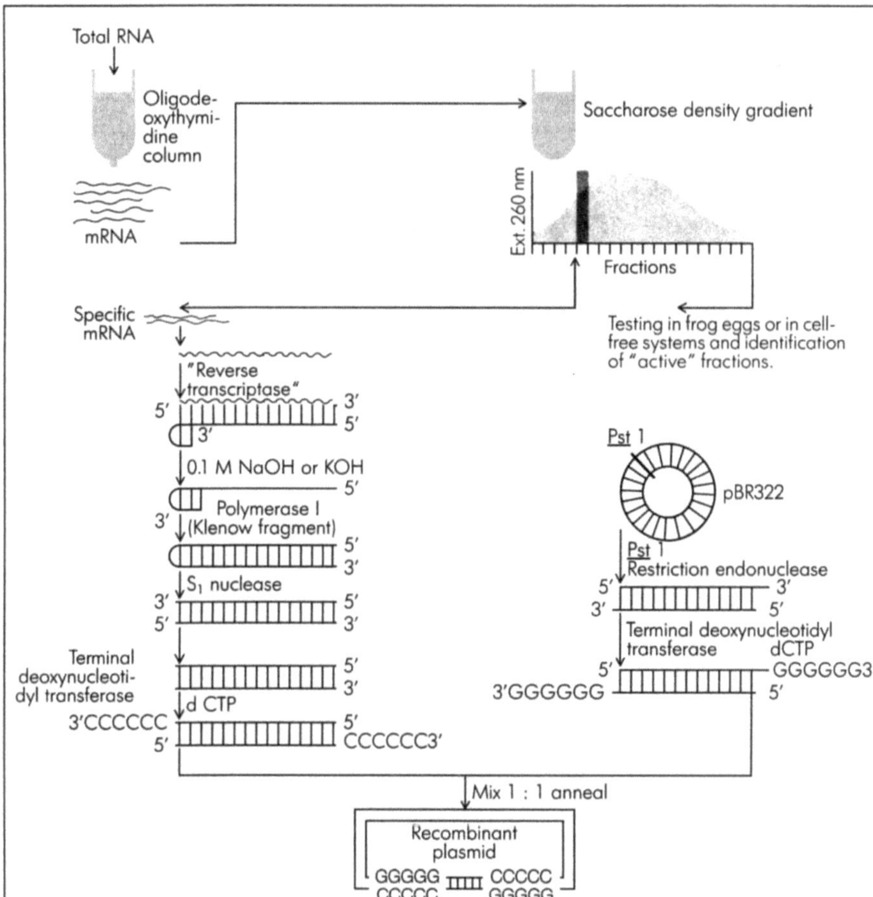

Figure 6.1. Procedure for cloning a lymphokine gene in a bacterial plasmid. On the basis of its content of 3'-oligoadenylic acid mRNA can be separated chromatographically from ribosomal and transfer-RNA on carrier material containing obligodeoxythymidine. The mRNA is then centrifuged using a saccharose gradient, and thereby separated into many different fractions depending on its sedimentation rate. The individual fractions are injected into egg cells from xenopus laevis or tested in cell-free, protein-synthesizing systems. The fraction that stimulates synthesis of the desired protein, e.g. gamma-interferon, i.e. the fraction which contains the specific mRNA, is copied by reverse transcriptase into complementary DNA strands. After digestion of the RNA strands the single DNA strands are prolonged by polymerase 1 to double strands. These "hairpin loop" double strands are split by S_1-nuclease into double strands with free ends. After modification of the ends by the addition of oligodeoxycytidylic acid residues the DNA fragment is ready to be incorporated into a plasmid which has been cleaved by a restriction enzyme and whose ends have been modified by the addition of complementary oligodeoxyguanylic acid residues. Because of the base complementarity the DNA fragment can now fit into the plasmid. The plasmid can then be closed by means of DNA ligase to form a covalent ring molecule again.

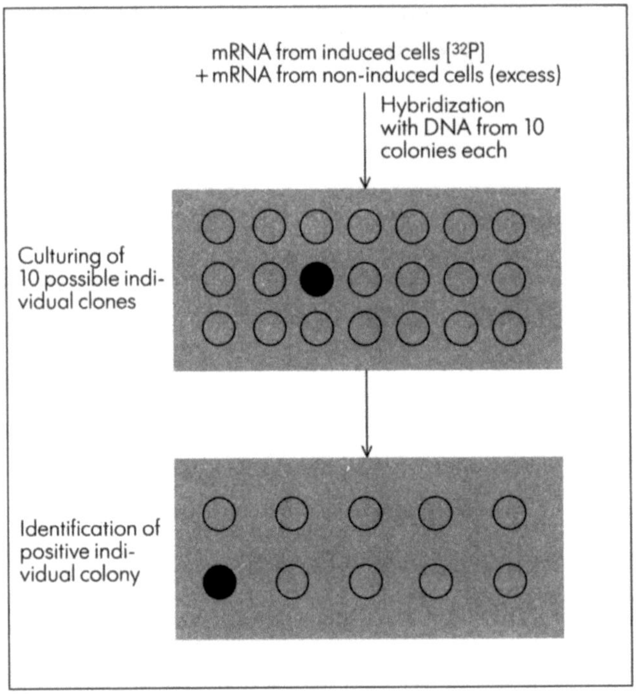

Figure 6.2. Identification of the bacterial colony containing the desired gene. [^{32}P]-labelled mRNA from "induced" cells and an excess of non-labelled mRNA from non-induced cells are hybridized with DNA from several (10 in our example) transformed colonies. A positive reaction immediately indicates the colony with the desired gene or parts of the desired gene.

If the reaction is positive, the colony that reacts with the [^{32}P]-labelled mRNA can be rapidly identified and cultured in large quantities. It can now be determined by means of DNA sequencing whether the colony found contains the desired gene in full. If so, the question naturally arises as to whether and to what extent the gene is already being expressed. Expression often requires the integration of further regulatory elements into the DNA of the host organism.

In an alternative procedure one first hybridizes the total mRNA of induced cells against the cDNA from non-induced cells. In this situation, only mRNA species not represented in non-induced cells should remain single-stranded. These mRNA species can be isolated and tested for the presence of the required molecule by functional tests as described above or by hybridization with cDNA from induced cells.

The ability to clone, identify and express the genes of lymphokines in this way has been a great stimulus for both immunology and the immunopharmacology based on it. Since adequate amounts of extremely pure lymphokines can be made available, the science of immunopharmacology has now reached a take-off point comparable with endocrine pharmacology in the 1950s and neuropharmacology in 1960s. The "protagonists" – in the present case the lymphokines, in the other two fields the hormones and neurotransmitters – are now present. Receptors are being sought, isolated and characterized. Subsequently, biochemical and molecular mechanisms of action of lymphokines and cytokines can be explored. In this way the basis for a new pharmacology of the immune system is created. Agonists and antagonists can be found for certain lymphokines and their receptors, as was the case in the past with hormones and neurotransmitters. These substances can be looked for on a "trial and error" basis, i.e. already existing substances are investigated to see whether they exhibit the properties of a receptor ligand. If such "leads" are found, their effects are optimized by selective modification of the molecules. The search can, however, be approached more "rationally" if lymphokines, their receptors or – ideally – the ligand-receptor complexes can be crystallized. If one obtains suitable heavy metal derivatives of such crystals the three-dimensional structure of the proteins or of the ligand receptor complexes can be determined by means of x-ray structural analysis. In this way the basis is obtained for the rational, i.e. systematic, synthesis of substances which – without being proteins themselves – mimic (peptidomimetics) or antagonize the biological effect of proteins.

6.2.2 Interferons

6.2.2.1 Definition and history

The question as to why higher organisms cannot suffer concurrently from more than one viral infection prompted the two virologists A. Isaacs and J. Lindenmann in 1957 to carry out what proved to be a very significant experiment. They infected amnion cells from chicken eggs with influenza virus. They then investigated the influence of the medium in which the infected cells were suspended on the infection of fresh cells with another virus. They found that cellular supernatants of virally infected cells from which cells, cell components and viruses had been removed protected other cells against infection from a broad spectrum of unrelated viruses. They designated the substance they considered responsible for this phenomenon "interferon". It was subsequently shown that the interfering activity could be traced back to a protein, or to be more exact, a glycoprotein. Interferon also proved to be not virus-specific but species-specific: it was found that interferon from one animal species protected only cells of the same species against viral infections and was less effective, or not effective at all, against cells of other species. Isaacs and Lindenmann had themselves observed that killed influenza virus also induced the formation of interferon. The next few years witnessed the discovery that not only viruses but also other microorganism, components of microorganisms and synthetic substances induced the formation of interferon. Many interferon inducers are polyanions: nucleic acids, synthetic polynucleotides, pyran-copolymer and lipopolysaccharides. The fact that so many substances gave rise to the formation of interferon was an early indication that the physiological role of this substance was not confined to warding off viral infections. However, it was almost twenty years before it became clear that interferon was a pleiotropic substance and that the antiviral effect was only one of a whole spectrum of phenomena that were triggered by it. The early realization that there were several species-specific interferons, i.e. mouse, chicken and human interferon, was followed by the discovery in the mid-seventies that chemically and biologically distinct interferons existed within any one species.

Human interferon was obtained largely from virally infected leucocytes or from human fibroblasts induced with polynucleotides. The two interferons differ in many respects and it was therefore necessary to make a distinction between leucocyte interferon and fibroblast interferon. Soon a third human interferon was added, which was formed in lymphocytes and monocytes under the influence of antigens and mitogens. This interferon, which, unlike leucocyte and fibroblast interferons, is destroyed at pH 2, was designated immune interferon.

Further differentiation was eventually achieved with the help of genetic engineering. As already mentioned, this technique makes it possible to establish gene banks and to identify and characterize those genes which code for proteins with interferon activity. According to the present state of knowledge, we can define interferons as a family of different proteins or glycoproteins that exert antiviral, antiproliferative, immunomodulatory and differentiation-promoting effects.

6.2.2.2 Classification

Three classes of human interferon which differ basically in structural and functional terms are known today: α-, β- and γ-interferons. These designations correspond to the earlier standard classification of type I (α and β) and II (γ) interferons. As already mentioned, this older classification refers to the origin of the different interferons in leucocytes or lymphoblastoid cells, fibroblasts or lymphocytes. *Table 6.2* provides an overview of the different classes of human interferons, their origin, and their previous designation. α-, β- and γ-interferons differ with respect to antigenicity, amino-acid composition and amino-acid sequence, α- and β-interferons consist (with one known exception) of 166 amino acids, while γ-interferon (immune interferon) comprises only 146 amino acids.

There are at least sixteen different α-interferons the synthesis of which is specified by the same number of genes. The α-interferons are structurally very similar: differences between them affect not more than 20% of their 166 amino acids. Biologically, however, there are considerable differences within this group.

Table 6.2. Survey of the three main groups of interferons

Designation	Former synonyms	Properties (size)	Origin	Spec. activities (IU/mg protein)
Alpha-interferon Alpha IFN	Leucocyte interferon Type 1 interferon "virally induced"	pH2 stable heterol. active (bovine cells) 166 a.a.	Leucocytes Lymphoblastoid cells	$>10^9$
Beta-interferon Beta IFN	Fibroblast interferon Type I interferon "virally induced"	pH2 stable heterol. inactive (bovine cells) 166 a.a.	Fibroblasts	10^9
Gamma-interferon Gamma IFN	Immune interferon Type II interferon "mitogen-induced"	pH2 labile 146 a.a.	Lymphocytes Macrophages NK-cells	$>>10^6$

a.a. = amino acids

Contrary to earlier assumptions, most human α-interferons do not possess carbohydrate components although they all contain a fundamentally glycosylatable asparagine molecule. According to the calculations of Weissmann and his colleagues, β-interferon went its separate evolutionary way from the α-interferons about 500 million years ago, while the differences within the α-group could have developed in a period of about 33 million years.

In contrast to the heterogeneous nature of the α-interferons, only two human genes for β-interferon have been identified so far. β-Interferon is normally found as a glycoprotein; in SDS-PAGE electrophoresis its molecular weight is 23,000 daltons. When genetically engineered and expressed in *E. coli*, β-interferon does not carry carbohydrate moieties and has a molecular weight of 18,000 daltons. The homology of its amino acid sequence with those of the α-interferons is about 30%. Since the literature reports varying sizes of mRNA species coding for β-interferon, the likelihood of there being as yet undiscovered β-interferons cannot be excluded entirely. But the β-interferons are certainly very far from being as heterogeneous as the α-interferons. Neither the β-interferon gene nor the α-interferon genes contain introns.

In contrast, the only γ-interferon gene known to date contains several introns. The γ-interferon molecule is glycosylated at two sites. In highly purified preparations of γ-interferon three activity peaks have been found at molecular weights of 45,000, 25,000 and 20,000 daltons. All these activities are unstable at pH 2. These differences can be accounted for by three phenomena: in the first place γ-interferon molecules can aggregate to form dimers which may even represent the biologically active form of this lymphokine. Secondly, shorter forms of γ-interferon, lacking several amino acids at the carboxyl end, may occur spontaneously. Such forms retain full biological activity as long as the deletion is not longer than ten amino acids. In fact, these shorter molecules are up to ten times more potent than native γ-interferon. Thirdly, different degrees of glycosylation may account the observed molecular heterogeneity of native γ-interferon. The non-glycosylated, genetically engineered γ-interferon produced in *E. coli* has 146 amino acids and a molecular weight of 17,000 daltons. There is no homology with α- or β-interferons. The genes for α- and β-interferons are located on chromosome 9 while the γ-interferon gene is on chromosome 12.

6.2.2.3 Properties

All interferons have antiviral properties, i.e. they can put cells that are non-infected but nevertheless susceptible to viral infection in a state in which they are resistant to a broad spectrum of pathogens – the "antiviral state". Biochemically this state is characterized by changes in a number of parameters which can be correlated not only with antiviral effects but also with toxic manifestations. Each interferon has its own individual spectrum of cells on which it exerts its effects. All human interferons can convert human cells to an antiviral state. The α-interferons also act effectively on bovine and cat cells, while β-interferon influences rat cells. γ-Interferon does not have an effect on the cells of any of these species. Within the group of α-interferons, recombinant, genetically engineered α_1-interferon is 100 times as effective against bovine cells as against human cells. Hybrid interferons produced by gene fusion, e.g. α_1/α_2-interferon, have a much better effect on murine cells than any of the two original substances.

Besides the antiviral activity of the interferons, particular interest has been focused on the antiproliferative properties of these substances, which were first investigated by Ion Gresser in France during the 1960s. Efforts were initially concentrated on the effect of interferon on tumours experimentally induced in animals with oncogenic viruses. The animals treated with interferon developed fewer tumours and lived longer than the controls. Interferons later proved to offer protection against tumours of demonstrably non-viral origin as well. It was also found that interferon inhibited *in vitro* growth of normal and malignant cells, i.e. it has a direct cytotoxic effect. It was, however, already evident in 1972 that the direct antiproliferative activity alone could not explain curative effects of interferon in animals with tumours: interferon was also effective *in vivo* against experimentally induced leukemia (L 1210), although *in vitro* the tumour cells showed resistance to interferon. We now know that a number of individual effects make up the antitumour activity of interferon observed in clinical practice and in experiments.

The immunomodulatory effects, which will be discussed below, seem to play as important a role as the antiproliferative properties in clinical and experimental cancer therapy. In terms of units of antiviral activity, γ-interferon is more potent than the α- and β-interferons with regard to direct cytotoxic and immunomodulatory effects. It has a synergistic effect with α- and β-interferon in a number of study designs; this synergism is observed in both the antiproliferative and the antiviral effects.

All interferons influence a number of immunological parameters. The effects often depend on the trial conditions: while large doses of interferon prolong survival of skin and organ transplants, small doses often have the opposite effect. The time of administration also seems to influence certain reactions: when administered 24 hours before the sensitizing or DTH (delayed type hypersensitivity) triggering antigen, interferon inhibits the development of such reactions, but if it is administered simultaneously with the antigen, it can intensify them. This effect is possibly due to inhibition of suppressor cells. Similar phenomena are observed with *in vitro* antibody formation in response to sheep erythrocytes: given at the same time as the antigen, interferon inhibits antibody formation, whereas if it is given 48–72 hours after the antigen, it promotes antibody production. The effect of interferons on *in vivo* antibody formation is inconsistent. A clear reduction in circulating B-cells has been observed in patients during treatment with α-interferon, but antibody formation was not directly impaired.

The effects of interferon on the functions of cytotoxic T-cells, T-suppressor cells and T-helper cells have not been clearly defined. They depend too much on the experimental conditions to permit any general conclusions.

In fact, the physiological significance of the interferons does not seem to reside in modulation of the specific B- or T-cell dependent immunity. Rather, it is associated with that primitive, endogenous system of defense against acute threat, of which granulocyte, macrophage and NK-cell functions are also parts. The effects of interferons at this level are actually more distinct than the effects on T-

and B-lymphocytes outlined here only briefly. The effects of interferons on a number of different parameters are remarkably complementary in functional terms: the activity of macrophages is enhanced by interferons; surface adhesion and spread of these cells also increases as does their ability to phagocytose inert particles. The number of Fc receptors on the cell surface also increases. As a result of these changes, Fc receptor-mediated phagocytosis is enhanced six to twelve hours after peak concentrations of interferon in the blood have been attained.

Interferons also enhance the ability of murine macrophages to kill tumour cells. Similarly, the effect of β-interferon on human monocytes enhanced their ability to bring about cytolysis of an SV 40-transformed cell. In connection with antitumour effects, especially of γ-interferon, particular interest has been directed at the effects of interferon on NK-cells. The enhancement of NK-activity against tumour cells that has been described by many authors is presumably based on an accelerated maturation of NK-precursors rather than on enhancement of the cytotoxic potential of mature T-cells. Here too, the activity of γ-interferon seems to be much higher than that of α- and β-interferon if the proteins are compared at doses which have equal antiviral activity. The rather premature designation "immune interferon" therefore seems to be justified after all.

Another essential property of all interferons is the ability to enhance expression of class-I and -II histocompatibility antigens. In this context, too, γ-interferon is much more effective than α- and β-interferons. In connection with enhanced expression of HLA-A, B and C antigens interferons bring about a rise in the formation and release of β_2-microglobulins. This rise can also be determined clinically as a typical interferon effect. As a result of enhanced expression of HLA antigens, foreign cells, such as allogeneic tumour cells, become "more foreign" and therefore more readily recognizable as such. The evolutionary significance of this effect is not immediately apparent, especially since autologous tumour cells do not carry foreign HLA antigens. In fact, NK-cells under the influence of interferon do not exhibit increased activity against autologous tumour cells: possibly this enhanced expression of HLA antigens was originally a defence mechanism for warding off cells of animal or parasitic origin. The enhanced expression of class-II (Ia) genes may be understandable when viewed in the framework of more efficient communication between antigen-presenting cells and lymphocytes.

To sum up, interferons tend to stimulate mainly those functions of the immune system that serve the nonspecific defences. This applies to the phenomenology of the antiviral state as well as to the enhancement of macrophage activity and the more rapid mobilization of NK-cells. The enhanced expression of Fc receptors and histocompatibility antigens of both classes can also be understood in this context, although the latter reactions should achieve a closer association of the "primitive" effector functions with the – in evolutionary terms – younger mechanisms of specific antigen recognition.

In addition, a number of interferon effects have been described which could be classified as "differentiation-promoting" or developmental effects, e.g. the conversion of immature muscle cells to mature, myoglobin-producing cells, inhibition of expression of the globin gene in cells in Friend virus-induced erythroleukemia, stimulation of the methylation of transfer RNA and enhanced expression of carcinoembryonic antigen on tumour cells. This list is by no means complete. The last-mentioned effect, like enhancement of expression of MHC-I genes, might possibly be a means of "demasking", and thus more effectively eliminating, tumour cells. Interferons are also able – as Gresser showed – to convert radiologically transformed cells back to a normal phenotype. There are occasional reports of changes in the motility of cells, which could have an inhibitory influence on the development of tumour metastases.

6.2.2.4 The interferon receptors

In order to exert their physiological or pharmacological functions, interferons must first react with their receptors. According to our present knowledge there are two such receptors: one which binds α- and β_1-interferons and another one for γ-interferon. β_2-Interferon, which is identical with Il-6 binds to its own receptor and is not considered in this context. Cells which are responsive to α- or β-interferon carry between 2×10^2 and 6×10^3 α/β-receptors on their surface. The binding of α- or β-interferon to its receptor is temperature and concentration dependent. At 4°C the binding reaches its maximum after two and a half hours and is saturatable. At 37°C the bound interferon is internalized as measured by the decreasing sensitivity of bound material to trypsin or acid over time. The dissociation constants for the interaction of α- and β-interferons with the corresponding receptor, were found to range from 10^{-9} to 10^{-11} M. So far, no indications of receptor heterogeneity have been found. Cells which do not carry the α/β-receptor are insensitive to α- and β-interferons. The presence of the receptor, on the other hand, does not automatically confer sensitivity to a particular cell: resistant cell lines which carry the receptor have been identified. The species specificity of α- and β-interferons appears to be a consequence of receptor specificity. Some 'irregularities' concerning the interaction of the α/β-receptor and the corresponding interferons remain unexplained. Some cells, e.g. bovine cells, bind α-interferon but not β-interferon. As one would expect, β- and γ-interferon do not compete for binding since they occupy different receptors. There are, however, some reports indicating the contrary. The reasons for these discrepancies are not obvious. Gangliosides have been linked with the binding of interferons – as a matter of fact, for some time they were thought to constitute the receptor or at least part of it. Possibly their unequal representation on the surface of different cells can account for some of the observed irregular phenomena. In most sensitive cells, interferon is internalized after receptor binding. Again, however, there are exceptions: in mouse L1210 cells and in Raji cells, α-interferon was shown to exert biological effects without being internalized. Thus, there is no stringent proof that internalization is a prerequisite for the biological activity of interferons. On the other hand, experiments with liposomes have shown that γ-interferon which is brought to the cell interior via liposome fusion, bypassing the receptor, can also be biologically active. This does not seem to be the case for α- or β-interferons.

The human α/β-receptor gene is located on chromosome 21. The apparent Mr of the receptor is 130,000. The receptor of α/β-receptors on cell surfaces can be down-regulated by α- or β-interferons but not by γ-interferon.

The γ-receptor occurs on cells which are sensitive to γ-interferon at a density of about 10^3 – to 10^4 molecules per cell with dissociation constants ranging from 10^{-9} to 10^{-11} M. The species specificity of interferon γ resides in the structure of its receptor. As is the case with α-interferon, the induction of cellular functions by γ-interferon occurs already at rather low receptor occupancy. The molecular weight of the γ-interferon receptor amounts to 90,000; since the molecule obtained by gene cloning comprises only 500 amino acids, corresponding to a molecular weight of approximately 55,000, the receptor must be heavily glycosylated. In humans, the gene for the γ-interferon receptor is located on chromosome 6. At present, it is not yet clear whether the receptor gene on chromosome 6 is sufficient for inducing all biological functions of interferon γ. Animal cells containing the human chromosome 6, expressing the human γ-interferon were still infected with and destroyed by vesicular stomatitis virus. In experiments with mouse-human and hamster-human cell hybrids both human chromosome 18 and chromosome 21 have been inferred to be essential for the induction of HLA antigen expression by γ-interferon. In mouse B-cells, expressing the human receptor, however, MCH class-I antigen expression was adequately stimulated by γ-interferon without the presence of additional genetic material from human cells.

In view of these somewhat contradictory findings, it is not yet clear whether the γ-interferon receptor alone suffices to transmit all γ-interferon effects or whether additional gene products are needed.

6.2.2.5 Biochemical and molecular changes induced by interferons

A number of biochemical effects, induced by interferons, have been observed in sensitive cells. Some of these changes can be interpreted in connection with important functional alterations such as the antiviral state. Others are not yet understood.

Two enzyme systems which are induced by interferons in sensitive cells have received much attention: the 2′–5′-oligoadenylate synthetase system and the P1/eIF-2α protein kinase system. Since both of these systems, especially the second one, has been linked with the antiviral state induced by interferons, they shall be discussed here in some detail.

2′–5′-oligoadenylate synthetase, which is induced by interferons, catalyses the formation of oligoadenylate molecules with the unusual phosphodiester linkage 2′–5′ instead of 3′–5′, using ATP as the substrate. It is interesting to note that the levels of 2′–5′-oligoadenylate are not increased if cells are treated with interferon alone. Significant increments in the intracellular concentrations of these molecules can only be observed if interferon-treated cells are infected with viruses such as EMC, VSV, influenza virus or vaccinia concomitantly with or shortly after interferon treatment. The reason for this phenomenon relates to the fact that the synthetase activity depends strictly on the presence of double-stranded RNA. Interferon induces the formation of 2′–5′-adenylate synthetase. The newly formed enzyme, however, remains inactive until it binds to double stranded RNA, which can either be provided by the replicative forms of infecting virus or by other forms of double-stranded RNA. 2′–5′-oligoadenylate in turn activates an endonuclease which attacks messenger RNA and to an even greater extent ribosomal RNA. 2′–5′-synthetase has been cloned. The gene specifying the synthesis of this enzyme is located on human chromosome 11. The number of messenger RNA molecules coding for the enzyme increases in response to interferon with kinetics similar to those observed for the synthetase itself. Differential splicing of the primary transcripts leads to the synthesis of mRNA molecules of different lengths, which in turn give rise to synthetases of different size – without obvious consequences for their enzymatic or biological activity.

2′–5′-Oligoadenylate molecules are metabolically quite unstable. They are degraded into AMP and ATP by a phosphodiesterase which occurs in non-induced as well as in interferon-induced cells. In a few cell lines, interferon leads to an increase in the activity of this enzyme. This, however, is not a general phenomenon. The degradation of 2′–5′-oligoadenylate is rapidly followed by a reversion of the oligoadenylate-activated endonuclease to an inactivated state.

The second enzyme, which is induced by interferons and which is also dependent on double stranded RNA, is a protein kinase which specifically phosphorylates the ribosome associated protein P1 and the eukaryotic initiation factor 2 α. Evidence exists that the P1/eIF2α kinase is ribosome associated; in fact, the kinase activity could never be separated physically from P1. Therefore, the conclusion appears justified that P1 and the kinase are identical – and that P1 phosphorylates itself. The purified P1/eIF2 kinase depends on double-stranded RNA for activation just like the 2′–5′-adenylate synthetase. The enzyme is highly specific: it phosphorylates only itself and initiation factor-2α. Other factors involved in protein biosynthesis are no substrates for this enzyme. O-Phosphoserine is the main phosphoester linkage produced by eIF-2α kinase. Interestingly, this enzyme is induced by α- and β-interferons to a much higher degree than by γ-interferon. There is evidence indicating that the inhibition of protein synthesis produced by phosphorylation of the α-subunit of eIF-2 is more essential for the induction of the antiviral state than the 2′–5′ adenylate synthetase. Both systems, the synthetase and the protein kinase, however, seem to be instrumental in the inhibition of protein synthesis and consequently in bringing about the antiproliferative effect *(Fig. 6.3)*.

A phosphoprotein phosphatase present in non-treated as well as in interferon-treated cells is responsible for removing the phosphate moieties from P1 and the α subunit of eIF-2.

Other well known proteins which are induced in interferon-treated cells include metallothionine II, thymosin B4, the major histocompatibility complex genes and the so-called protein Mx. All of these proteins seem to be augmented by transcriptional activation.

All three interferons, α, β and γ, induce the expression of class-I genes in a variety of cells. As one might expect, the expression of the β2-microglobulin gene is also stimulated by interferons. Interferon γ – but not interferon α – is a potent stimulator of the expression of class-II and class-III MHC genes, including some complement components like C2 and factor B.

The increased expression of MHC class-I genes may facilitate cytotoxic reactions and may be responsible for part of the antiviral and antiproliferative responses observed after interferon treatment. The stimulation of class-II expres-

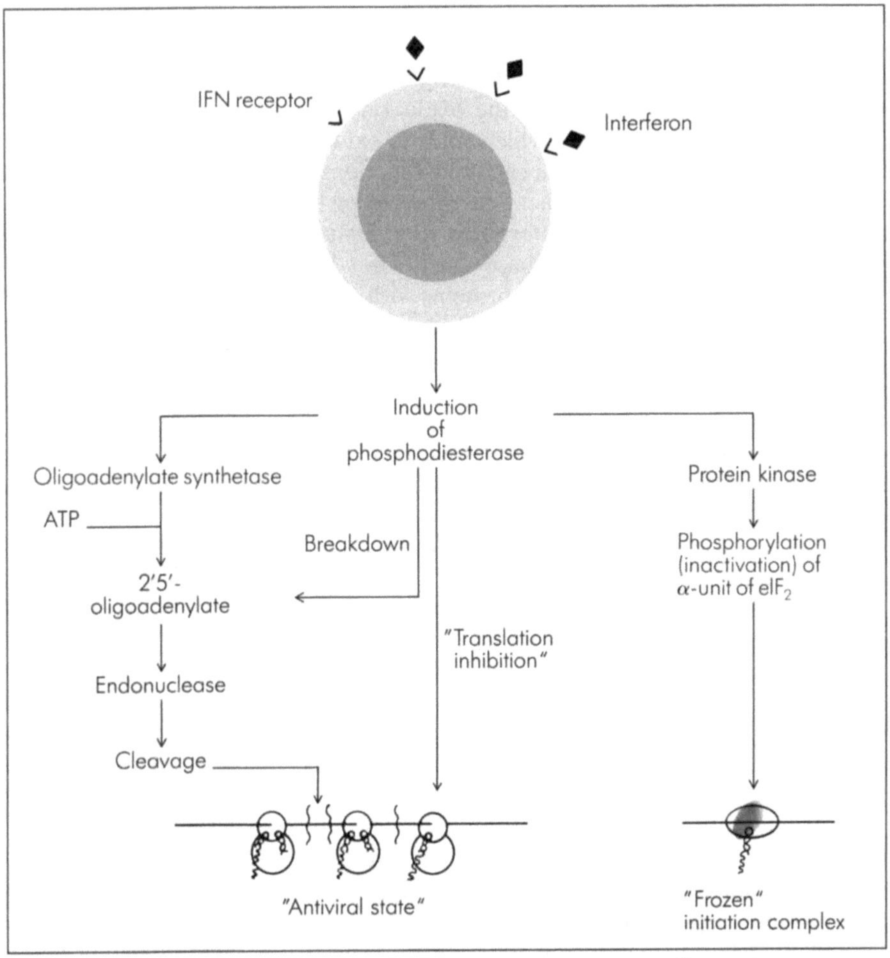

Figure 6.3. Biochemical characteristics of the "antiviral state" produced by interferon.

sion on the other hand, could be a more general prerequisite for interaction between immune cells, e.g. between antigen presenting cells and various subsets of T-cells. The fact that the expression of class-III genes is also enhanced as a consequence of interferon action points to the general immune-stimulating properties of interferons.

Recently a protein called Mx was described, which can be induced by α-interferon in a mouse strain, which is intrinsically resistant to influenza virus infections. γ-interferon does not induce the formation of this 75 kd protein which accumulated in the cell nucleus in mouse cells. An analogous protein occurs in human cells after interferon induction. This protein is also inducible by α- and β-, but not by γ-interferon. Unlike the mouse protein, the human Mx protein is located in the cytoplasm. The protein seems to be important in conferring upon cells resistance against influenza viruses: Mx-mouse cells are sensitive to influenza infections, but can be made resistant, if transfected with DNA which contains an intact copy of the Mx gene.

A number of additional peptides are induced in interferon-treated cells: xanthine oxidase which catalyses the oxidation of xanthine and hypoxanthine, and indolamine 2,3 oxygenase which leads to oxidative cleavage of indole rings, are two important enzymes with catabolic functions.

Of particular interest is the fact that γ-interferon induces some peptides which are not seen after α- or β-interferon. For instance, γ-interferon induces a polyamine-dependent protein kinase which is not dependent on double-stranded RNA and phosphorylates cellular proteins with molecular weights of 68,000 and 72,000 daltons. These findings are difficult to interpret at present, but they illustrate the differences between α- and β-interferons on the one hand, and γ-interferon on the other.

Interferons stimulate the synthesis of prostaglandins. The antiviral effect induced by interferon can be reversed by cyclooxygenase inhibitors. There have also been reports that certain side effects of interferon such as fever can be reduced by intrathecal administration of indomethacin.

It is as yet uncertain which biochemical effects of the interferons are causally related to their antiproliferative effects. The possible role of 2′5′-oligoadenylic acids and the P1/eIF2α system have already been mentioned. Recent flow cytometry investigations have showed that tumour cells in the G_0 and G_1 phases were those most affected by the antiproliferative activity.

Interferons inhibit ornithine decarboxylase, the enzyme that catalyses the first rate-limiting step in polyamine synthesis and is involved in many cellular regulatory processes. Perhaps this finding represents a biochemical correlate for the effects of interferons on differentiation.

Under the influence of interferons, cells develop a more rigid membrane of lower fluidity. The glycoproteins are redistributed on the cell surface. The enzyme that catalyses the synthesis of N-acetylglucosaminyl-dolichyl-phosphates from uridine disphosphate-N-acetylglucosamine and dolichyl phosphates is inhibited. Interferon-treated cells thus release viruses that lack important glycoproteins and are therefore no longer infective.

6.2.2.6 Physiological role of the interferons

An important step towards achieving an understanding of the physiological function of the interferons is the assessment of the role played by these substances in healthy and infected individuals.

In normal, uninfected animals or humans, interferons in the plasma occur only in traces and are hardly measurable. Basically, interferons are substances which are secreted in a paracrine or autocrine fashion. Their occasional classification as 'hormones' reveals neglect of this fact. Interferons, like other cytokines, are mainly formed in lymphatic tissue, which is closely associated with body surfaces – like the gut, associated lymphoid tissue, the thoracic duct associated tissue, the bronchial-associated tissue and the skin-associated tissue. The intimate contact of immune cells and mainly microbial antigens at these interphases leads to frequent or even constant activation of the cells which 'defend' such surfaces. The presence of α- and of γ-interferon in such tissues is much higher than the low plasma levels might indicate. As a matter of fact, interferons are typical substances which act locally: their concentration in the lymph is low. After draining of the lymph into the blood-stream, it can hardly be measured, even with sensitive assays which detect a few units per ml (equivalent to about 10^{-13} M). In acute and generalized infections, however, the picture can change dramatically.

In some experimental and clinical infections there is an early rise in blood interferon levels. In clinical mumps the titres reach a peak on the first day of the illness and decline thereafter. In the first few days of an influenza infection the increase in titre is due largely to a change in α-interferon. Subsequently, another interferon dominates that is not identical with α-interferon. The physiological relevance of the rise in blood levels of interferon in virally infected experimental animals or in patients seems to be confirmed by experiments in which mice were given specific interferon-neutralizing antisera before being inoculated with herpes virus, Semliki Forest virus or with the causative organism of chronic lymphocytic choriomeningitis. In all these cases the disease followed a more severe course and virus titres were higher than in the controls.

In the late stages of AIDS, α-interferon levels in the plasma can be distinctly elevated. As a matter of fact, some of the symptoms of this disease, such as fatigue, fever, malaise and myalgia could be attributed to elevated interferon levels. It is, however, not normal α-interferon which is increased, but an atypical α-interferon which is acid-labile like γ-interferon. This material appears to be produced by NK-cells.

The same type of interferon was also found in patients with systemic lupus erythematosus. Some clinical significance can probably be attributed to the ability of peripheral mononuclear cells to form and secrete interferon in vitro as a response to mitogens or antigens. In certain types of immune deficiency, such as in the early stages of the acquired immune deficiency syndrome (AIDS), this ability is greatly reduced with respect to both α- and γ-interferon. This deficiency, which cannot be compensated by Il-2, may be an important correlate of the breakdown of immune defences in this disease.

6.2.2.7 Clinical uses of interferons

The interferons which are in current clinical use (1989) can be divided into several major groups: the partially purified natural interferons, the highly purified natural interferons and the highly purified genetically engineered interferons. For a long time the interferon which was obtained from leucocyte supernatants from door blood and which was made available by Kari Cantell in Helsinki was the only one that could be used for clinical purposes. Only 1% of it consisted of interferon, i.e. different α-interferons, while almost 99% comprised auxiliary substances. It was later purified to an interferon content of over 90% with the help of monoclonal antibodies. A preparation containing mostly α-interferons was also obtained from lymphoblastoid cells, the "Namalva" cells. This preparation sometimes contained rather large amounts (5–10%) of β-interferon. Fibroblast interferon consists almost entirely of β-interferon. Most clinical trials were carried out with preparations of about 10% purity. In the meanwhile, however, highly purified genetically engineered β-interferon has been made available; it differs from natural β-interferon in not possessing a carbohydrate portion.

Clinical trials were also being performed until recently with an approximately 10% γ-interferon from human lymphocytes. In the meantime, there has been an increasing shift of interest to the highly purified recombinant interferons (which include several α- as well as β- and γ-types).

Pharmacokinetics. The pharmacokinetics of interferons often vary quite considerably. Since β-interferon cannot be taken up in sufficient amounts from an intramuscular depot, it has to be administered intravenously. α-Interferons, on the other hand, are quantitatively absorbed from the site of injection when given i.m. or s.c. The pharmacokinetics of the most commonly used recombinant α_2-interferons are similar to those of natural α_2-interferon. This is not true of all interferons. Recombinant α_1-interferon, for instance, disappears from the circulation more rapidly than natural α_1-interferon despite comparable invasion times. Peak plasma levels are generally found two hours after i.m. and four hours after s.c. injection. Therapeutically effective plasma levels are still demonstrable 24

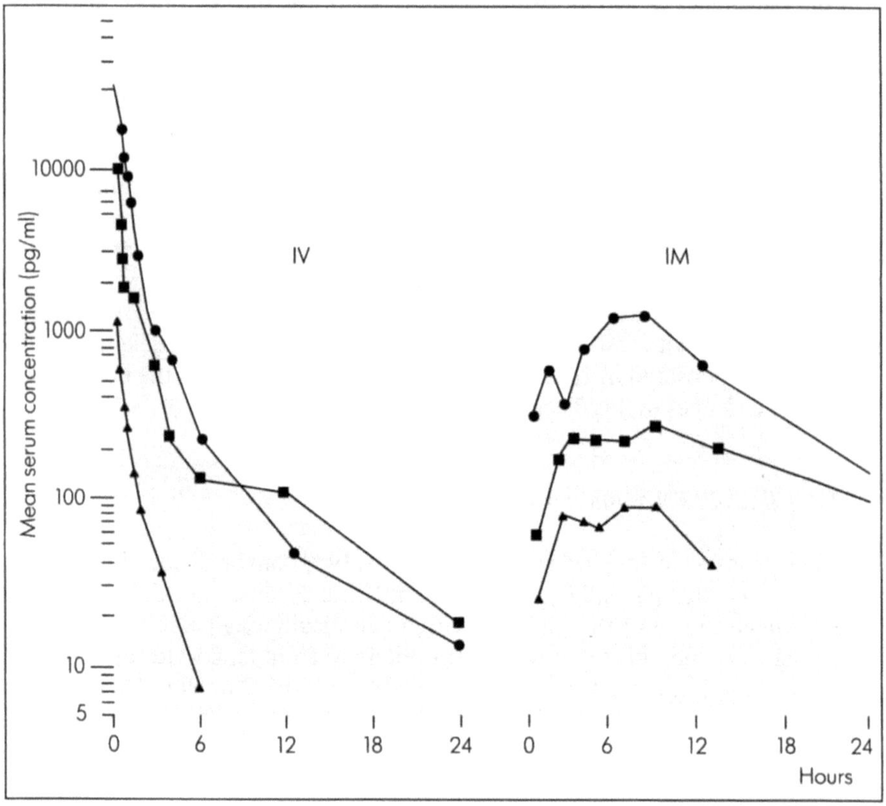

Figure 6.4. Mean concentration of recombinant leukocyte interferon in serum after intravenous or intramuscular administration of 3 (▲), 9 (■) or 18 (●) × 10^6 units. Every point is the mean value of 3 subjects.

Table 6.3. Side effects of treatment with alpha (lymphoblastoid) and beta (fibroblast) interferons (22 patients per group). Incidence as percentage (Doses in megaunits).

Symptom of finding	Alpha IFN 0.3–30 i.m.	Beta IFN 3–30 i.v.
Fever	86.3	90.9
Chills	54.5	63.6
Fatigue	50.0	63.6
Loss of appetite	45.4	31.8
Nausea	13.6	4.4
Headache	9.0	9.0
Pain	9.0	9.0
Dizziness	4.5	9.0
Diarrhea	3.6	–
Leucocytopenia	22.7	22.7
Thrombocytopenia	18.1	13.6
Hepatotoxicity	4.5	40.4

hours after administration of higher doses (9–18 $\times 10^6$ units). *Fig. 6.4* shows the mean interferon concentrations after i.v. or i.m. injection of recombinant α_2-interferon (which is identical with 2a) in 9 healthy volunteers. The half-lives derived from this example are between 0.75 and two hours on intravenous administration, and between 2.6 and 5 hours on intramuscular administration. Despite the range of individual values, these figures show that parenteral interferon therapy with practicable dosage intervals is possible. Though absorption, distribution and elimination must be thoroughly investigated, as things stand today, the kinetic parameters do not in principle constitute limiting factors for the success or failure of interferon therapy. The latest findings suggest that interferons are mainly broken down in the kidneys.

Adverse reactions. When the first – scarcely purified – leucocyte interferons were investigated, it was observed that they caused fever and a number of other effects that were often designated "flu-like" symptoms in the Anglo-Saxon literature. There were initial doubts as to whether these symptoms (fever, maylgia, malaise, chills and fatigue) were caused by the interferon itself or, as was thought more likely, by the large amounts of impurities that were administered with the interferon. It is now known that interferon is the cause of these adverse reactions. What is more, in view of the modulation of important biosynthetic functions, such toxic phenomena are not particularly surprising.

Table 6.3 summarizes the adverse reactions observed in Japanese clinics in phase-1 studies of α- and β-interferon. The incidences of toxic symptoms are probably more or less in line with those observed in Europa and the USA. It should, however, be pointed out that dizziness, with an incidence of 4.5 and 9%, must be regarded as a manifestation of neurotoxicity of interferons. This toxicity also manifests itself in confusion, depression, an impaired sense of taste and smell and reversible EEG changes. Sudden death has also been observed under interferon therapy, particularly in France. Fortunately, further investigations in the US have not conformed this finding. On the other hand, cardiac arrhythmias have occasionally been seen in patients given high-dose therapy.

Therapeutic properties. The hopes placed in the interferons were for a long time unrealistically high. But on account of the heterogeneity of the preparations and differences in the dosages and modes of administration used, both their use and the assessment of their value have proved to be much more complicated than was originally expected. A further complicating factor – particularly in the field of oncology – was the heterogeneity of the clinical situations in which the interferons were used.

Only recently have precisely defined indications emerged in the fields of viral infections and tumours. These indications are discussed below.

Encouraging results have been obtained in the treatment of chronic hepatitis B. The Stanford group in particular repeatedly reported rapid and reproducible reduction of virus-associated antigens in the blood. Interferon therapy brings about a fall in the Dane particle, a decline in the DNA polymerase activity associated with this particle, and a drop in the HBs-antigen and Hbe-antigen titres. In about 60–100% of the groups treated with interferon, virus-associated markers disappeared from the blood. These findings were obtained with leucocyte interferon but have been reproduced elsewhere with other natural and recombinant interferons.

In a recent study 34 male hepatitis B carriers with active viral replication were treated with up to 10 megaunits of lymphoblastoid interferon/m^2 body surface daily for six months. In all interferon-treated cases viral DNA polymerase became detectable. Of the 23 treated patients, 11 experienced a 'hepatitis-like illness' between eight and twelve weeks after the initiation of treatment. In this study, the amino aspartate transferase levels during this illness correlated with permanent cure of the affected patients from their chronic hepatitis. Only the 6 patients in which the AST levels rose to ten times the normal values or higher experienced complete and permanent remission with disappearance of Hbs and Hbe antigens and development of anti-Hbe antibodies. Five patients who had only moderately increased AST levels became positive again towards the end or after cessation of treatment. In all patients who did not experience a 'hepatitis-B-like illness', the DNA polymerase was substantially inhibited but never became negative. The immune mechanism underlying the acute illness is not clear. One could speculate that activation of cytotoxic T-cells and subsequent lysis of infected liver cells occurred in some patients and that this mechanism is involved in the clearance of infectious particles from the liver.

Very promising results have also been obtained with interferon in patients with certain virally induced tumours. Interferon even seems to be the treatment of choice in juvenile papillomas of the larynx: more recent results show that cure can be expected in over 50% of patients.

Condylomata acuminata of the genital organs caused by human papilloma virus (HPV) have been shown to respond very well to administration of relatively low doses of α-interferon. The daily doses of α-interferon which proved effective in this sexually transmitted disease ranged between 0.5×10^6 and 3×10^6 daily as i.m. injection units. These doses are usually given i.m. for one month and then t.i.d. for up to fifteen weeks of total treatment. The response rates of this and similar schedules have been in the range of 60–80%. Relapses, however, occur in up to 45% of all patients. β- and especially γ-interferon have also been shown to be effective. In refractory cases, cryosurgery followed by systemic and local treatment with interferon α is often used successfully. Less favourable cure rates of, still, 20% have been reported for treatment of warts and condylomata lata.

Local α-interferon administered (as a nasal spray) at an early stage during rhinovirus infection seems to alleviate the subjective and objective symptoms of the ensuing rhinitis. This experience, which has been confirmed by a number of authors, provided the basis for the development of a corresponding pharmaceutical formulation. Treatment must continue for several days and the total dosage must amount to about 15 million units. Nasal congestion and bleeding can occur as a side-effect and may turn out to be prohibitive for this route of administration.

Recurrent varicella zoster infection represents another indication for interferon therapy. Early initiation of therapy, i.e. on the appearance of the first lesions, with daily dosages of 5×10^5 units per kg can influence the course of the illness. Patients treated with interferon develop fewer vesicles at the primary dermatome, less pain, fewer post-therapeutic neuralgias and fewer visceral complications. In addition, acute varicella infections in children with leukemia respond to interferon.

Herpes simplex keratitis also seems to respond to local administration of interferon. The daily dosage should amount to about 10^6 units. Treatment must be continued for at least seven days.

As one might expect, interferons have been and are being tried in the acquired immune deficiency syndrome. While there is no unequivocal evidence for a role of interferons in the retroviral infection itself, good results have been obtained in the treatment of Kaposi's sarcoma, which is one of the most frequent manifestations of frank AIDS. Up to 60% (on average around 25%) of all patients with Kaposi's sarcoma experience a major response which means that the tumour will disappear or shrink by at least 50%.

More recently, low doses of α-interferon are also being tested in conjunction with reduced doses of AZT in patients with AIDS or with the AIDS-related complex (ARC). The data available at the time of writing do not suffice to draw any conclusions; tentative evidence, however, seems to indicate that clinical improvement as measured by an increase in CD4 cells can be achieved with this combination.

Some attempts to cure cytomegalovirus infections in immunosuppressed patients with interferon have proved unsuccessful: although a fall in virus titre was observed in several cases, an unequivocal clinical improvement was not obtained.

The great, and probably somewhat irrational, hope that interferons would be a major addition to cancer therapy – on a level, say, with surgery, irradiation and chemotherapy – has not been fulfilled. Interferons have so far been a disappointment in the treatment of solid tumours such as bronchial carcinoma, colorectal carcinoma, and breast and ovarian carcinoma.

In 1983 Priestman reported on a series of clinical studies in which patients with advanced solid tumours were assessed according to standardized criteria. A total of 150 patients were involved, with renal cell carcinoma (47), melanoma (51), breast carcinoma (23), small-cell bronchial carcinoma (10) and non-small-cell bronchial carcinoma (19). All patients were given intramuscular alpha-interferon at daily doses of between 3 and 50 million international units for at least 28 days. Patients who reacted to the therapy with an objectifiable reduction of at least 50% in the measurable tumour mass over a period of four weeks were rated as responders. According to this criterion, which of course does not mean "cure", a response was seen in 7–10% of all patients with renal cell carcinoma, 3–6% of melanoma patients and 22% of patients with breast carcinoma. But not a single patient with bronchial carcinoma responded to the therapy. The results in the treatment of malignant melanoma and of renal cell carcinoma have since been improved: The response rates are in the order of 8–20% for metastasizing malignant melanoma (depending on the stage of disease) and between 20 and 30% for renal cell carcinoma.

With these reservations, however, we must confirm that the generally negative results obtained with interferons in the treatment of solid tumours have not been improved. Kaposi's sarcoma, which develops in 50% of all patients with the acquired immune deficiency syndrome (AIDS), is a positive exception.

Interferon has been investigated in treatment of osteogenic sarcoma (osteosarcoma), particularly in Sweden. But although the results obtained since 1972 with local resection and concomitant interferon therapy seemed to be better than those obtained earlier with radical surgery alone, these early results were not confirmed. The same applies to interferon treatment of glioblastomas. Positive reports have been published. They have, however, never been extensively verified.

In malignant systemic diseases, on the other hand, the general picture is much more positive. Hairy cell leukemia is a rare condition which is characterized by an uncontrolled chronic proliferation of atypical B-cells, splenomegaly, anemia and an increasing proneness to infections. This disease may go into permanent remission after splenomectomy. α-Interferons have proved to be very effective in this condition, inducing partial or complete remissions in more than 80% of all patients. The doses employed so far have varied greatly, ranging from less than 3×10^6 units three times a week to 12 million units daily for several months up to more than one year. In spite of these encouraging results, important questions regarding this therapeutic approach remain open: first, we do not know the optimal dosage regime. Secondly, the optimal duration of therapy has not been defined. Thirdly, and perhaps most importantly, we do not know whether combinations of α-interferon and other cytostatic drugs, e.g. deoxycoformcyin may not allow for even better results. Non-Hodgkin lymphomas represent another sensitive target for therapy with α-interferons. For cutaneous T-cell lymphomas the response rates have been between 40 and 60% even in cases with advanced disease. Clearly lymphomas with a slow proliferation rate and low degree of malignancy react better to interferon treatment than highly malignant lymphomas. In the latter, the response rates are in the range of 10–15%.

Chronic lymphatic leukemia is a diffusely proliferating lymphoma with a low degree of malignancy. Response rates to α-interferons have been disappointingly low, in the range of 10–20%. Similar rates have been obtained in multiple myeloma. Remissions or partial remissions in 20% of all cases can be observed after six to ten weeks of treatment.

Another, more encouraging, chapter of α-interferon therapy is represented by chronic myelogenous leukemia. No satisfactory cytostatic therapy has so far been developed. Therefore an attempt with α-interferon appeared particularly justified. Results available so far indicate that a normalization of blood leucocytes lasting from a few months to more than two years can be achieved within six to twelve weeks of therapy.

Chronic myelogenous leukemia is characterized by an abnormal chromosome, the Philadelphia chromosome (Ph 1). In molecular terms the abnormality, which can be morphologically recognized under the light microscope, results from translocation of a protooncogene c-abl from chromosome 9, where it is normally located, to chromosome 22. On chromosome 22, the c-abl gene is inserted in the direct vicinity of the so-called bcr region. A new mRNA is then transcribed from the 'bcr-abl' rearrangement site, which gives rise to the synthesis of a fusion protein. This protein has a tyrosine kinase activity which is similar to that of the tyrosine kinase specified by the viral analogue of c-abl. In some cases, interferon treatment leads to the disappearance of all cells carrying the Ph 1 chromosome. In view of these results, it appears likely that α-interferons, perhaps in connection with cytotoxic agents yet to be selected, will be part of the future therapy of this disease.

An interesting, though somewhat exotic, clinical indication has recently been identified for the use of γ-interferon. Certain forms of x-linked chronic granulomatous disease are due to a low expression rate of the 91 kd glycosylated heavy chain of the cytochrome b of phagocytes. This enzyme, in turn, is part of a membran-associated NAPH oxidase which produces superoxides and related toxic oxygen metabolites (see also Chapter 2). γ-Interferon has been shown to partially correct the low levels of gene expression and to improve and even normalize oxygen radical formation and bactericidal potential in granulocytes. The effects were observed after subcutaneous infection of γ-interferon (0.1 mg/m^2 of body surface) on two consecutive days. Further clinical studies of this effect seem warranted.

6.2.2.8 Synopsis, prospects

From the therapist's viewpoint more than 30 years after the pioneering publication of Isaacs and Lindenmann, the therapeutic results with interferons have, perhaps, been somewhat disappointing. Enormous efforts have been made over many years to isolate, characterize, purify and produce interferon in large amounts for therapeutic purposes. Despite the success of these efforts, the results so far achieved are not in proportion to the efforts or the hopes that have been invested in interferon. A failure, then? Far from it. Such a verdict would be in line with the short-term utilitarian thinking of a marketing manager. In the first place, research cannot be judged from the viewpoint of short-term therapeutic usefulness alone. Secondly, interferon research has made a great contribution to our understanding – vastly increased compared with 1957 – of the function of the immune system and hence has provided a basis for the development of future therapeutic approaches. And, after all, the therapeutic potential of interferon therapy is only beginning to be exploited! Dealing with these proteins is far more complicated than was originally anticipated. But were the hopes placed in them ever realistic? Interferons are substances which, administered in low doses, exert defensive activity within a complex network of cell-mediated and humoral functions. We have seen that its primary effect is enhancement of nonspecific defences. Can such substances which are administered in unphysiologically high doses – without simultaneously influencing other immune functions – be expected to exert the full therapeutic potential that they possibly carry ? There is no answer to this question at the moment, though the implications are negative. But comparison with glucocorticosteroid therapy shows that physiological concentrations are not always therapeutic concentrations. Several pathways warrant exploration: continuation of high-dosage therapy with individual interferons, particularly in cases of fresh, previously untreated tumours; secondly, combination of interferons with interleukins, cytostatics or, for that matter, other interferons; thirdly, the exploration of interferon administered in low doses alone or in combination with other agents.

Does γ-interferon really complement the effects of α- or β-interferons? Are hybrids produced by gene fusion from α- and γ-interferons or from other interferons more effective and better tolerated than the parent substances?

Some of these questions can already be answered in part. Combination of α_2-interferon with acyclovir or with adenine arabinoside has been shown to be effective in both clinical and experimental viral infections. Interesting results are also available on the effects of α_2-interferon and α-difluoromethyl ornithine, an inhibitor of ornithine decarboxylase and thus of polyamine synthesis. Renal adenocarcinomas of human origin which were transplanted to the thymectomized (nude) mouse were more markedly inhibited by a combination of the two substances than by either of the substances on their own. Attempts have, of course, already been made to incorporate interferon into chemotherapeutic regimens but even an interim judgment in this respect would be premature. Combination of γ-interferon and interleukin 2 in immunocompromised patients is, of course, an obvious approach in view of the functions of the two lymphokines. But, so far, there is a complete lack of relevant clinical experience.

Preliminary experimental results with α-interferon and interleukin-2 have shown true synergy of the two compounds which could be represented in typical isobolograms. Some of these surprisingly synergistic effects have also been seen in humans. Clinical studies, now on the way, will tell whether the combined application of these lymphokines will work on human tumours. Since the synergics observed so far allow a reduction of the doses of both agents as compared with monotherapy, the combined use of Il-2 and α-interferon is bound to be better tolerated than any of the two agents alone. Interferon-α has been shown to 'sensitize' certain solid tumours like colon carcinomas for the action of 5-fluorouracil. This synergism is currently being studied clinically.

Research in the fields of molecular biology and immunology in the last few years have opened up broad channels of access to the interferons for pharmacologists and clinicians. It is now up to the therapeutically orientated sciences to exploit the newly gained territory. After unjustified optimistic expectations and an equally unwarranted pessimism, the pendulum of medical judgment is now swinging back into a position of reason. Miracles are not to be expected but steady progress is likely to be made. A reassessment of the situation in five years' time may show that the therapeutic advances which the interferons will then have constituted can be very substantial.

6.2.2.9 Interferon inducers

Interferon is induced not only by viruses but also by double-stranded RNA, synthetic double-strand polynucleotides and, for that matter, by a number of polymeric polyanionic substances such as lipopolysaccharides (LPS), pyran-copolymer and many others. Induction of interferon by these substances is probably always a pleomorphic reaction that includes activation of macrophages and a great many other functions associated with nonspecific defences.

At a time when interferons were not available in unlimited amounts and with a high degree of purity, the idea of synthesizing endogenous interferon in the infected or tumour-bearing organism had a certain attraction. But now that interferons can be produced in any amount and degree of purity by genetic engineering, the idea has lost some of its appeal. The amounts of interferon that can be obtained in the body by means of interferon inducers are much lower than what can be supplied exogeneously.

The experimental and, particularly, the clinical studies carried out with many interferon inducers have proved to be disappointing. The results have failed to come up to expectations, even lagging behind the therapeutic effects of the interferons themselves. In addition, both poly I:C and pyran-copolymer have proved to be highly toxic compounds. Poly I:C was administered mainly to patients with advanced tumours in doses ranging from 0.3 to 75 mg per m^2 body surface. Fever, chills, nausea, vomiting, weight loss and cytopenia occurred as side effects. Remissions were not obtained in this groups of patients and were very rarely seen in patients with less advanced disease. Poly I:C stabilized with poly L-lysine also proved to be extremely toxic in man. The same applies to pyran-copolymer and even to double-stranded RNA: in animal experiments these substances, administered in therapeutic doses, proved to be associated with increased acute lethality, pyrogenic effects, suppression of hematopoiesis, coagulopathies and direct cytotoxicity. Unfortunately, the side effects observed in experiments also occurred in clinical use.

On the assumption that the toxicity of double-strand and, in some cases, stabilized polynucleotides is due at least in part to their stability towards nucleases and their long sojourn in the body, Ts'o and his colleagues, and Carter and his colleagues produced polynucleotides with "mismatched" bases, e.g. $rI_n{:}r(C_{12}U)_n$. These "mismatched" polynucleotides proved to be virtually as effective in the mouse as poly I:C but caused much fewer side effects. One such preparation named "Ampligen" was tested clinically in cancer patients and in patients with AIDS. Apparently the drug was well tolerated. However, the clinical results obtained so far have been disappointing. While the final judgement on this agent cannot yet be made, its further clinical development appears rather unlikely.

6.2.3 Interleukin 2

6.2.3.1 Definition and history

In 1976 Morgan, Ruscetti and Gallo discovered that T-cells from human bone marrow could be cultured in vitro over a period of months under the influence of supernatants of mitogen-stimulated lymphocyte cultures. Gallo and his colleagues designated the biological activity underlying the phenomenon "T-cell growth factor" or TCGF. This factor had already figured in the literature under a variety of names, but its existence and activity had never been so precisely described. It was agreed in 1979 to name this factor interleukin 2 (Il-2), and it is under this designation that it has since been described and characterized. Interleukin 2 plays an indispensable role in the mobilization of the immune response. If a resting T-lymphocyte encounters a foreign antigen which it recognizes by virtue of its specific receptor in association with histocompatibility antigens on antigen-presenting cells, then the lymphocyte expresses the interleukin 2 receptor on its surface within eight to twelve hours. This receptor, a heterodimer comprising the tac subunit of 55,000 daltons and a 75,000 dalton subunit has a very high affinity for interleukin 2 (see Chapter 2). As far as we know today, it is expressed exclusively on activated T-lymphocytes and never on resting cells. More recent findings suggest that interleukin 2 is also needed for clonal expansion of B-cells, a fact which suggests that activated B-cells can also express an Il-2 receptor (see Chapter 2).

Expression of the interleukin-2 receptor, which can be triggered by an antigen or by T-cell mitogens such as concanavalin A, is designated step one of T-cell activation. The same antigenic or mitogenic stimulus brings about the synthesis and release of interleukin 2 in the T-helper cells, a subpopulation of T-lymphocytes. These cells also express the interleukin-2 receptor. Whether a cell expresses only the interleukin-2 receptor and becomes a T-suppressor cell or a cytotoxic cell, or whether it also produces interleukin 2 (helper cells) depends, according to some authors, only on the histocompatibility "environment" in which the antigen is presented to the lymphocyte. Recognition of the antigen in association with class I histocompatibility antigens leads to the development of suppressor T-cells or cytotoxic T-cells. On the other hand, a T-lymphocyte to which the antigen is presented in association with a class-II antigen develops into a T-helper cell. It should, however, be borne in mind that a growing number of authors question whether the production of interleukin 2 is restricted to T-helper cells. More recent data suggest that cytotoxic T-cells also produce interleukin 2 and at the same time react to it. This situation is known as "autocrine stimulation". In addition, it is assumed that production of interleukin 2 requires a second stimulus, i.e. recognition of interleukin 1. Il-1 is a cytokine formed by stimulated monocytes or other antigen-presenting cells. During the interaction of an antigen-presenting cell with a T-lymphocyte, Il-1 is secreted by the former and provides the "second stimulus" to the T-cell. The synthesis of interleukin 2 by T-helper cells is designated the second phase of T-lymphocyte activation. The third phase of T-cell activation, the actual proliferation of T-cell clones, stems exclusively from the interaction of interleukin 2 with its receptor, regardless of whether the T-cell is a cytotoxic, helper or suppressor cell.

Interleukin 2 is a protein with 153 amino acids. There seems to be only one gene for interleukin 2; in man it is located on chromosome 4. It has one short intron and two larger introns which comprise more than two kilobases each. Until genetically engineered interleukin 2 became available in 1984, the most important source of the substance had been the Jurkat cell, a T-lymphoma cell growing in cell cultures. On stimulation by a lectin, the Jurkat cell produces large amounts of interleukin 2, and the yield can be considerably boosted by simultaneous stimulation with lectin and 4-phorbol-12-myristine-13-acetate. An alternative, though less productive, source are human mononuclear cells stimulated by concanavalin A. The human interleukin-2 molecule is glycosylated on a threonine in position 3. The heterogeneous behaviour of different types of interleukin 2 in electrophoresis is very probably due to differences in the degree of glycosylation. When obtained from genetically engineered clones of *E. coli,* Il-2 is, of course, non-glycosylated. In this form the molecule is very lipophilic and only weakly soluble in water. In the early days of its production, this fact caused difficulties in providing suitable and fully active dosage forms. These problems, however, have been overcome.

6.2.3.2 Properties

Il-2 can induce proliferation of all T-cells that have been activated by contact with an antigen and Il-1 or with mitogens. Purified and unpurified Il-2 have been used to clone individual T-cells and bring about clonal expansion of these cells. Large amounts of T-cells with helper or with cytotoxic properties can be produced in this way.

Like γ-interferon, Il-2 promotes the maturation of NK-cells. The effect observed with Il-2, however, considerably surpasses the activity of γ-interferon. The two lymphokines have a synergistic effect in NK-cell activation. γ-Interferon seems to play an initiator role in the maturation process, while Il-2 controls its later stages. Cyclic AMP antagonizes the synergistic action of Il-2. Il-2 triggers the formation and secretion of γ-interferon in T-lymphocytes. Therefore the above-mentioned synergism may come into play even if Il-2 is added to lymphocytes alone. It is still uncertain whether the macrophage activation which has also been observed under the influence of Il-2 is only due to the Il-2-induced γ-interferon or whether it represents an independent effect of this lymphokine. Apparently, Il-2 also induces in T-cells the formation of lymphokines, which promote the proliferation of B-cells (B-cell growth factor?). The lymphokine thus appears to play a key role as a growth and differentiation signal in the immune system *(Fig. 6.5).*

The ability of Il-2 to expand cytotoxic lymphocytes became the basis of so-called adoptive immunotherapy. In principle, this experimental therapy is carried out as follows: mice are initially immunized in vitro with syngeneic or allogeneic tumour cells. Consequently the animals generate cytotoxic lymphocytes against the antigens of these tumour cells. These cytotoxic lymphocytes are then culti-

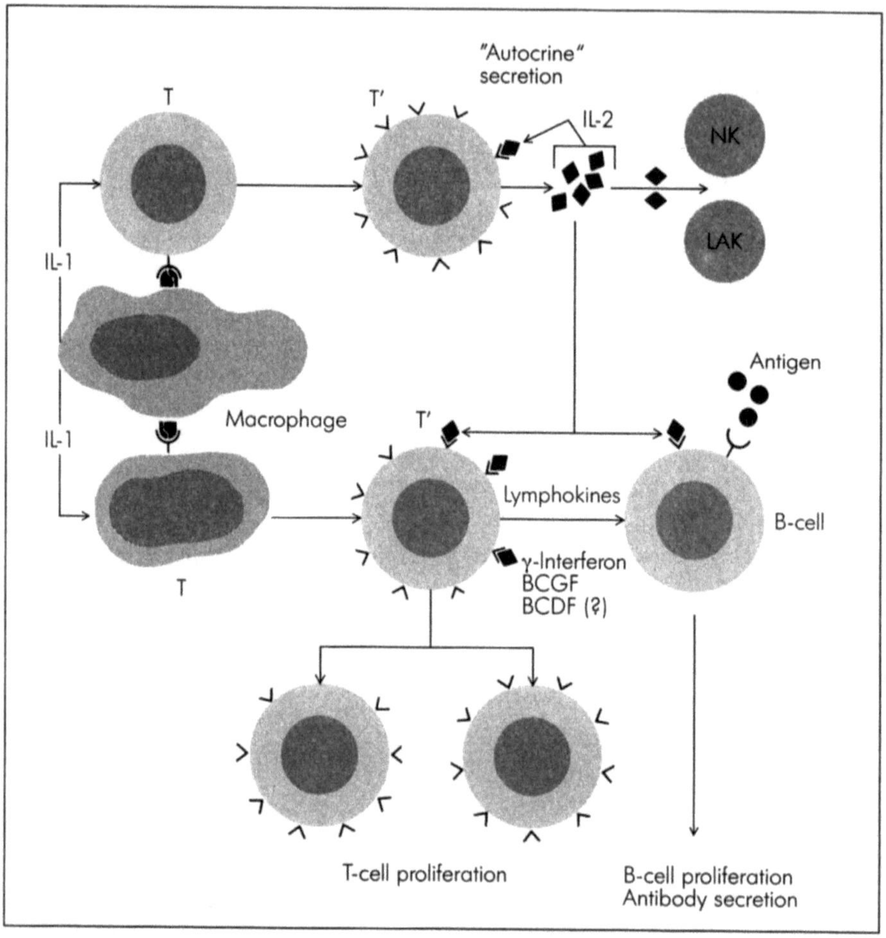

Figure 6.5. Diagram of the main functions of IL-2 in the immune system. The antigen presented by an accessory cell is recognized in association with a histocompatibility antigen by the T-cell receptor of a T-lymphocyte. The T-lymphocyte (T) is "activated" by this process and by a humoral stimulus. It forms IL-2 receptors and begins to secrete IL-2. IL-2 now brings about clonal expansion of activated T-cells. In addition, IL-2 induces recruitment and activation of NK and LAK cells and also influences the proliferation of B-cells after contact with antigen.

vated and expanded with Il-2 in the presence of the tumour cells that have been used for the immunization. Since only those cells that have reacted to the tumour antigens will have expressed their Il-2 receptors, these are the only cells that react to Il-2. Thus, cytotoxic T-cells directed against the tumour cells undergo clonal expansion; these can then be re-infused into tumour-bearing mice *(Fig. 6.6)*.

This therapy can be used on its own or in combination with chemotherapeutic measures. In experiments involving a syngeneic murine lymphoma (FBL-3) that disseminates rapidly throughout the body, the following results were obtained: 11 out of 66 animals were cured with a single dose of 180 mg cyclophosphamide per kg (a cure rate of 17%). With cyclophosphamide and an injection of normal lymphocytes given five days later, 3 out of 47 animals were cured (6%). In two separate experiments, cells which had been taken from *in vivo* immunized animals were resensitized *in vitro* and expanded, thus bringing about cure in 41 of 50 (82%) and 44 of 61 (72%) mice. The cytotoxic lymphocytes responsible for these effects can be kept in culture for months without any great loss of cytotoxicity. Even more impressive results have been obtained in similar experiments with allogeneic tumours.

Peripheral human lymphocytes or splenic lymphocytes from the mouse can, however, be activated without tumour cells by Il-2 alone. Prolonged incubation of these cells with Il-2 *in vitro* give rise to activated lymphocytes, which consist largely of activated NK-cells and non-MHC restricted cytotoxic lymphocytes. Human cells of this type contain a subset which resembles T-cells (CD3 positive, CD19 negative) and a second population which is phenotypically closer to NK-cells: $CD3^-$ but $CD19^+$! These "LAK" cells (lymphokine activated killer cells) lyse fresh, autologous, syngeneic and allogeneic, primary and metastatic tumour cells. In a typical experimental protocol, LAK cells were generated by incubating 10^8 normal splenic lymphocytes from C57/B1 mice for 72 hours in 175 ml of a "complete" cell culture medium, i.e., in the presence of amino acids, fetal calf serum and 250,000 IU of recombinant Il-2. 3×10^5 cells from a syngeneic pulmonary sarcoma (MCA 105) were injected on day 0 into C57/B1 mice. On days 3 and 6 the animals received an i.v. injection of about 10^8 LAK cells or of normal lymphocytes. They also received on days 3–8 daily intraperitoneal injections of 25,000 IU of Il-2 in 0.5 ml saline or – for control purposes – only the saline solution. On day 13 after inoculation of the tumour, the pulmonary metastases were counted. Each group consisted of 5 animals. The results are given in Table 6.4.

From these values, which were obtained in a very similar fashion with two other syngeneic sarcomas, it can be seen that combined therapy with LAK cells and Il-2 produces far better results than treatment with LAK cells alone. The readily obtainable LAK cells presumably require constant stimulation by Il-2 in order to maintain their state of activation.

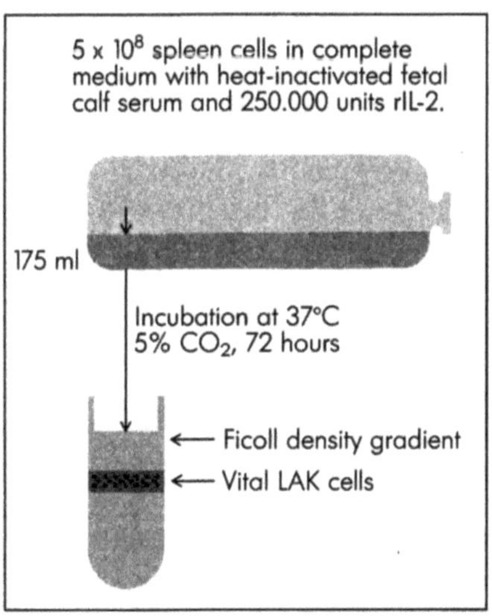

Figure 6.6. Induction of LAK cells (lymphokine-activated cells) by incubation of spleen lymphocytes with IL-2.

Table 6.4.

Treatment	Number of metastases on day 13 of study (mean of 5 animals)
Saline solution	141
Il-2	115
Normal lymphocytes and saline solution	215
Normal lymphocytes and Il-2	138
LAK cells and saline solution	75
LAK cells and Il-2	13

A third approach utilizes the cytotoxic properties of tumour infiltrating lymphocytes (TIL). These cells can be isolated from tumour tissue by growing single cell suspensions of the tumour, in the presence of Il-2. Under these conditions, the cytotoxic lymphocytes which have infiltrated the tumour will selectively expand while the tumour cells are gradually destroyed. After several weeks of incubation such cultures consist of pure populations of lymphocytes which can be further expanded in Il-2 containing media without losing their specific cytotoxicity. In the elimination of micrometastases TIL appear to be 50–100 times more potent than LAK cells when the comparison is made on a cell per cell basis. TIL are cytotoxic lymphocytes which bear CD3 and CD8 antigens. They act specifically against the tumour from which they were isolated. This is in contrast to LAK cells which are derived from NK cells or from null cells and therefore carry a much broader specificity.

6.2.3.3 Mechanism of action

As with the interferons, some growth factors and peptide hormones, the effect of Il-2 is linked to interaction with its receptor. A very low dissociation constant is typical of this binding: for human T-cells it is (Kd) $3\text{–}5 \times 10^{-12}$ M! An average of 4,000–12,000 receptors are found on activated T-cells. The amino acid sequence of the receptor is kown and the respective genes for the Il-2 receptor have been cloned. The primary gene product of the small subunit has a molecular weight of 35,000 daltons. The "mature" p55 subunit emerges after to glycosylation steps: an N-glycosylation, which is sensitive to tunicamycin, and an O-glycosylation, which is sensitive to monensin. The carbohydrate components are not directly involved in the binding of the Il-2 molecule, but it is possible that they have a bearing on the affinity of the molecules for one another.

Two findings argue that the binding of Il-2 to the known Il-2 receptor is indeed the first step in a sequence of signals leading to cell proliferation: the Il-2 concentration-binding curve follows exactly the kinetics of DNA synthesis, measured by the incorporation of [^{3}H] – or [^{14}C] – thymidine. It could be argued that this need not necessarily be the case, since Il-2 binding is a gradual, concentration-dependent process, while the onset of cell division should follow "all or nothing" kinetics. The number of receptors per cell does, however, vary greatly. Because the intensity of signal transmission (number of messenger molecules) depends on the number of occupied molecules, it is understandable that only with higher Il-2 concentrations do cells with a relatively low number of receptors have a sufficient number of them occupied to generate enough messenger molecules for initiation of cell division. Secondly, it can be shown that the capacity for cell proliferation induced by Il-2 declines in proportion to the blockade of Il-2 receptors by monoclonal antibodies and the ensuing reduction in the number of Il-2-occupied receptors.

6.2.3.4 Changes in Il-2 production in vivo

Since interleukin can be measured by sensitive biological methods or, more recently, by very exact, direct antibody-mediated methods such as radioimmunoassay (RIA) and enzyme linked immuno-assays (Elisa) tests in body fluids or cellular supernatants, interesting results have been published on fluctuating Il-2 concentrations in body fluids which could be correlated to distinct clinical situations. Following autologous or allogeneic bone-marrow transplants the cell-mediated and humoral immune responses of the recipients continue to be deficient for about two years. This immune deficiency manifests itself in an enhanced susceptibility by transplant patients to bacterial, fungal and viral infections and is presumably due to a lack of Il-2. During this period peripheral mononuclear leucocytes from patients show less response than normal lymphocytes to mitogens such as phytohemagglutinin or concanavalin A. In this connection *in vitro* cultures show a greatly reduced ability to form Il-2. If the cells which react poorly to mitogens are enriched with purified exogenous Il-2, they exhibit blast transformation rates which are within the range of normal cells.

Peripheral lymphocytes of patients with autoimmune diseases such as rheumatoid arthritis or systemic lupus erythematosus also displayed a low rate of Il-2 synthesis and a diminished reaction to exogenous Il-2 *in vitro* after mitogen stimulation.

Similar findings have been obtained in patients with various forms of leukemia. In T-cell leukemia, a reduction in Il-2 production may even have the effect of slowing down the progress of the disease. At all events, adult T-cell leukemia in two patients whose leukemic cells showed a normal response to Il-2 proved to have a dramatic and rapidly fatal course. Dutch authors, however, have subscribed to the theory that deficient production of Il-2 and a reduced response to this lymphokine could be signs of a differentiation block. Reduced ability of the peripheral lymphocytes to synthesize Il-2 and react appropriately to Il-2 is also found in solitary and metastasizing tumours.

6.2.3.5 Therapeutic uses of Il-2

Preclinical studies:

The principle of adoptive immunotherapy and the LAK cell approach have already been described. Il-2, however, it also effective in many experimental tumour models when given by itself. Some important insights could be derived from therapeutic animal experiments which have not always been applied rigorously to the clinical situation.

In the first place, Il-2 seems to work better against immunogenic tumours than against tumours which are of little or no immunogenicity. While immunogenicity is often defined as the expression of class-I antigens on the surface of tumour cells one must understand that this definition is only true with respect to allogeneic tumours and not for syngeneic tumours.

Since Il-2 works through the activation of T-cells or NK-cells the integrity of the immune system of the host is a prerequisite for its efficacy. Radiation, pretreatment with steroids or with cytostatics but also genetic defects concerning immune functions tend to interfere with the effectiveness of Il-2.

As mentioned also in conjunction with activated macrophages the tumour burden is a critical parameter for the efficacy of Il-2. This may have to do with the basic inaccessability of large tumours to activated lymphocytes but it also relates to the limitations in the numbers of cells that can be recuited even under optimal conditions to attack existing micrometastatic foci.

As one might expect, the efficacy of Il-2 can be enhanced by the simultaneous, subsequent or prior application of other lymphokines such as α-interferon and TNF. Especially in the case of the latter, the sequence of administration seems to be important: the application of TNF before Il-2 treatment is more successful than the reverse sequence. There is at least some theoretical reason why the use of monoclonal antibodies directed at tumour markers may benefit from the prior administration of Il-2 – many cells which are induced by the lymphokine carry Fc receptors and could function in an ADCC reaction against the tumour if armed with the appropriate antibody.

Finally – Il-2 seems to be more effective if available at low plasma concentrations over prolonged periods of time. Intraperitoneal or subcutaneous regimens have been more successful in animals than regimens based on intravenous application. As described below this finding is not fully supported by the clinical evidence obtained so far.

Clinical studies. Il-2 is at present being quite extensively investigated as an anticancer agent. Some clinical studies were designed to define the therapeutic potential of Il-2 alone, while others are structured around the use of Il-2 activated killer cells and tumour infiltrated lymphocytes together with Il-2. More recently, Il-2 has also been studied in combination with α-interferon. In most of the protocols, Il-2 is first given for four to five days as a bolus injection every eight hours. The doses initially used ranged between 10,000 and 100,000 units/kg but amounted to 10^5 units/kg in most trials. This course of therapy is followed by a rest period of approximately one week and is then repeated. Several such courses, interrupted by rest periods, can be administered. When Il-2 treatment is combined with the application of LAK cells the lymphocytosis occurring after the first course of Il-2 treatment is exploited for five consecutive days of leukapheresis, starting two or three days after completion of the first round of Il-2 injections. Approximately $0.5–1.2 \times 10^9$ lymphoid cells are recovered at each leukapheresis. These cells are then incubated for three to four days in a suitable medium containing 1,000 U/ml Il-2. Subsequently the cells are washed and re-infused into the patients. During the entire period of LAK cell treatment the patients received Il-2 according to the same dosage pattern as that used at the initiation of therapy.

When Il-2 is given as a bolus injection a high plasma level is rapidly obtained. Most of the Il-2 is cleared from the plasma within six to eight minutes after injection. After this period a more prolonged clearance rate becomes apparent. This second clearance rate is even more prolonged if Il-2 is applied by infusion and of Il-2 concentrations are measured after several infusions. These findings clearly indicate that the lymphokine distributes into a deep compartment from which it is gradually released.

Considerable toxicity was observed during the initial studies conducted at the NCI in which bolus injections had been used. In subsequent trials an attempt was made to eliminate some of this toxicity by infusing Il-2 continuously at doses of 3×10^6 units/m^2/day for a total of four to five days.

From the first studies it seemed that infusions were about as effective as bolus injections but less toxic. This impression, however, had to be corrected when equal daily doses administered either as bolus injections or as continuous infusions were compared in the context of one study. Surprisingly, continuous infusions turned out to generate more side effects. At least in terms of the degree of lymphocytosis following Il-2 therapy they were also more effective. The issue of bolus injections versus infusions is still not settled although most authors now advocate the former.

Undoubtedly Il-2 alone exerts clinically significant antitimour effects in humans. In cases of malignant melanoma treatment with Il-2 alone allowed for response rates of about 25%. While this figure is roughly equal to the results of combined LAK and Il-2 treatment in this disease, it represents almost exclusively partial responses. After LAK cell treatment at least 30% of the total number of responses tend to be complete. In renal cell carcinoma Il-2 alone induces responses in about 20% of all patients with one third being complete and two thirds incomplete.

More data have become available from studies in which LAK cells were administered along with Il-2. The overall figures emerging from these studies representing complete and partial responses are as follows: renal cell carcinoma 30%, melanoma 20–30%, colon carcinoma 15–20%, non-Hodgkin's lymphoma 60%.

More recently Il-2 has also been used in combination with α-interferon and with TNF. Both combinations seemed to be very effective, although the numbers of cases treated do not yet allow binding conclusions.

Early studies in which tumour infiltrating lymphocytes were administered together with Il-2 have demonstrated the clinical feasibility of this approach. There is evidence to suggest that at least in some tumours this aproach may be more effective than the use of LAK cells.

Conceptually, the combined use of Il-2 and α-interferon makes sense for several – speculative – reasons. Interferon induces the expression of HLA class-I antigens on tumour cells, thus making them more immunogenic to HLA-restricted lymphocytes. The second, perhaps more plausible, reason is that α-interferon provides a direct attack on the viability of the tumour cell, which is effectively complemented by activation of immune cells. These cells have the capacity to attack tumour cells and may achieve a higher "kill rate" if their targets have been predamaged by an independent mechanism.

Il-2 is a pleotrophic substance which, when applied in pharmacological doses, causes a wide spectrum of side effects. Chills and fever are common symptoms. This is not unexpected: activated lymphocytes will form increased amounts of γ-interferon which in turn will activate macrophages. These cells will then secrete large amounts of Il-1, which is the endogeneous pyrogen. A very typical toxicological effect which is regularly seen after Il-2 administration concerns the cardiovascular system: within minutes after injection of Il-2, peripheral vascular resistance falls, while heart rate and cardiac output increase. Leakiness of the microvascular bed, followed by massive extravasation of serum and edema formation, is the underlying cause of the hemodynamic changes. The reduction of intravascular volume is followed by oliguria. The pathophysiological mechanism of the capillary leak syndrome remains to be elucidated. A number of possibilities deserve consideration. Among these are histamine or prostaglandin-mediated effects, direct effects of Il-2 or of other lymphokines induced by Il-2 on the vascular endothelium, or damage to endothelial cells by an increased number of activated neutrophils adhering to the endothelium and releasing toxic oxygen radicals. It has also been shown that Il-1 and γ-interferon can act on endothelial cells, with resulting generation of oxygen radicals. Oxygen scavengers like methylthiourea have been shown to provide protection against such effects. In experimental animals, prior irradiation, cyclophosphamide treatment or the use of steroids can mitigate or even prevent the vascular leakiness associated with Il-2 treatment. Central nervous effects like hallucinations, delusions, confusion or disorientation are frequent. The underlying mechanisms are not clear, although cerebral edema as a consequence of the vascular leak may at least offer a partial explanation for these symptoms.

Patients receiving Il-2 almost invariably develop malaise and anorexia. Most likely the complete loss of appetite is due to TNF, which is induced by Il-2 and which is identical to cachectin, the protein which inhibits appetite and which causes shock.

Immediately after the start of Il-2 treatment, lymphocytopenia develops which, after cessation of therapy, is followed by a rebound lymphocytosis. Upon prolonged treatment with Il-2 anemia and thrombocytemia appear. The extent of these deficiencies may necessitate blood transfusions. Eosinophilia is a fairly common event after prolonged treatment.

All of these changes which often require additional therapy in the course of treatment with Il-2 are completely reversible when Il-2 is discontinued.

In summary one can state that Il-2 has proved to be an effective agent in the treatment of several cancers, most notably melanoma, renal cell carcinoma, non-Hodgkin's lymphoma and to a lesser extent colon carcinoma: The compound has considerable toxicity. However, both the toxicity and the still limited clinical efficacy must be seen as representing initial results which can and will be improved upon. Il-2 is likely to become part of a great number of therapeutic regimens which will comprise other lymphokines as well as more conventional cytostatic drugs. It appears at least possible that the true therapeutic potential of Il-2 has not yet been uncovered, owing to the fact that the clinical use of biological response modifiers has so far been dominated by concepts which are clearly derived from cytoreductive chemotherapy and which may be inadequate in conjunction with compounds which are powerful regulators of immune function at very low concentrations.

6.2.4 Colony stimulating factors

All blood cells, erythocytes, granulocytes, lymphocytes, monocytes and platelets develop from a common ancestor: the bone-marrow stem cell. The various dcevelopmental pathways leading from a pluripotent stem cell to committed stem cells, precursor cells and on the mature terminal cells are controlled by a number of proteins, some of which have been identified, cloned and characterized. The factors which control erythropoiesis or the development of megakaryocytes and blood platelets are of little concern in the context of this book because they do not influence immune functions. Likewise there does not seem to be a role for these factors in the treatment of disorders of the immune system. All the other factors which are known to stimulate the development of leucocytes, however, could have a role as immunopharmacological agents. Il-1 (hematopoietic) and Il-6 seem to play a role in the early stages of hematopoiesis, including perhaps the expansion of stem cells or early precursor cells. Il-4 or BSF-1 not only has a role in B-cell development but also in regulating the proliferation and activation of mast cells.

As mentioned in the second chapter, Il-5 appears to be the single most important factor in the generation of eosinophils. Only four colony stimulating factors, however, can at this time be discussed in therapeutic terms: Il-3, GM-CSF, G-CSF and – with certain limitations – M-CSF; of these four CS-factors GM-CSF and G-CSF have been studied extensively in animals and in man. Therefore these proteins which are only months away from their official introduction into clinical practice will be described below in greater detail. Interleukin 3, also first described as multi-CSF, has a broad spectrum of activities: it stimulates the formation of eosinophils, neutrophils, and monocytes. GM-CSF is also a multilineage factor with a preferential effect on the generation and activation of granulocytes and monocytes. G-CSF and M-CSF are very lineage specific for stimulating granulocyte and monocyte formation, respectively. The latter factor, however, does not exert a strong proliferative effect on monocytes. Its function may rather lie in the activation and maintenance of monocytes and macrophages.

The detection of the hematopoietic factors became possible after the method of growing cells in soft agar had been established in 1966. If 10^5 bone-marrow cells are suspended in soft agar all cells will die unless at least one of the growth factors is present. Depending on the number and the concentration of the hematopoietic factors in such soft agar cultures, precursor cells continue to proliferate and form colonies of mature granulocytes or monocytes. With human bone-marrow cells the formation of such colonies, each comprising between 50 and 5,000 cells, takes seven to fourteen days of culture.

The advent of recombinant DNA technology enabled scientists to clone the genes for all of the factors mentioned above, to express these genes in suitable vectors and to study the structure and function of each factor in detail. In pursuing this goal different strategies were applied. G-CSF and M-CSF were first purified to homogeneity and submitted to structural analysis. From the partial amino acid sequences of each of the factors nucleotides could be derived according to the rules of the genetic code which were used as hybridization probes to identify the cDNAs of the two factors. The sequences obtained were then expressed in suitable vectors.

In the case of Il-3 and GM-CSF a different strategy had to be used. Both factors have an extremely high intrinsic biological activity. Apparently "rich" sources of the factors contain in reality only trace amounts of the factor proteins. Therefore cDNA clones were expressed in mammalian cells, in this case COS-1 cells from monkeys. On account of the high intrinsic activity of the factors very small amounts are detectable by bioassays. For two reasons Il-3 proved to be the most elusive colony stimulating factor. First it is expressed in peripheral blood lymphocytes at very low levels and secondly gibbon and human Il-3 turned out to have relatively little structural homology with the murine factor (49% at the nucleotide level and 29% at the amino acid level).

Each of the colony stimulating factors has four distinct effects on responsive cell populations: they are necessary for the maintenance (survival) of cells; secondly they induce proliferation; thirdly, they control differentiation, and lastly, they activate mature differentiated cells. These basic functions are not equally represented in each factor: GM-CSF and Il-3, for instance, stimulate so many cell lineages apart from granulocyte and monocytic cells that they can hardly be classified as very selective differentiation signals. G-CSF, on the other hand, can be regarded as representing a rather specific differentiation signal. M-CSF may under most conditions not exert very powerful stimuli of differentiation or proliferation. This factor, however, appears to be rather active in enhancing the function of already differentiated monocytes and macrophages. The hematopoietic factors which we know today act in sequence: Il-1 and Il-6 are active at early stages of the hematopoietic cascade, Il-3 and GM-CSF are still multilineage factors although they already show a preference for the stimulation of myeloid and monocytic cells. G-CSF and M-CSF are active late in the hematopoietic cascade, displaying a rather narrow spectrum. The preferential effect of GM-CSF on granulocytes and monocytes is the result of multiple points of attack: GM-CSF acts at three or four different levels of differentiation. It stimulates a precursor cell which is the common ancestor of erythrocytes, platelets, monocytes and neutrophils as well as eosinophils. However, it also acts on the committed precursor cell of each of these lineages and moreover strongly affects the direct precursors of granulocytes and monocytes. The overlapping specificities of the hematopoetic factors open interesting possibilities for their combined use in therapeutic situations *(Fig. 6.7)*.

Each of the CSFs binds to its own specific receptor, which has no capacity to bind other CSFs. These receptors are all monomeric polypeptides They range in molecular mass from 50 kd to 165 kd. The largest receptor is the one for M-CSF. It is identical to the c-fms proto-oncogene product. The receptors are expressed on bone-marrow cells in relatively low numbers: these cells carry between 70 and 350 receptor molecules for GM-CSF and 50–1,000 for Il-3, 1,500–10,000 for M-

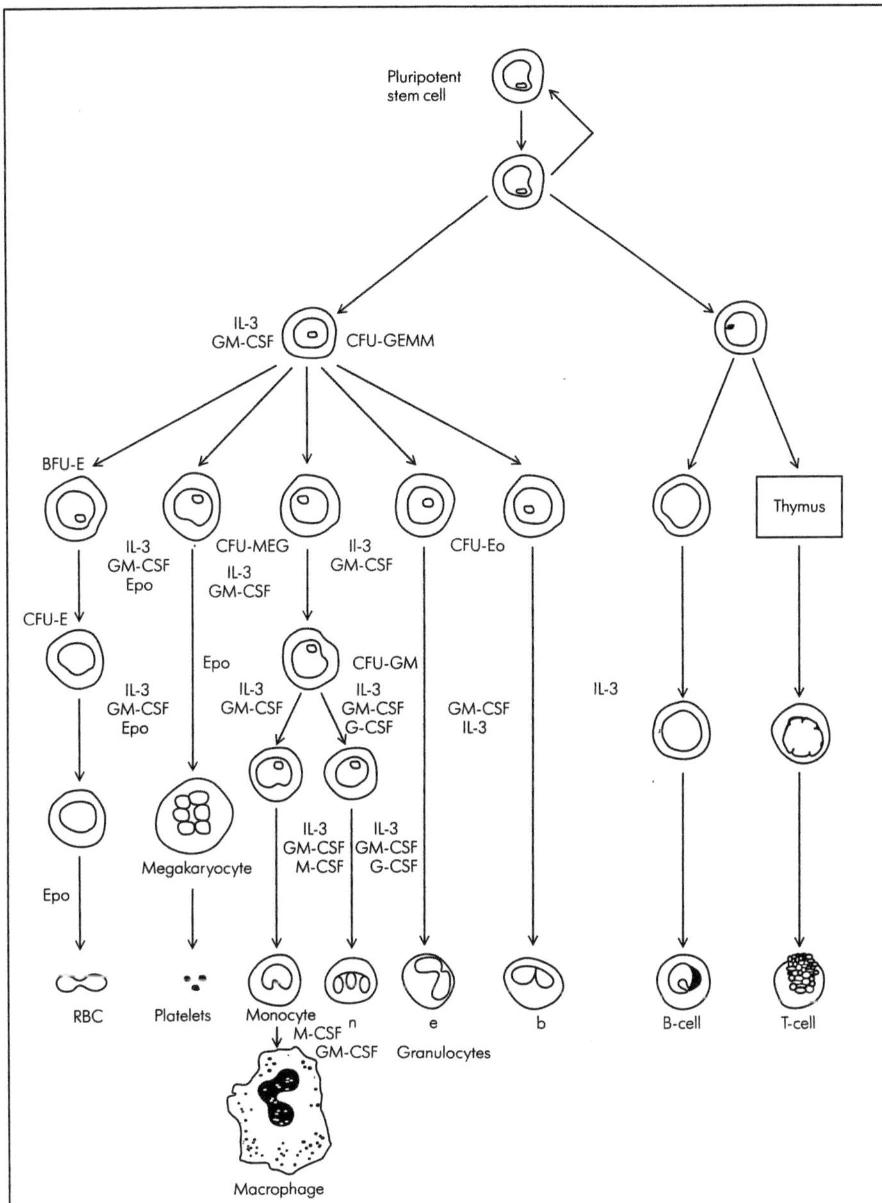

Figure 6.7. Scheme of blood cell differentiation from a bone-marrow stem cell. Interactions of colony stimulating factors with cells at various stages of development.
Abbreviations: CFU: colony forming unit. BFU: burst forming unit. EO = eosinophil. meg = megakaryocyte. GEMM = granulocyte, erythrocyte, monocyte, megakaryocyte. E = erythroid. Epo = erythropoietin. GM = granulocyte, monocyte. M = monocyte. n, e, b = neutrophil, erythrocyte, basophil.

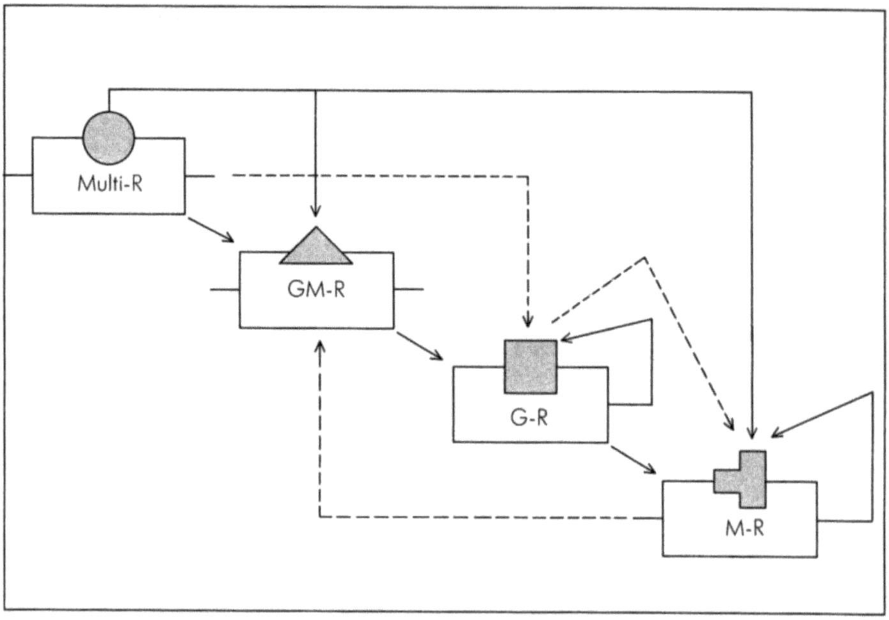

Figure 6.8. Sequence of down-regulation of CSF receptor types following occupancy. The solid lines describe down-regulation at low (physiological) concentrations. Dotted lines indicate additional mutual relationships which can only be observed at high factor concentrations.

CSF and 50–500 for G-CSF. In spite of the low number of receptors a low receptor occupancy suffices to drive cells into proliferation or differentiation or to activate them functionally. The CSF receptors are subject to up- and down-regulation. Like other hormones, CSFs down-regulate their own receptors. This is mainly due to rapid internalization of occupied receptors as compared with unoccupied ones. In contrast to this isologous receptor down-regulation there is a trans-down-modulation between various factors which follows a "hierarchical" pattern. At concentrations which induce half-maximum effects (200 U/ml) Il-3 down-regulates GM-CSF and M-CSF receptors, GM-CSF down-modulates M-CSF receptors, while G-CSF and M-CSF do not down-regulate any receptors other than their own. However, at higher concentrations (1,000–4,000 U/ml), Il-3 and GM-CSF also down-regulate G-CSF receptors, G-CSF reduces the number of M-CSF receptors and M-CSF down-modulates GM-CSF receptors *(Fig. 6.8)*. These regulatory effects occur only on bone-marrow cells and are not seen on leukemic or factor-dependent immortalized cells. The biological significance of these regulatory events is not yet clear. At first sight one would assume that a cell loses responsiveness to a factor whose receptor had been down-modulated. One would, for example, expect a loss of sensitivity to M-CSF if GM-CSF had led to reduction of the number of M-CSF receptors on the surface of a particular cell. In many cases, however, this expectation is not in line with experimental observations. In fact, myeloid precursor cells whose G-CSF receptor is down-modulated by large concentrations of GM-CSF or Il-3 still differentiate into granulocytes. This observation and similar ones have led some authors to suggest that occupancy of the GM-CSF or Il-3 receptor would send a strong proliferation signal to the cell but that, in addition, internalization of unoccupied G- or M-CSF receptors would induce subsequent differentiation, as if these receptors had been occupied by their isologous ligands *(Fig. 6.9)*.

Human colony stimulating factors are formed by a large variety of cells; such T-lymphocytes, monocytes, fibroblasts and endothelial cells. Recent studies have shown that the release of CSFs often occurs as part of a regulatory cascade in which LPS or other microbial cell wall constituents activate monocytes which in turn secrete I1-1, TNF as well as G and GM-CSF. TNF produced under such conditions will cause endothelial cells as well as fibroblasts to secrete GM and G-CSF, while M-CSF appears to be produced constitutively by all three cell types: monocytes, fibroblasts and vascular endothelial cells. Il-1 has been shown to cause stromal cells from mouse bone-marrow to secrete GM and G-CSF *(Fig. 6.10)*.

M-CSF and G-CSF can be demonstrated in the serum of animals, G-CSF in particular after bacterial infections. GM-CSF is present at much lower concen-

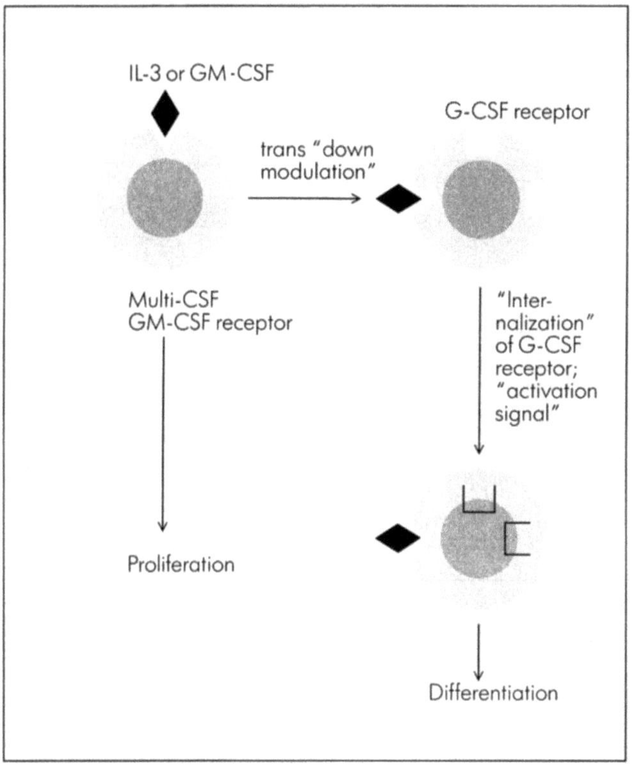

Figure 6.9. Model of the receptor "trans-down modulation" concept according to N. Nicola. An IL-3 or GM-CSF molecule delivers a proliferative signal to a hematopoietic cell via occupying its corresponding receptor. This occupancy of receptors causes down – modulation of empty G-CSF or M-CSF receptors. It is assumed in the model that this "internalization" of unoccupied receptors delivers a differentiation signal to the respective cells. In this way "overproliferation" of cells in the presence of an oversupply of GM-CSF or IL-3 could be avoided. The coupling of proliferation and differentiation in normal progenitor cells is provided by receptor down-modulation and hence activation of lineage-specific receptors. A failure in receptor trans down-modulation could disrupt this balance and lead or at least contribute to leukemia.

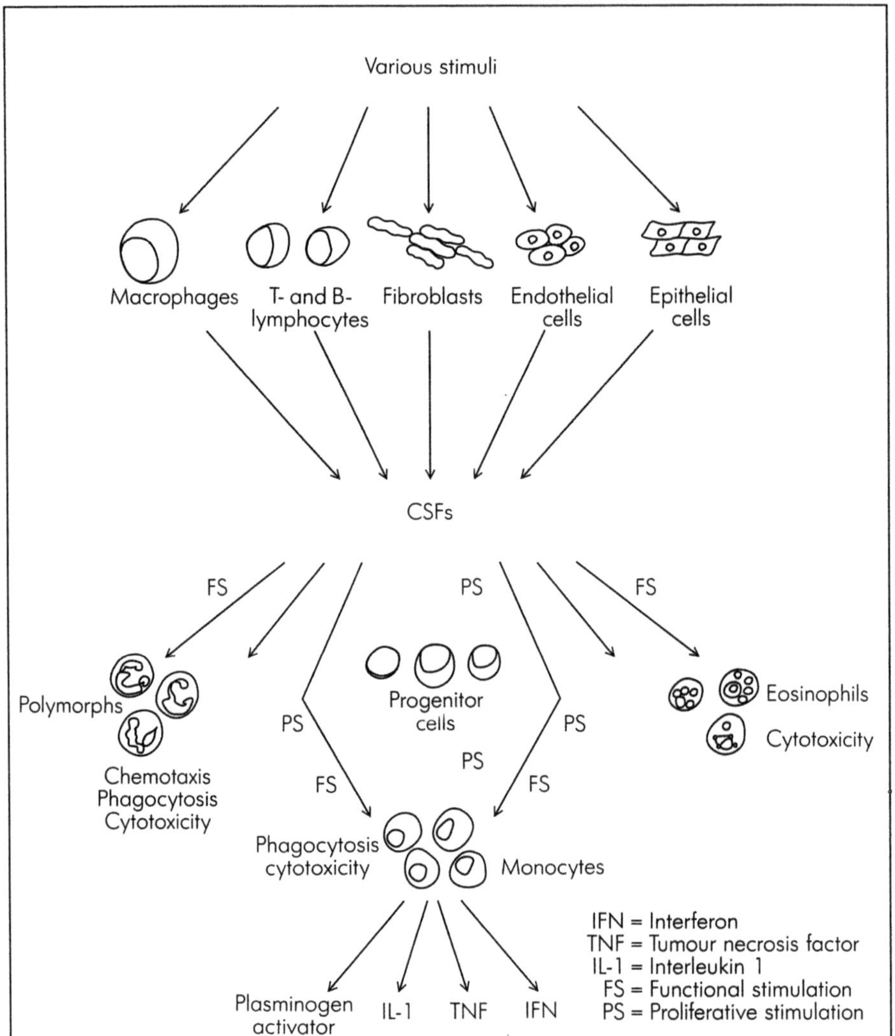

Figure 6.10. Sources and functions of colony stimulating factors. CSFs are formed in a large variety of cells as a response to a multitude of (chemical) stimuli. The main effects of CSFs in their target cell populations are illustrated.

trations. Il-3 has not been detected in the serum. The only CSF occurring in human urine is M-CSF.

6.2.4.1 GM-CSF

Properties and origin. Mature human GM-CSF contains 127 a.a. If expressed in *E. coli,* the protein has a molecular mass of 14,000. The molecule contains two sites for N-glycosylation. When GM-CSF is expressed in COS cells, these sites are glycosylated. Consequently the protein secreted from these cells has a molecular mass of 19,000. Depending on the cells in which GM-CSF is made, the degree of glycosylation and as a consequence the molecular weight of the glycoprotein can vary. Glycosylation, however, is not necessary for biological activity: the non-glycosylated factor is fully active.

The precursor protein of GM-CSF has 144 a.a., corresponding to a cDNA open reading frame of 432 nucleotides. 17 a.a. are cleaved off during secretion. The mature GM-CSF molecule contains 4 cysteine molecules. All four seem to be involved in SH linkages which contribute essentially to the correct conformation of the molecule; treatment with reducing agents like mercaptoethanol leads to inactivation.

The human gene for GM-CSF contains four exons separated by three introns. It is located on the long arm of chromosome 5 in the vicinity of the genes for Il-3, M-CSF, the M-CSF receptor (c-fms) as well as Il-5. The location of these genes spans the distal region of the deletion seen in the so-called 5q-syndrome, which is associated with a clonal proliferative disorder of granulocytes and macrophages and which is a common disorder in secondary acute myeloid leukemia.

Based on granulocyte-macrophage colony formation in bone-marrow cultures, native GM-CSF has a specific activity of 12×10^8 units/mg. (50 units/ml is the concentration stimulating half-maximum numbers of colonies to develop in cultures of mouse bone-marrow cells.) Recombinant GM-CSF synthesized in *E. coli* has a specific activity of 5×10^8 units/mg and the material expressed in COS cells was reported to have a specific activity of 4×10^7 units/mg.

Biological effects in vitro. GM-CSF stimulates the formation of neutrophils, monocytes, platelets and eosinophils in bone-marrow cultures. Half-maximum stimulation of culture formation can be obtained at concentrations between 5 and 20 pM, depending on the origin of the material and the experimental conditions. 50–250 pM, corresponding to 1–5 ng/ml, is needed for maximum stimulation. The molecule has 70% homology with the murine factor at the nucleotide level and 60% homology with mouse GM-CSF at the a.a. level. Its activity, however, is restricted to humans and primates.

Besides its proliferative effects, GM-CSF also induces functional changes in mature cells. It inhibits migration of mature granular sites and activates neutrophils and eosinophils, as judged by increases in their phagocytic activity, degranulation, lysozyme production and superoxide generation. GM-CSF also enhances antibody dependent cytotoxicity of neutrophils, monocytes and macrophages.

Pharmacological effect. When infused into cynomolgus monkeys at a rate of 50 units per minute per kg of body weight, GM-CSF (expressed in COS cells, specific activity $1–2 \times 10^7$ units/mg) caused an immediate increase in neutrophils, bands and monocytes followed by a somewhat delayed increase in eosinophils. During continuous infusion at the doses indicated, peak levels of blood cells were reached within one week.

Immediately after discontinuation of GM-CSF infusions over a ten-day period leucocyte counts fell off but did not quite revert to normal during an observation period of twelve days. Prolonged administration of GM-CSF in primates for up to 28 days produces elevated leucocyte levels in the range of 30,000–90,000 cells/ μl during the whole infusion period without apparent adverse effects.

After an intravenous bolus injection 35S-labelled GM-CSF pepared from COS cells disappeared from the circulation of cynomolgus monkeys in two phases: during the α-phase the biological half-life was approximately seven minutes. Subsequently, during the so-called β-phase, the material was eliminated at a much slower rate (half-life approximately 80–90 minutes).

It is, however, doubtful whether continuous infusion represents the most efficient way of administering GM-CSF. A total daily dose of 84 μg of glycosylated GM-CSF/kg administered in three s.c. injections produced white cell counts which were twice as high as those elicited by an i.v. infusion of the same daily dose. The fact that neutrophil counts started to increase immediately (within the first 24 hours) after the first dose of GM-CSF indicates that this factor also enhances the release of mature cells from the bone-marrow pool. GM-CSF also stimulates neutrophil functions *in vivo*: white cells obtained from primates as little as three days after the first dose of GM-CSF showed an eightfold increase in their ability to kill *E. coli* bacteria *in vitro* and an approximately threefold increase in their production of superoxide anions.

An interesting finding relating to the biological effects of GM-CSF was obtained from transgenic mice expressing the GM-CSF gene which they obtained together with a retroviral promotor. These animals exhibited strongly elevated levels of GM-CSF in the blood (2,000 units/ml), in the urine, in the peritoneal cavity and in the eye. A striking abnormality in these animals was a pronounced bacterial opacity in their eyes, which went along with retinal damage and the presence of great numbers of enlarged macrophages in the vitreous as well as in the anterior and posterior chamber, in the retina and in the iris. The peritoneal and pleural cavities contained the same cells as those which also infiltrated striated muscle. The animals usually die at the age of two to four months as a result of muscle wasting, possibly the consequence of the infiltration of their musculature by activated macrophages.

Clinical applications. GM-CSF has been studied quite extensively in clinical settings. The main thrust of the investigations carried out so far was directed at three clinical problems: hematological reconstitution after autologous bone-marrow transplantation, myelodysplastic syndromes, and amelioration of bone-marrow toxicity during and after treatment with cytostatic and/or antiviral agents.

Patients with advanced malignancies (breast cancer or melanoma) who had been treated with high-dose combination chemotherapy and had received autologous bone-marrow transplantations responded favourably to GM-CSF when the lymphokine was administered by daily infusions during periods of two weeks, starting immediately after the injection of bone-marrow cells. Doses of 2.0, 4.0, 8.0, or 32 μg/kg resulted in recovery of leucocytes and granulocytes which was significantly accelerated in comparison with historical controls matched for age, diagnosis and treatment. At the end of the treatment period blood leucocyte counts showed a distinct dose-dependent increase over control values. Even the lower dose range (2–8 μg/kg/day) resulted in average leucocyte counts of 1,500, which was almost twice the value of the historical controls. In patients who had received 16 μg/kg of GM-CSF the mean leucocyte count was 2,600 and in those treated with 32 μg/kg the corresponding figure amounted to 3,120. No consistent effect on platelet counts was detected in this study. At doses between 2 and 16 μg/kg side effects observed in connection with the administration of GM-CSF were mild and not clearly dose-related. Myalgias or arthralgias, edema, generalized weight gain, hypotension and plural effusion occurred in several patients. These side effects are reminiscent of the toxic side effects associated with the clinical use of Il-2 which were characterized as "capillary leak syndrome".

It is at present not clear whether and in what way the special status of patients having undergone cytoreductive chemotherapy and bone-marrow transplantation contributed to the generation of this syndrome.

Interestingly, these side effects were not observed in individuals suffering from AIDS or ARC. Patients who met the diagnostic criteria for this disease were male, 18–50 years old, had a total peripheral-blood leucocyte count of 3,000 per μl or less, and did not receive myelosuppressive therapy or suffer from any acute complications. Such patients were divided into five dosage groups with 1.3×10^3, 2.6×10^3, 5.2×10^3, and 2×10^4 units per kg per day and were treated for two weeks. As already observed in non-human primates GM-CSF induced an acute increase in total peripheral-blood leucocytes within 24 hours of the first dose. Most likely this increase is due to release of preformed leucocytes. Subsequently, total white cells increased during the first week of treatment. After this point in time a more moderate increase which could largely be attributed to the appearance of eosinophils and neutrophilis was observed. After discontinuation of treatment, cell concentrations decreased acutely within 24 hours and subsequently decreased more gradually to levels which, two weeks after cessation of treatment, were still well above the initial values. The absolute number of lymphocytes also increased in some patients during treatment. However, the ratio of CD4 to CD8 cells remained unaltered. Similarly, the ability to culture virus from blood cells did not change. This group of patients experienced only mild side effects like back pain, myalgia, chills, nausea or headache. Fever seems to be an occasional complication of therapy with GM-CSF, as is reversible elevation of liver transaminases after prolonged treatment periods with higher doses of the hematopoietic factor.

GM-CSF has also been used in cases of myelodysplastic syndromes and in aplastic anemia. After one or two courses of treatment, each lasting two weeks, distinct clinical effects were observed. Most patients responded with an increase in cellularity of their bone marrow and with marked elevation of peripheral-blood neutrophils, monocytes, lymphocytes and eosinophils. Granulocytes isolated during or after treatment with GM-CSF exhibited higher levels of H_2O_2 production when stimulated *in vitro* with chemotactic agents.

Patients with AIDS who are treated with azidothymidine regularly experience myelosuppression. In studies which at the time of writing have been going on for nine to ten months, GM-CSF administered three times a week at moderate doses prevented this complication at the expense of very mild untoward effects.

In a similar vein, GM-CSF has been studied for its ability to alleviate the myelosuppressive effects of cytoreductive chemotherapy in patients with advanced malignancies. Results obtained so far indicate that GM-CSF given immediately after a course of combination chemotherapy can significantly shorten the period of hematological recovery and significantly reduce the risk of opportunistic infections. Relevant clinical studies have shown that daily doses of up to 32 μg/kg of GM-CSF are well tolerated by patients undergoing cytoreductive chemotherapy. The optimal dosage schedules for GM-CSF in relation to various patterns of myelosuppressive chemotherapy have not yet been established.

By serendipity it was found that GM-CSF at doses between 4 and 65 μg/kg per day can lead to a pronounced reduction of serum cholesterol levels. The mechanism of this phenomenon is not yet understood. It was found that the fall in serum cholesterol concentration did not always coincide with a rise in peripheral-blood leucocytes. However, the data currently available do not exclude the possibility that the dramatic increase in cell formation seen as a consequence of GM-CSF treatment leads to increased utilization of newly synthesized cholesterol for the formation of new membranes. Other mechanisms such as inhibition of cholesterol formation or an increased shift of cholesterol carrying LDL particles into monocytes and macrophages also seem possible.

6.2.4.2 G-CSF

Physico-chemical properties – origin. G-CSF is a lineage-specific hematopoietin. This property puts it into the same group as M-CSF. In contrast, GM-CSF and Il-3 have been classified as pluripotent or multilineage factors. Occasionally the latter two factors have been called "class 1 factor", while G-CSF, which selectively stimulates the generation of neutrophils, is listed as a "class 3 factor". Two subtypes of human G-CSF have been described; they differ by three amino acids in positions 36–38 which are deleted in the shorter version of the protein. G-CSFa, the longer protein, contains 177 amino acids. It is first synthesized as a protein comprising 207 amino acids, including a leader sequence of 30 hydrophobic amino acids. The shorter version, G-CSFb, has 204 amino acids as a precursor and 174 amino acids as the mature protein. The difference between the a and the b form of G-CSF results from alternative splicing pathways; the gene for G-CSF contains 5 exons and 4 introns, and there are two donor splice sites at the 5′-end of intron 2. Interestingly, the two versions differ with respect to their biological activity, the shorter peptide being significantly more potent than the longer one. In the following sections the term G-CSF will therefore always relate to the more active shorter protein. In its natural, O-glycosylated form, G-CSF has a molecular weight of 19,600. When treated with neuraminidase and O-glycosidase the molecular weight shifts to 18,600. The recombinant protein synthesized in *E. coli* carries an N-terminal methionine and is, of course, unglycosylated. There appears to be no difference whatsoever in the biological activity of glycosylated versus non-glycosylated material.

In contrast to other hematopoietins, G-CSF is not species-specific. There is a 69.3% nucleotide sequence homology between human and murine G-CSF, while at the amino acid level the degree of homology is even higher: 73%.

Human and murine G-CSF show almost complete cross-reactivity with respect to receptor binding and biological activity. There are only 100–500 receptors for G-CSF on progenitor cells or on mature neutrophils. Half-maximum effects are already elicited at only 5–10% of receptor occupancy.

The G-CSF receptor is a single chain protein of Mr 150,000. At 0 °C, G-CSF associates with this protein very tightly. The binding is virtually irreversible. There is no direct evidence for internalization of the ligand-receptor complex. At 37 °C, however, the complex decays with a biological half-life of approximately four to six hours.

The murine G-CSF gene is located on chromosome 11. Its human counterpart maps to a site on human chromosome 17, just proximal of the breakpoint which is found in the 15:17 translocation. This translocation is a frequent anomaly in promyelocytic leukemia. It has recently been shown that the coding sequence of G-CSF is not structurally affected by the translocation.

G-CSF is formed by essentially the same cells as those which synthesize GM-CSF: monocytes, fibroblasts, stromal cells of the bone marrow, vascular endothelium and T-cells. It was first isolated from the supernatants of two squamous carcinoma cell lines.

In vitro activity. When introduced into human bone-marrow cultures at a concentration of approximately 500 U/ml, G-CSF from a bladder carcinoma cell induces the formation of various colonies which can be classified as CFU-GM, BFU-E and CFU-GEMM. The effect on the generation of the latter colony-type which represents a granulocyte-erythrocyte-megakaryocyte and macrophage precursor mixture is very weak. The effect on the other two colony types is about equal. The GM colonies can be classified as representing mainly granulocyte precursors on the basis of their biochemical characteristics: they are chloroacetate esterase positive and α-naphthyl esterase negative, which is consistent with their granulocytic nature.

Recombinant human G-CSF supports the generation of early erythroid precursors (BFU-E) only in the presence of small amounts (1 μg/ml) of erythropoietin. Maximum colony formation is induced by G-CSF within seven days. Half-maximum stimulation occurs at 5×10^{-12} mol/l (approximately 100 pg/ml).

G-CSF has profound effects on mature granulocytes. The formation of superoxide anions in response to the chemotactic peptide f met-leu-phe is greatly enhanced by the factor as is phagocytosis. Furthermore, G-CSF stimulates the ability of mature granulocytes to participate in antibody-dependent cytotoxic reactions against tumour cells (ADCC). On the basis of these *in vitro* results G-CSF can be characterized as a selective growth and differentiation factor for granulocyte (neutrophil) precursors as well as a powerful priming factor for mature neutrophils.

In contrast to GM-CSF, G-CSF is a potent inducer of terminal differentiation on a number of myeloid leukemia cell lines such as WEHI-3B, HL-60 M1 and others. The most striking effect of G-CSF has been observed on the WEHI-3BD mouse myeloid leukemia cell line. These cells when exposed to G-CSF develop into mature granulocytes and monocytes. More importantly, G-CSF can suppress self-generation of leukemic stem cells and can therefore lead to complete extinction (clonal deletion) of this leukemic cell population.

However, it is not yet certain to what extent this effect of G-CSF can be exploited clinically. So far, a reliable screening method for myeloid leukemic cells that is capable of predicting which cells can be suppressed by G-CSF or other CSF types does not exist. There is, on the other hand, an inherent danger of a proliferation response of a leukemic cell population, since most immature precursor cells carry G-CSF receptors. Further laboratory studies will have to be carried out before clinical trials addressing "differentiation therapy" could be justified.

In vivo activity. When injected into healthy mice, G-CSF causes a rise in neutrophil counts which – depending on the dose and duration of treatment – can amount to approximately 10^5 cells/μl, which is one hundred times the normal level.

After six days of injections with 3×12 ng of G-CSF, neutrophil counts of 3,000/μl were measured, 3×50 ng of G-CSF over the same period resulted in 8,000 neutrophils/μl, and 3×200 ng during six days produced granulocytemia of 22,000 cells/μl. The injection of G-CSF into mice also causes marked expansion of stem cells, myeloid progenitor cells as well as erythopoietic cells in the bone marrow. In view of the selectivity of G-CSF in vitro these effects must be interpreted as representing secondary phenomena.

In cynomolgus monkeys, G-CSF has effects similar to those seen in mice. The neutropenia and bone-marrow aplasia which can be induced in these animals with cyclophosphamide (doses ranging from 60–200 mg/kg) requires about four weeks after the cessation of cyclophosphamide treatment for complete restoration. With G-CSF injections of 10 μg/kg/day started before or immediately after the toxic insult to the bone-marrow and continued over ten to fourteen days, animals have been shown to recover normal or even above normal neutrophil values within seven days. Since human G-CSF is not species-specific, it may not be surprising that this agent can alleviate an autosomal recessive disorder which occurs in certain gray Collie dogs and is characterized by neutropenic episodes at fortnightly intervals. This animal disease can be viewed as a model for human cyclic neutropenia, which has also been shown to respond positively to G-CSF.

Neutropenic mice have been shown to be very sensitive to certain microorganisms, even to gram-negative opportunistic pathogens which must be injected into healthy animals in high numbers in order to produce lethal septicemias. Mice become severely neutropenic four days after an i.p. injection of 200 mg/kg cyclophosphamide. During this period of neutropenia they easily succumb to experimental infections with gram-positive and gram-negative bacteria. Daily injections of G-CSF (1–2.5 μg) per animal for four days provided complete or nearly complete protection against subsequent experimental infections with *S. aureus, S. marcescens, P. aeruginosa, E. coli* and *C. albicans.* These studies are in line with older investigations which had demonstrated a positive relationship between the induction of endogenous CSFs by macrophage activating agents and survival of experimental infections in animals made neutropenic by treatment with cyclophosphamide.

Pharmacokinetic studies. There are at present only few data available which describe the pharmacokinetic behaviour of G-CSF in humans. When the material was infused intravenously over 40-minute time periods into patients, the serum levels remained relatively constant for a period of about 40 minutes. Thereafter, G-CSF disappeared with an average biological half-life of 5½ h as determined by radioimmunoassay. Trials in which G-CSF was infused over somewhat shorter time periods and in which the activity was subsequently measured in the serum by different bioassays gave somewhat conflicting results: G-CSF was found to be eliminated from the serum in a biphasic manner with a rapid first phase lasting 30–60 minutes, characterized by a half-life between five and ten minutes. During a second phase the remaining activity disappeared with a half-life of approximately 100 minutes.

Clinical studies. There are four major indications for the potential clinical use of G-CSF:

1) Restoration of hematopoiesis, thereby accelerating recovery from disease-related or iatrogenically induced neutropenia. This indication could also include cases in which G-CSF is administered in order to prevent functional damage to myelopoiesis, e.g. during prolonged administration of cytostatic or antiviral agents.
2) Augmentation of host defences against infection.
3) Stimulation of functionally primed effector cells with antitumour activity.
4) Clonal extinction of hematopoietic tumour cells by differentiation induction.

So far there is good clinical evidence documenting the safety and efficacy of G-CSF in the first group of indications. There is reasonable experimental evidence suggesting that G-CSF might have a place in the treatment of infections and in the elimination of tumour cells. Finally, there is only limited experimental evidence that G-CSF could become an important tool in the induction of differentiation in leukemias.

Several clinical studies have shown that G-CSF can significantly shorten and mitigate the neutropenic episodes connected with cytostatic therapy in cancer patients *(Fig. 6.11)*. In a study of 27 patients with advanced transitional cell carcinoma of the urothelium who received several cycles of combined chemotherapy, G-CSF had pronounced beneficial effects: treatment with G-CSF at doses between 1 and 60 μg/kg/day before chemotherapy resulted in a dose-dependent increase in the absolute neutrophil counts. When given after chemotherapy, G-CSF (recombinant material) reduced the number of patient days on which the absolute neutrophil count was 1,000/μl or less by 90%! Similarly, the number of patient days on which antibiotics had to be given to treat fever and neutropenia was reduced from 35 (controls) to one. Finally, the percentage of patients who would be exposed to a new cycle of chemotherapy as planned increased from 29% for the controls to 100% for the treatment group. Similar results were obtained with patient groups undergoing cyclic chemotherapy because

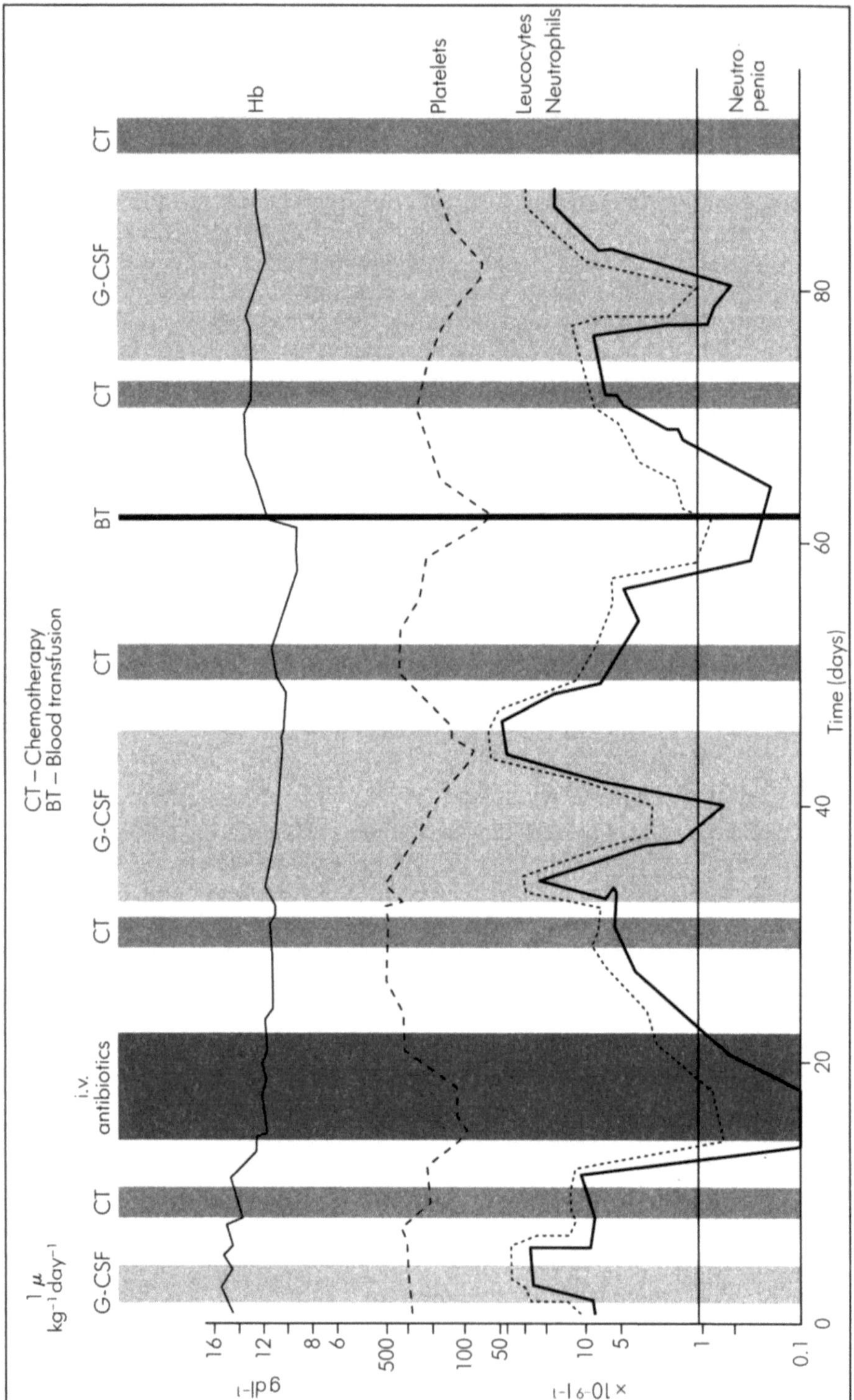
CT – Chemotherapy
BT – Blood transfusion
1 μ kg⁻¹ day⁻¹ G-CSF
CT
i.v. antibiotics
CT
G-CSF
CT
BT
CT
G-CSF
CT
Hb
Platelets
Leucocytes
Neutrophils
Neutro-penia
g dl⁻¹
16
12
8
6
× 10⁻⁹ l⁻¹
500
100
50
10
5
1
0.1
Time (days)
0
20
40
60
80

of small-cell lung carcinoma and in groups comprising different types of malignancies.

The only therapy currently available for the treatment of AIDS and of the AIDS-related complex (ARC) is azidothymidine (AZT). The drug has been estimated to extend the life span of AIDS patients and of patients with ARC by 9–12 and by 14–18 months respectively. The single most severe side effect of AZT which limits its application in the two indications mentioned and prevents its use in HIV-positive patients is myelosuppression. Preliminary data indicate that the application of G-CSF in low doses can prevent or mitigate myelosuppression when given parallel to AZT. There is justified hope that G-CSF may add a new dimension to the use of AZT in AIDS, in AIDS-related complex and perhaps even in HIV-positive patients.

Toxicity and side effects. Cynomolgus monkeys who were infused with recombinant G-CSF at doses of 10, 50, 250 and 1,000 mg/kg/day over a two-week period showed no effects which could be attributed to specific toxicity of the compound. Hypercellular bone marrow, neutrophilia and extramedullary hematopoiesis were consistent compound-related changes.

In humans the only clinical side effect noted regularly after treatment with G-CSF was mild to severe bone "medullary" pain occurring in 22% of all patients. Usually this symptom did not require treatment. In rare more severe cases the side effect was found to respond well to indomethacin. Laboratory evaluations showed marked increases of leucocyte alkaline phosphatase, serum alkaline phosphatase and lactate dehydrogenase. In addition, a mild increase in uric acid was recorded in patients treated with 30–60 μg/kg per day. All these changes were transient and returned to normal within one week after discontinuation of G-CSF treatment.

6.2.4.3 Interleukin 3

This multilineage hematopoetin is still in very early stages of clinical trials. The pharmacological information available today is still very limited.

Properties and origin. Il-3 was first cloned from a gibbon T-cell line. It is a small polypeptide which comprises 152 a.a. The first 19 a.a. of this polypeptide include a very hydrophobic sequence which is typical of a leader sequence. The mature protein contains 133 a.a. and has a molecular mass of 14.6 kd. The molecule contains two N-glycosylation sites, which could account for the molecular heterogeneity found in native Il-3 which was isolated from T-cell lines and from WEHI-3B cell supernantants.

The nucleotide sequence of the gibbon Il-3 gene is almost identical to the human gene which was subsequently isolated from a human gene library. The

Figure 6.11. G-CSF reduces neutropenia following chemotherapy.

human polypeptide shows only a 29% sequence homology with the murine material.

The gene for human Il-3 contains five small exons separated by one large and three small introns. It is located on chromosome 5, close to the gene for GM-CSF. The Il-3 sequence is lost in the 5 q syndrome.

Il-3 mRNA is expressed in T-cells. In gibbon T-cells the abundance of this mRNA is between 0.01% an 0.1%. In human peripheral blood lymphocytes this mRNA is even less abundant.

Il-3 is species specific. It binds to a large variety of precursor cells consistent with its multilineage function. Cross-linking experiments with labelled Il-3 have shown that Il-3 attaches with equal affinity to two single chain receptor molecules having molecular weights to 60 and 75 kd, respectively. It is at present not clear whether the two molecules are distinct Il-3 receptors or a single receptor showing different patterns of glycosylation or other modifications. Il-3 receptors are expressed on the surface of target cells in relatively small numbers ranging from 50–1,000 molecules per cell.

Biological activities. In human bone-marrow cultures Il-3 or multi-CSF gives rise to mature granulocytes, monocytes, eosinophils, megakaryocytes and mast cells. In the presence of small amounts of erythropoietin, Il-3 also stimulates the generation of erythroid cells.

If Il-3 is injected into animals it shows effects commensurate with its multilineage function. Recombinant murine Il-3 injected into mice i.p. at doses of 200 ng for up to six days produced a variety of changes, all indicative of general stimulation of blood cell formation and activation. The spleens of mice injected with Il-3 showed an 50% increase in weight, elevated levels of maturing granulocytes, eosinophils, nucleated erythroid cells, megakaryocytes and mast cells. The frequency of progenitor cells in the spleen was elevated 6–18 fold. Similar changes were observed in the peritoneal cavity. In one mouse strain, increased numbers of infiltrating hematopoietic cells were also found in the liver. Rises in mast cells were observed in the mesenteric lymph nodes, skin and intestines.

Potential clinical uses. Il-3 given alone or in combination with other hematopoietins may find its most important use in the reconstruction of hematopoietic tissue after damage induced by radiation or chemotherapy, or in disease-related situations like myelodysplasia. In preliminary experiments in mice and in primates, pretreatment with Il-3 specific for the animal species followed by G-CSF treatment led to much higher and more sustained elevation of neutrophils than the use of either hematopoietin alone. It may turn out that optimal management of hematopoiesis and blood cell activation will require the use of several factors given in parallel or – perhaps more logically – applied sequentially. It is likely that – for the time being – Il-3 will be used in autologous and allogeneic bone-marrow transplantation and in attempts to reduce neutropenia following cytoreductive treatment in various malignant conditions.

6.2.4.4 M-CSF

Properties and origin. Like G-CSF, M-CSF is a class-2 hematopoietin, acting mainly on monocytes and myelo-monocytic cell lines. Human M-CSF occurs in the urine. It is a dimer comprising two identical subunits which carry no biological activity of their own. The molecular weight of the native material found in human urine ranges between 47 and 76 kd. Murine M-CSF isolated from L-cell supernatants has a molecular weight of 70,000 and dissociates into subunits of 35–38 kd under reducing conditions. Digestion of both murine and human M-CSF subunits with endo-β-N-acetylglucosaminidase D yields subunits of 16.0 kd, of which the polypeptide portions account for 14.5 kd.

Oligonucleotide probes derived from the amino terminal sequence of human M-CSF were used to isolate several clones from a human genomic library. One of these clones was subsequently employed in the screening of a human cDNA library which had been prepared from 1.5–2.0 kd mRNA extracted from a human pancreatic tumour cell line. This approach led to the isolation and expression of a clone in COS 7 cells. The protein was active in stimulating monocytic precursor cells. Its effect was neutralized by an antibody against human urinary M-CSF. Hybridization analysis of M-CSF mRNA from a variety of human cells subsequently showed that a 4.0 kb transcript is the predominant mRNA coding for M-CSF. A detailed comparison of the two mRNA species revealed that the longer sequence contained an insert of 894 nucleotides within the coding region as well as a longer 3′-non-coding sequence. These differences result from alternative splicing of the primary M-CSF transcript. Since the insertion of 894 nucleotides does not distort the reading frame, the two mRNAs specify the synthesis of two related but not identical M-CSF molecules which are processed post-translationally to yield two different final forms of M-CSF, a 70–90 kd protein comprising a homodimer of 35–45 kd (containing 224 aa) and a 40–50 kd glycoprotein containing subunits with a molecular mass of 20–25 kd and 145 aa. There is, however, only one M-CSF gene which contains many exons spread over a range of 22 kb of DNA. The gene is located on chromosome 5 close to the genes which encode Il-3, GM-CSF and the M-CSF receptor. The receptor is a single chain protein of 16.5 kd. It is identical to the c-fms proto-oncogene.

M-CSF is formed by monocytes, fibroblasts and endothelial cells. In mice the pregnant uterus is an abundant source of M-CSF.

Biological activities. In human bone-marrow cultures, M-CSF elicits the formation of predominantly macrophage colonies although some effect on neutrophil formation has also been reported. It is believed that M-CSF may participate in maintaining a reserve of progenitors for neutrophils but that GM- or G-CSF are needed to drive these cells on to become mature neutrophils. M-CSF seems to stimulate blood monocytes to secrete large amounts of TNF, G-CSF and interferon. M-CSF has been shown to synergize strongly with hematopoietin (Il-1) in the generation of monocytes.

Potential clinical uses. The most likely clinical application of M-CSF would be in situations in which activation of macrophages might help to overcome infections, especially intracellular bacterial or fungal infections. Secondly, one might consider the use of this cytokine for the elimination of micrometastases in malignant conditions.

6.2.5 Thymic hormones

6.2.5.1 Definition and history

As already mentioned in Chapter 2, the thymus plays a crucial role in the development of T-lymphocytes and thus of the immune system – a discovery that was made only some decades ago. It was already assumed towards the end of the last century that the thymus was an organ with endocrine activity, and this probability was substantiated by the experiments of Abelous and Billard in which reduced muscle tone in thymectomized frogs was restored by means of thymus extracts. Subsequently, a number of physical functions came to be associated with the thymus gland. Our interest is confined to the lymphopoietic effects stemming from the thymus, first reported in 1940 by Bomskov and Sladovic.

An endocrine function of the thymus essential for the immune system was predicated on the following conditions:

1. The removal of the thymus had to lead to characteristic disturbances which were reversed by re-transplantation of thymus tissue. This condition has long since been fulfilled. Mice thymectomized shortly after birth are unable to form an immune response to T-cell dependent antigens. Such animals can survive for any period of time only in sterile surroundings. Implantation of thymus tissue into the thymectomized animals can reverse the immune deficiencies observed.
2. It had to be proved that the immunorestorative function of thymus tissue in thymectomized mice was mediated by humoral factors secreted by thymus cells. The evidence was obtained by implanting thymus cells that were enclosed within Millipore chambers. These implanted cells were also able to offset the immunological deficiencies of thymectomized or congenitally athymic mice.
3. Cell-free extracts from thymic glands had to be able at least temporarily to take over the function of the intact organ. This prerequisite has also been satisfied.
4. The last precondition was the identification of the thymic hormone(s), their isolation and purification from thymic extracts, the elucidation of their structure, and determination of the efficacy of the pure substances or of synthetic copies.

Efforts are still in progress to satisfy this last requirement. Several peptides with effects on the formation, development and function of T-lymphocytes have been isolated. Their structures have been determined and their biological function confirmed and elucidated in detail. Comparably precise knowledge of other substances found, or assumed to be present, in the thymus has still to be obtained. It is theoretically possible that immunologically active peptides found in the thymus do not stem from the thymus at all but are simply transported there. At least for thymosin $alpha_1$ (see below) its thymic origin is demonstrated by the fact that mRNA from the thymus was translated into authentic thymosin $alpha_1$ in a cell-free, protein-synthesizing wheat-germ system.

Research on the thymic hormones, their physiological functions, pharmacological properties and therapeutic value is still in progress. However, some of the enthusiasm surrounding this area has faded since, on the one hand, fully convincing clinical results with thymus peptides have not yet been forthcoming while, on the other, the clinical importance of other substances, e.g. the colony stimulating factors, has been impressively documentated. In the present context only those substances will be discussed for which pharmacological or even clinical findings have been obtained or at least suggested.

6.2.5.2 Thymosins and related peptides

Thymosin fraction 5 contains a number of immunologically effective peptides. They and some of the polypeptides they contain are already objects of large-scale clinical studies. The isolation of this fraction from calf thymus and the designations of the relevant polypeptides should therefore be described in brief.

A homogenate obtained from calf thymus is centrifuged at 14,000 *g*, passed through a glass wool filter and finally heated to 80 °C. After acetone precipitation the material is redissolved and subsequently fractionated with $(NH_4)_2SO_4$ in a stepwise fashion. The fraction which is saturation precipitated between 25 and 50% is then subjected to ultrafiltration and finally desalted on Sephadex G 25. The resulting material is designated thymosin fraction 5. An analogous procedure is used with the protein which precipitates at 50–95% saturation; after ultrafiltration and removal of salt, it yields fraction 5A.

If fraction 5 is subjected to isoelectric focusing, the peptides which it contains form discrete bands corresponding to the relative number of their carboxyl and amino groups in the pH gradient. The acidic proteins with isoelectric points (pI) below pH 5 are designated the alpha fraction, while the weakly acidic peptides with isoelectric points between pH 5 and pH 7 are designated the beta fraction and those above pH 7 the gamma fraction. Their suffixes 1, 2, 3 etc. identify individual peptides or proteins within these three groups. The individual peptides have been named in order of isolation as alpha, beta or gamma 1, 2, 3, etc.

Bovine thymosin $alpha_1$: this peptide, which accounts for about 0.6% of thymosin fraction 5, consists of 28 amino acids and has a molecular weight of 3108 daltons. The amino acid sequence has been elucidated. The terminal amino group is blocked by an acetyl moiety. The peptide is derived from a longer peptide with a molecular weight of 16,000 daltons as a result of specific cleavage or degradation. Chemically synthesized or cloned thymosin $alpha_1$ exhibits the same biological activity as the material isolated from thymus tissue. Thymosin $alpha_1$ from human thymus has the same primary structure as thymosin $alpha_1$ from calves, pigs or sheep; it has a consistently uniform structure.

Other thymosins: The peptides alpha$_5$ and alpha$_7$ are markedly acidic (pI of 3.5) and have no lipid or carbohydrate portions. The molecular weight of alpha$_5$ is 3000 and of alpha$_7$ 2200 daltons. A peptide beta$_1$, isolated from fraction 5A, is made up of 74 amino acids and has a molecular weight of 8451 daltons. It is apparently not a thymic hormone but a nucleoprotein which was inactive in immunological tests. The situation is different with thymosins beta$_3$ and beta$_4$, also derived from fraction 5A. The former has an isoelectric point of 5.2 and a molecular weight of 5500 daltons, the latter a pI of 5.1 and a molecular weight of 4982 daltons.

The full amino acid sequence of beta$_4$ has been elucidated and seems to be largely identical with that of thymosin beta$_3$. The only differences between the two peptides are in their carboxyl terminal portions.

6.2.5.3 Immunological effects of thymosin

The non-fractionated thymosin fraction 5 is, however, the most closely investigated thymic hormone preparation with which the greatest clinical experience has been gained. The most important action of this peptide mixture, from which all or most other effects stem, is the stimulation by thymosin of the development of stem cells from bone marrow to reactive T-cells. *In vitro,* thymosin increases the number of T-cell rosettes, the sensitivity of peripheral blood lymphocytes or spleen cells to antigens or mitogens, and the formation of cytotoxic T-cells in the mixed lymphocyte reaction. Thymosin induces stem cells to form terminal deoxyribonucleotidyl transferase, an enzyme which is possibly connected in some way with the development of immunological differentiation during antigen-dependent maturation of T-cells in the thymus. Under the influence of thymosin, thymocytes express the T-cell antigens Lyt 1^+, 2^+, 3^+ and the Thy-1 antigen. Likewise, the formation of a 5′-exonucleotidase is induced in human thymocytes.

In vivo experiments have shown that thymosin stimulates lymphocytopoiesis, especially in thymectomized or athymic mice kept in pathogen-free conditions. Evidence pointing in the same direction has, however, also been found in healthy and in adrenalectomized rats and mice. Thymosin increases the number of rejection reactions to allotransplants in both normal and thymectomized animals. Resistance to virally induced tumours (Moloney's viral sarcoma in the normal mouse) is increased by thymosin fraction 5. A similar situation exists for resistance of healthy mice to allogeneic or xenogeneic tumours. NZB (New Zealand Black) mice develop an autoimmune disease similar to lupus erythematosus, most probably as a result of a maturation defect affecting thymus cells, which leads to a deficit of specific T-suppressor lymphocytes. Thymosin fraction 5 can eliminate the maturation block, facilitate the formation of T-suppressor cells and in this way slow down the development of the autoimmune disease. T-cells are induced by thymosin, in the presence of antigen, to synthesize lymphokines such as interferon and migration inhibition factor (MIF). In older mice thymosin fraction 5 can restore the reduced ability to synthesize hemagglutinating antibodies to the levels found in young animals. When combined with chemotherapeutics, thymosin fraction 5 has proven to be effective in treatment of a number of experimentally induced tumours, and this combined therapy has been found to be superior to therapy with chemotherapeutics alone.

6.2.5.4 *Clinical findings with thymosin*

In children with primary immune disease, e.g. the Di George syndrome, mucocutaneous candidiasis, the Wiskott-Aldrich syndrome or other diseases associated with thymic hypoplasia or dysplasia, thymosin fraction 5 appears to be therapeutically effective. In trials which were carried on for almost ten years, both immunological and clinical parameters improved under therapy. The number of lymphocytes increased and their function improved, while the patients suffered from fewer intercurrent infections, gained weight and generally showed an improved clinical picture. The dosage schedule for the first two to four weeks was 400 mg per m^2 body surface s.c., followed by maintenance therapy of 60 mg per m^2 body surface. The total number of patients with primary immunodeficiency who received thymosin fraction 5 has in the meantime risen to about 100. However, the numbers of patients for each clinical entity are still too small to allow statistically relevant statements. In view of the good tolerability shown by thymosin fraction 5, many specialists believe that this therapy is indicated in primary immune deficiency whenever the lymphocytes of the child in question respond *in vitro* to thymosin fraction 5.

The first randomized phase-II trial with thymosin was conducted in 55 patients with inoperable bronchial carcinoma (oat-cell type). Thymosin fraction 5, in a daily dosage of 60 mg per m^2 body surface, was administered for six weeks in conjunction with intensive chemotherapy. The results seem to demonstrate that thymosin fraction 5 raises the average survival time of patients who had been rendered tumour-free by preceding chemotherapy from 240 days (placebo and chemotherapy) to 450 days. The analysis of this trial showed that thymosin exerts no direct activity on tumour cells and that its limited, but clearly positive, clinical effect is due to its immunostimulatory properties.

The side effects of therapy with thymosin fraction 5 were relatively mild in view of the impurities in the preparation employed. In a recently published summary of the results of therapy in 82 children with primary immune deficiency, only 9 cases were reported in which treatment had to be withdrawn on account of adverse reactions. Four patients exhibited local reactions after the injection (marked redness, swelling or the Arthus reaction). In 2 cases the drug had to be withdrawn because of hemorrhagic diathesis; expiratory stridor, progressive thrombocytopenia associated with eosinophilia, acute encephalopathy and lymphoma were each observed in one patient. Even in the thymosin-treated tumour patients, only few serious side effects were seen.

Biological activity of various peptides from thymosin fraction 5. Thymosin $alpha_1$, both *in vitro* and *in vivo*, produces most, if not all, changes known to be caused by thymosin fraction 5. In terms of weight, thymosin $alpha_1$ is about one hundred times more effective than the entire fraction 5 with respect to the increase in the number of T cell rosettes. In healthy persons, the proportion of lymphocytes which can form "autologous" rosettes with erythrocytes from the same source is about 26%. In cancer patients this figure may be considerably reduced. "Normal" conditions can be restored within a short time by incubating these lymphocytes with thymosin $alpha_1$. Tumour patients also occasionally exhibit a shift in the ratio of T-helper to T-suppressor cells. Under normal conditions this ratio is 3:1, but in the presence of a tumour the T-suppressor cell population may grow substantially so that the ratio is 1:1 or even less. Incubating the blood lymphocytes of cancer patients with thymosin $alpha_1$ may help restore a normal T-helper/T-suppressor ratio. Clinical trials with thymosin $alpha_1$ in tumour patients have, however, not produced any convincing results. Little is known as yet about the remaining thymosin components. Thymosin $alpha_5$ seems to enhance the function of T-helper cells or to promote the differentiation of these cells. Conversely, thymosin $alpha_7$ apparently possesses immunosuppressive (i.e T-suppressor cell-inducing) properties. The thymosins $beta_3$ and $beta_4$ appear to be responsible for earlier stages of T-cell differentiation. It is under their influence that bone marrow stem cells give rise to prothymocytes, which already express terminal deoxynucleotidyl transferase but are still negative with respect to Thy 1 and Lyt antigens. No clinical findings with these peptides are available.

6.2.5.5 Other thymic hormones

A large number of peptides obtained from thymus tissue have also been described. Only a few of them, however, have been chemically and biologically characterized so that we can draw at least tentative conclusions about their function. They will be described here only in brief.

THF (thymic humoral factor): This peptide (pI 5.6 and molecular weight 3220 daltons) was isolated from calf thymus, by means of methods largely similar to those employed in the isolation of thymosin fraction 5. However, the heat inactivation step was omitted in obtaining THF. THF has a number of properties reminiscent of thymosin fraction 5 or thymosin $alpha_1$. Spleen cells from mice thymectomized immediately after birth differentiate under the effect of THF to cytotoxic lymphocytes, which may bring about the rejection of an allotransplant or be involved in a graft versus host reaction. T-helper cells also develop in neonatally thymectomized mice under the influence of this peptide. It is quite possible that THF is a component of thymosin fraction 5, although it has no structural similarity with thymosin $alpha_1$. The substance is now undergoing clinical testing.

Thymopoietin: This general term encompasses two peptides TP I and TP II, now known to be closely related and, as shown by analysis of the amino acid sequences, differing in only two positions. Both peptides have 49 amino acids. The molecular weight of TP II is 5562 and the isoelectric point of both peptides is 5.5. There are no biological differences between TP I and TP II. Thymopoietin accelerates the development of prothymocytes to thymocytes and increases intracellular cAMP concentrations in thymocytes. Early stages of B-cell differentiation are inhibited, while late stages are accelerated. On granulocytes, TP I and TP II promote the expression of complement receptors. The *in vivo* action of TP II observed in rodents concerns the differentiation of prothymocytes to thymocytes in nude mice (nu/nu).

Thymopentin (TP-5): Thymopentin (TP-5) is a pentapeptide, which corresponds to the sequence of amino acids 32–36 in thymopoietin. It has been reported to exert all the effects of thymopoietin itself. Initial studies have shown it to be necessary for the maturation of prothymocytes to thymocytes. Under its influence prothymocytes acquire the TL and Thy-1 surface antigens. TP-5 has also been reported to enhance the function of mature lymphocytes as measured by the intensity of allogeneic responses. In mice, rejection of allogeneic transplants can be enhanced by TP-5. The immunostimulatory effects last two weeks. Very high doses of TP-5 can obviously exert immunosuppressive effects.

At parenterally administered doses of 0.1 mg/kg TP-5 can partially protect guinea pigs which were immunosuppressed by 20% body surface burns from the lethal effects of subsequent infections with *Pseudomonas aeruginosa*. Similar effects were observed with other animal models, characterized by trauma and caloric malnutrition on the one hand and experimental infection with opportunistic microbes on the other. It is not clear whether the therapeutic effects of TP-5 are entirely T-lymphocyte mediated or whether they involve other mechanisms as well. The phagocytic activity of neutrophils and macrophages, measured as "bactericidal index", from TP-5-treated animals was distinctly enhanced. TP-5 did not, however, stimulate phagocytosis and intracellular killing in neutrophils or macrophages when these cells were exposed to the peptide *in vitro* over a wide range of concentrations (1 pg – 1 mg/ml).

Parameters of cellular immunity (cell-mediated immunity against dinitrofluorobenzene) which are impaired as a result of trauma, thermal injury of malnutrition can apparently be partially restored by TP-5, at least in some animal species.

Human studies with TP-5 have provided evidence that the peptide when applied i.m. at 50 mg/day (3× a week for a total of three weeks) can restore response to a hepatitis B vaccine in previously unresponsive patients with renal failure. There have also been positive reports on the effects of TP-5 on the frequency of herpes simplex infections in predisposed populations and on the duration of ongoing herpes infections. *Most other clinical reports on TP-5 are anecdotal and refer to immunocompromised patients suffering from fungal or intracellular bacterial infections. Although many observations seem to indicate the potential usefulness of TP-5, conclusive clinical evidence is still lacking.*

Thymulin: Thymulin is a nonapeptide hormone produced by thymic epithelial cells. Its biological activity is strictly dependent on the presence of the metal zinc in the molecule. Effects similar to those described for TP-5 though not as extensive have been reported for thymulin. Like thymosin, thymulin seems to be able to modify the course of the lupus erythematosus-like disease in NZB mice.

6.2.6 Transfer factor

This factor consists of dialysable material derived from homogenized lymphocytes which has the ability to elicit delayed-type hypersensitivity to various antigens in anergic individuals. There is some evidence that this form of passive sensitization is antigen-specific, i.e. reactivity is transferred only to those antigens against which donor lymphocytes can also react. The arguments against such specificity are not easy to refute in view of the none too clearly defined nature of the transfer factor. It cannot be excluded, for instance, that at least certain transfer factor preparations themselves contain small amounts of the antigen against which they mediate hypersensitivity. Injection of TF would then be tantamount to sensitization with these antigens.

The essential functional components in transfer factor compounds are a purine base, ribose, a phosphodiester group and a peptide. The active substance in transfer factor might therefore be a short ribonucleotide, perhaps even a mononucleotide, which is protected against further breakdown by a non-covalently bound peptide. The function of the peptide residue might be to help the nucleotide effect more efficient transport into the cell; the analogy with synthetic isoprinosine is obvious in this case (see below).

Most of the clinical studies performed with transfer factor do not allow any far-reaching conclusions. Many positive findings were anecdotal. In other cases, controls were inadequate or other therapies were given concomitantly. The available research is also not standardized: there is no animal model for the evaluation and quantification of transfer factor. The dosage was based on the number of leucocytes used for the manufacture of the administered amount. This practice gave rise to the concept of "leucocyte equivalents".

Transfer factor has been administered to patients with the Wiskott-Aldrich syndrome for periods of up to five years, resulting in temporary clinical improvement in 14 out of 32 cases. At the end of the trial, however, not clear correlation was established between treatment and clinical course. Patients with chronic mucocutaneous candidiasis exhibited improved responses to antifungal chemotherapy after prior treatment with transfer factor. Apparently the best results were obtained with leucocyte dialysates from patients who had been sensitized to *Candida* antigens.

Transfer factor may also be effective in viral infections. In a randomized, double-blind trial, 61 children with acute lymphoblastic leukemia (ALL) were assigned to two groups. One group received transfer factor from five donors who had just recovered from a chickenpox infection and whose lymphocytes exhibited extraordinarily high reactivity to varicella-zoster antigen in vitro. In half the patients in this group, skin reactions to varicella-zoster virus were negative before treatment and positive thereafter. Sixteen patients in the group treated with transfer factor and 15 in the placebo group were in contact during the clinical trial with children who were infected with the varicella virus. In the piacebo group 13 of the 15 exposed children came down with chickenpox, while only one of the children treated with transfer factor became infected with varicella.

Moreover, there is anecdotal, though well documented, evidence of the effectiveness of transfer factor in infections due to rare mycobacteria. In all cases reported, treatment with transfer factor brought about positive skin reactions to antigens of the causative organism.

Despite some impressive evidence for the efficacy of transfer factor, the therapeutic importance of this mixture remains in doubt as long as it is not perfectly clear what the active component is and how it works.

It is perhaps rather symptomatic that since 1985 no paper has appeared which documents the clinical efficacy of transfer factor in an unambiguous fashion. Two lines of evidence deserve to be mentioned: the first one relates to the fact that "transfer factor" like other "immuno-modulators" appears to be able to restore or at least improve immunological parameters in certain groups of patients. There are reports on the reappearance of skin hypersensitivity reactions against a variety of antigens. In addition, an increase in the blastogenic response of lymphocytes from patients treated with transfer factor has been demonstrated in *ex vivo* experiments. However, the clinical significance of these findings is questionable.

The second line of evidence is even more disappointing. There seems to be an inverse relationship between the methodological solidity of clinical studies on the efficacy of transfer factors and positive outcomes. With few exceptions the studies which were well controlled and included adequate numbers of comparable patients gave negative or inconclusive results.

6.2.7 Tuftsin

Macrophages have two main functions in the immune system:

1. The uptake and destruction of bacteria and other microorganisms.
2. The presentation of antigens together with class-I or class-II histocompatibility antigens for activation of lymphocytes.

Both functions depend on the most efficient possible uptake of the particular antigen. This uptake is greatly accelerated by opsonization of the antigen and binding of the immune complexes to the macrophage Fc receptors. The accelerated uptake stems from activation of the macrophages or of the polymorphonuclear leucocytes through occupancy of the cell Fc receptor. Several years ago, Victor Najjar reported the following finding: after the binding of antigen, IgG antibodies which had attached to Fcγ receptors of macrophages or other Fcγ carrying cells released from their CH_2 domains a tetrapeptide with the following sequence: NH^2-Thre-Lys-Pro-Arg-COOH. A membrane-bound enzyme, leukokinase, was held responsible for cleavage at the amino terminal end of the tetrapeptide and an as yet undefined enzyme in the spleen for cleavage at the carboxyl terminal end. The new tetrapeptide was termed "tuftsin" because it had been discovered at Tuft's University. Researchers found that tuftsin developed whenever antigen-carrying IgG molecules reacted with their Fc receptors on macrophages or granulocytes. Splenectomized patients were unable to produce normal amounts of the tetrapeptide. Najjar and later other investigators were able to show that tuftsin enhances phagocytosis and concluded from their experiments that this tetrapeptide is the physiological signal emitted by the Fc receptor for the uptake of antigens and that for this purpose it does not need the entire intact IgG molecule.

Some experiments indicate that tuftsin possesses such an amplifying function. One team from Israel incubated precultured peritoneal macrophages from mice with 50 μg/ml of a standard antigen (keyhole limpet hemocyanin) and with varying concentrations of tuftsin or its analogs. Subsequently, the cell layers were washed several times to remove any superfluous antigen. Fresh spleen cells were placed on the macrophages which had been in contact with the antigen and incubated with them overnight. After incubation, all non-adhering cells were collected, freed of adherent-cell contaminants and then killed by irradiation (x-rays). The cells were washed again and suspended, and 5×10^6 cells in 50 μl volume were injected into the rear paw of mice of the same species. On day 7 after injection, the popliteal lymph nodes were removed, suspended and, after elimination of all adherent cells, incubated together with the antigen KLH or with control substances. The proliferative response of the popliteal lymphocytes was then measured by incorporation of [^{3}H]-thymidine.

Lymphocytes from mice previously injected with cells which had been incubated with tuftsin-treated macrophages showed a one to seven-fold higher proliferative reaction to KLH antigens than did normal cells. The Israeli investigators interpreted their results as follows: they assumed that macrophages took up and presented more antigen in the presence of tuftsin than did control macrophages. Tuftsin-treated macrophages, when subsequently incubated with spleen cells, induced a greater number of specific T-helper cells than did control macrophages. The injection of T-helper lymphocytes generated under the influence of tuftsin, then in turn led to increased formation of cytotoxic T-lymphocytes in the adjacent popliteal region of the mice which had received the injection.

This experiments is not entirely convincing because the animals receiving the injection had only been in contact with killed T-helper lymphocytes which would be expected to elicit only humoral stimuli. However, it has been shown in numerous experiments that tuftsin and its synthetic analogs enhance phagocytosis in monocytes, macrophages and granulocytes. NK-cells have also been reported to respond to tuftsin. There can be little doubt about the validity of these experimental findings. Nevertheless, tuftsin has never demonstrated its inherent effectiveness in clinical studies so unequivocally as to become an accepted immunostimulant. Experiments with various analogs of the tetrapeptide have shown that the sequence Pro-Arg is the key to identification by the macrophage and to its activation. This dipeptide is, albeit in higher concentrations than tuftsin, effective as a macrophage activator. Threonine can be substituted for alanine in the tetrapeptide, and the analog is even more effective than tuftsin. This peptide and the pentapeptide NH_2-Thre-Lys-Pro-Arg-Gly-COOH do not increase the rate of phagocytosis, but do improve the "immunogenicity" of macrophages. These derivatives possibly also lead to increased secretion of Il-1 during antigen presentation, thus providing a second, strong signal for the activation of lymphocytes which have already "seen" their antigen in association with the MHC molecules.

Although neither tuftsin nor its analogs have achieved any clinical importance, the experimental path taken in the investigation of these peptides constitutes an original approach which should be pursued, even if no clinical success has yet been forthcoming.

6.3 Substances of microbial origin

Many immunostimulatory substances are of microbial origin: lipopolysaccharides, lipoteichoic acids, phospholipids, ubiquinones, glucans, etc. These substances, all of them antigens, have occasionally been classified as either T-cell dependent or T-cell independent. It was assumed that T-cell dependent bacterial antigens need the assistance of T-helper cells to trigger an immune response. Chemically, such antigens are, in the view of certain workers (e.g. D. Weir and C. Blackwell), "amphiphatic" structures, which have chemical groups of a characteristically different structure (e.g. hydrophilic and lipophilic portions). These T-cell dependent antigens contrast with T-cell independent antigens. Of the latter it has been postulated that they might, without the assistance of T-helper cells, bring about polyclonal activation, e.g. of B-cells, or exert a direct effect on accessory cells such as macrophages. Such T-cell independent antigens are generally substances with high molecular weights and multiple repetitive structures, which are relatively resistant to enzymatic breakdown. This category also includes lipopolysaccharides, glucans and peptidoglucans.

It is at least questionable whether this distinction is practical for *in vivo* experiments or, in particular, therapeutic settings. All substances of microbial origin – including preparations consisting of whole microorganisms – have an activating effect on the cells of the mononuclear-phagocytic system, i.e. monocytes, macrophages and antigen-presenting cells such as dendritic and Langerhans cells. This activation may be directed primarily at macrophages. This is particularly so with the β 1,3-D-glucans. On the other hand, activation of macrophages may take place primarily via activated T-cells, as with Bacille-Calmette-Guérin and Listeria monocytogenes. T-helper cells and macrophages form a functional unit in their reaction to certain antigens. This unit can be stimulated by either of the two components, but the emphasis or the primary stimulus at one time favours the macrophages, at another the T-helper cells *(Fig. 6.12)*. The decisive factor governing the effect is always the degree of activation of the total system. For defence against bacterial infection, this is equivalent to the degree of macrophage activity. Maximally activated macrophages can also lyse tumour cells, but for lysis of tumour cells and virally infected cells, the cytotoxic lymphocyte plays an important and perhaps dominating role. All microbial substances now being tested or occasionally used in clinical immunotherapy can be understood in this context.

6.3.1 Patterns of macrophage activation

The immune system of higher animals develops in an environment of microorganisms. Microbial parasites may be classified as extracellular, facultative intracellular and obligate intracellular, depending on the localization of their replication cycle. The first group includes gram-positive cocci and most gram-nega-

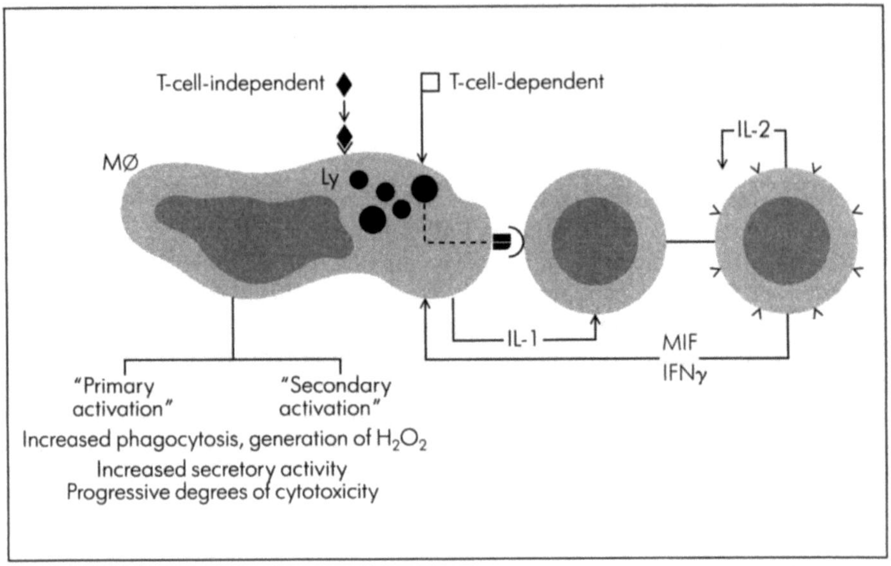

Figure 6.12. Diagram of activation of macrophages by T-cell-dependent and T-cell-independent antigens.
Ly: lysosomes
MIF: migration inhibitory factor.

tive rods. The parasitic behaviour of these bacteria is restricted to the extracellular spaces. They do not have biochemical means with which to resist the lytic mechanism within phagocytosing cells. The second group (facultative intracellular pathogens) includes *Mycobacterium tuberculosis, Mycobacterium bovis (BCG), Listeria monocytogenes, Brucella* sp., salmonellae, *Francisella tularensis* and the fungus *Histoplasma capsulatum.* These microorganisms can exist within mononuclear phagocytes just as easily as in the extracellular space. The third group is that of the obligate intracellular parasites, which can replicate only within the cell. The group includes chlamydias, rickettsias, viruses and the protozoa *Toxoplasma gondii, Besnoitia jellisoni* and *Trypanosoma cruzi.*

Resistance to extracellular pathogens extends to mechanisms which lead to their phagocytosis. This includes the formation of "opsonizing" antibodies, recruitment of neutrophilic granulocytes, activation of complement and, lastly, the phagocytosis of opsonized (i.e. covered with antibodies) microorganisms via the Fc or C3b receptors of the granulocytes.

The situation is different with regard to the facultative and obligate intracellular pathogens, which can replicate inside the cell. resistance to these pathogens can therefore not be achieved by opsonization of an invading organism, complement activation or phagocytosis, but only by critical changes in the intracellular milieu of the phagocytosing cells. The findings from a growing number of studies seem to prove that the production of oxygen radicals (detectable by the release of H_2O_2) is the biochemical mechanism which makes it possible to eliminate intracellular pathogens and probably also tumour cells. In 1936 Pullinger reported that mice infected with tubercle bacteria became resistant as a result of this infection to other, unrelated pathogens such as *Brucella abortus.* Since then, other examples have been reported in which infection with an intracellular pathogen grants protection against infections with other intracellular pathogens. Mackaness in 1964 called this phenomenon "acquired cell-mediated immunity". As already mentioned, it is based on the function of T-lymphocytes and macrophages. While certain (T-cell-independent) antigens can activate macrophages *in vitro*, the generation of completely bactericidal or even tumoricidal macrophages depends on the assistance of sensitized T-lymphocytes, more specifically T-helper cells. To express its full toxicity, a macrophage must receive at least two signals: an indirect signal mediated by T-cells and a direct signal through contact with the antigen. This "two signal theory" has been confirmed in a number of experimental models, but it must not be taken literally. While the transmission of a stimulatory signal through contact with a bacterial antigen constitutes a relatively well-defined event, the stimulus transmitted by T-cells can apparently contain several signals, mediated by different lymphokines such as gamma-interferon or CSF. It is not known, however, which signal frequencies and which type of signal produce maximum cytotoxicity.

It is also not known which biochemical cytotoxic mechanisms are responsible for the cytotoxicity in the various stages of macrophage activation. Activated macrophages secrete arginase, complement fragments, proteases, peroxidase, lysozyme and H_2O_2 or other reduced forms of oxygen.

Electron micrographs of activated macrophages attacking tumour cells show that close spatial contact is established between the target cell and the attacking macrophage. At the sites of contact on the cells, electron-dense pleomorphic particles with a granulated structure and a loosely enveloping trilaminar membrane are frequently observed. These structures are regarded as lysosomes that have been discharged by exocytosis from the macrophage to the immediate proximity of the tumour cell membrane. Labelling studies with dextran sulfate have shown that material from the cytotoxic cell is indeed transferred to the tumour cell. When homogenates of macrophages that had previously phagocytosed dextran sulfate were incubated with tumour cells, large amounts of dextran sulfate were subsequently found in the tumour cells. Another mechanism which has recently been held responsible for the cytotoxicity of macrophages for tumour cells is the secretion of tumour necrosis factor (TNF-α) by activated macrophages. This factor was described as early as 1975 and has since been cloned, sequenced and precisely characterized. It is found in the serum of rabbits, mice and rats which have been infected with BCG or *Corynebacterium parvum* and then treated with LPS two weeks later. A few hours after the last LPS injection the serum of these animals contains a protein that inhibits *in vitro* tumour cell growth and causes hemorrhagic necrosis of tumours *in vivo*. Synthesis of this factor can be inhibited by substances that impair macrophage function. Injection of hydrocortisone before the administration of LPS can completely suppress the release of TNF-α. This factor can also be obtained by *in vitro* incubation, together with LPS, of peritoneal cells from mice that have been previously infected with *Corynebacterium parvum* or BCG. Large amounts of TNF-α will then be released into the supernatant of the peritoneal cells. Human TNF-α can also be obtained from the supernatants of eight-day monocyte cultures. These findings suggest that TNF-α is a product of macrophages. A similar cytokine, TNF-β, is released from lymphocytes. It is a glycoprotein which in glycosolated form has a molecular weight of 20 kd. The pharmacological and therapeutic properties of TNF-α and TNF-β are currently under investigation. Partially purified murine TNF-α kills human tumour cells *in vitro* but not normal cells. Human TNF-α exhibits similar properties. The protein has a molecular weight of about 17 kd (see also chapter 2).

There is evidence to suggest that macrophages which have developed maximum activity against intracellular parasites and tumour cells will lose, at least in part, their ability to phagocytose and kill extracellular or facultative intracellular microorganisms. Thus microbicidal and tumoricidal properties are not necessarily identical. Mice chronically infected with *Toxoplasma gondii* or *Besnoitia jellisoni* are resistant to secondary infections with *Listeria monocytogenes* but are highly sensitive to streptococci or *Klebsiella pneumoniae.* Mice that have acquired an enhanced ability to destroy tumour metastases as a result of injections of pyran-copolymer or repeated BCG injections are just as sensitive as untreated animals to extracellular pathogens such as streptococci and staphylococci. On the other hand, granulocytopenic mice that have been treated with soluble glucans or ubiquinones are protected against extracellular bacteria but are completely susceptible to a metastasizing tumour such as the Lewis lung carcinoma. Zena Werb pointed out that resting macrophages and macrophages that have been activated by different stimuli can be classified on the basis of two biochemical characteristics: secretion of apoprotein E and H_2O_2. While the secretion of large amounts of H_2O_2 appears to be typical of tumoricidal macrophages, the secretion of apoprotein E was most marked in resting macrophages or in cells that had been stimulated only with thioglycolate *(Fig. 6.13).*

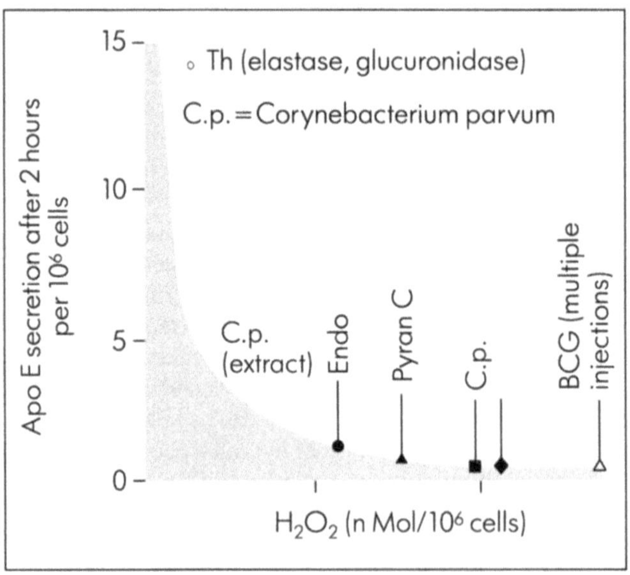

Figure 6.13. Relationship between secretion of apolipoprotein E and H_2O_2 in n Mol/10^6 cells. Points on the far right of the curve (high H_2O_2 production, low apolipoprotein secretion) are possibly typical of cytotoxic activity. C.p. = Corynebacterium parvum. Th = thioglycolate. Endo = endotoxin. Pyran C = pyran-copolymer.

Granulocytopenic mice that had been experimentally infected with different extracellular pathogens were protected against a fatal outcome of their infection only by substances that stimulated macrophages not only in their phagocytic but also in their secretory capacity. In this context, the secretion of colony stimulating factors appeared to be of particular relevance. Substances that only stimulated phagocytosis were ineffective in these models.

The phenomenon of acquired cellular immunity is perhaps the common denominator of all tumoricidal effects of microbial preparations such as *Corynebacterium parvum,* BCG, muramyl dipeptides and possibly even glucans and peptidoglucans.

It is not yet possible to say whether the functional state of a macrophage which protects against extracellular infection and is characterized by enhanced phagocytosis and secretion of CSFs represents a "lower" level of activation than that in which macrophages kill tumour cells, or whether we are dealing here with two qualitatively different states. It is possible that macrophage cytotoxicity develops as a result of different, complementary mechanisms. This would also explain why different stages of macrophage activation are characterized by typical biochemical patterns which permit varying degrees of antimicrobial activity and cytotoxicity.

6.3.2 Corynebacterium parvum and BCG

C. parvum can inhibit growth of a number of murine tumours on intravenous injection. Inhibition of growth is not complete, however, and there also tumours whose growth is, if anything, speeded up by *C. parvum.* Equally inconsistent results have been obtained with intravenous injections of BCG. Given such disappointing findings, it is rather surprising that so much attention has been focused on systemic administration of *C. parvum* or BCG. Clinical investigations have also since shown that presumably little can be expected from this type of immunostimulation.

The situation may be somewhat different with regard to local, i.e. intralesional, injection of these preparations. It has been demonstrated in a great number of animal models that this method produces regression of primary tumours and, what is more, eliminates lymphatic and hematogenous metastases.

BCG has been used a great deal in local treatment. McKenally injected BCG into the pleural cavity of patients following pneumonectomy for bronchial carcinoma and subsequently noted a reduction in the occurrence of tumours. Attempts to reproduce these results have often been disappointing, and therefore local administration of BCG in connection with thoracic surgery can by no means be considered a reliable procedure. The effect of local BCG injections into the lower limbs and the bladder lumen was investigated in patients with bladder carcinoma. Three clinical studies produced consistent results indicating a reduction in the tumour recurrence rate. More recent studies have corroborated the usefulness of BCG in the local treatment of bladder carcinoma. With completely resected tumours, BCG does not appear to offer distinct advantages over other intravesically used drugs, especially doxirubicin. For incompletely resected tumours the recurrence rate for BCG treated patients appears to be lower than for doxirubicin treatment. The particular merit of local treatment with BCG may therefore lie in the treatment of residual tumour after operation; other possible uses concern carcinoma *in situ* and superficial bladder cancer. Further positive findings have been reported for local injection of BCG in melanomas: 80% of the tumours treated disappeared temporarily or permanently. In addition, parallel to the animal experiments already mentioned, metastatic spread of the tumours regressed in 20% of these positive responders.

C. parvum and BCG probably have similar mechanisms of action which fit in with the theories already outlined. The involvement of T-cells in the development of the antitumour effect of *C. parvum* is particularly evident in studies of athymic mice. Though intralesional injection led to regression of several types of tumour such as fibrosarcoma or plasmacytoma in normal mice, this effect was not achieved in athymic mice. Likewise, the tumour regression resulting from intralesional injection of *C. parvum* does not occur in animals which have been depleted of their T-cells. All the evidence suggests that *C. parvum* not only exerts a direct effect on macrophages but also induces formation of T-cells sensitized to *C. parvum*. Through humoral signals these T-lymphocytes then bring about enhanced macrophage activity, including even the development of cytotoxity against tumour cells.

Intralesional injection of BCG induces tumour regression in athymic mice as well as in rats that are T-cell-depleted as a result of thoracic duct drainage. Under such conditions T-cells do not appear to be indispensable for the antitumour effect. On the other hand, intralesional BCG injections are more effective if the animals have been previously sensitized by systemic BCG immunization. T-cells reacting specifically to BCG can therefore actively contribute to the local effectiveness of this bacterial preparation.

In any comparison of *C. parvum* and BCG, it is evident that BCG is an antigen with a stronger direct effect on macrophages than *C. parvum,* and that the role of T-cells in BCG-initiated reactions is not so obvious as with *C. parvum*. Basically, however, macrophages are in both cases the main effector cells of antitumour effects and in both cases the macrophages are activated via direct contact with the antigen and through involvement of sensitized T-helper cells *(Fig. 6.12)*.

It has recently been shown that BCG vaccination of healthy individuals can lead to the formation of $CD4^+$ T-cell clones directed at mycobacterial antigen which specifically kill cells presenting mycobacterial antigen. These $CD4^+$ cells may therefore function as T-suppressor cells and prevent antibody formation against mycobacterial components.

6.3.3 Muramyl dipeptides

Mycobacteria are constituents of Freund's complete adjuvant. When an attempt was made to isolate and identify from these microorganisms the smallest chemical unit that, in an emulsion of mineral oil and water, would have the same effects as intact mycobacteria, it was first found that water-soluble peptidoglucan fragments can replace mycobacteria. Subsequently, N-acetyl-muramyl-L-alanine-D-isoglutamine or muramyl dipeptide (MDP) was discovered to be the minimum effective structure *(Fig. 6.14)*. This molecule has since been investigated very thoroughly by immunopharmacologists, and a large number of derivatives have been produced which vary considerably in the intensity and nature of their effects. Through this approach insights have been gained into the structural elements essential for the biological effect of MDP. The sugar ring cannot be opened or replaced by other molecules without the effect of MDP being lost. Likewise, the side chain with L-ala-D-isoglutamine is important for the effect of MDP, though certain changes are possible: L-ala can be replaced by L-aminobutyric acid and L-valine, and the peptide chain can be prolonged by insertion of a butyryl or octanoyl residue or of a butyl ester. Substitution is possible at positions 4 and 6 on the sugar molecule.

MDP itself has quite a large number of interesting properties. Water-soluble MDP derivatives in a water and mineral oil emulsion are effective as adjuvants, as are non-water-soluble derivatives in oily solutions with, for instance, long lipophilic residues in position 6. The adjuvant effect covers induction both of delayed-type hypersensitivity reactions, i.e. cell-mediated immune responses, and of humoral immune responses. However, no lipid vehicles are required for stimulation of antibody formation: water-soluble MDP derivatives can stimulate the formation of antibodies to human serum albumin and many other antigens in rodents without further additions. Injection of protein antigens and MDP together brings about an amplified primary response and – on renewed antigen exposure without repeated administration of MDP – an enhanced secondary response.

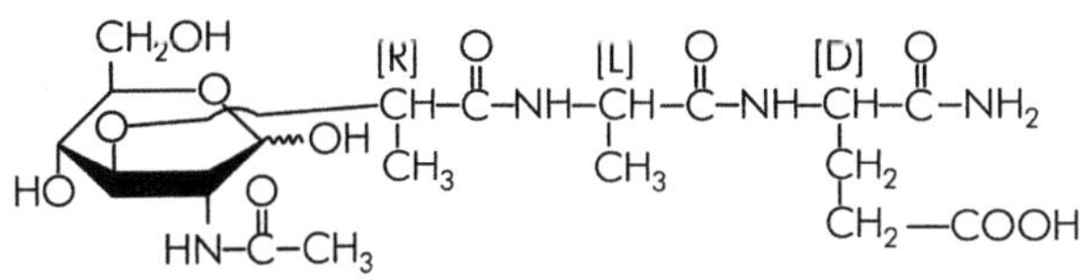

$C_{19}H_{32}N_4O_{11}$ N-acetylmuramyl dipeptide

Figure 6.14. Molecular structure of muramyl dipeptide.

As a result, MDP derivatives can increase non-specific resistance in mice, guinea pigs and other rodents. This effect probably depends on direct stimulation of neutrophilic granulocytes and macrophages. MDP activates macrophages *in vitro* without involvement of other cells. It was very soon found that macrophages thus stimulated release a factor that stimulates lymphocytes; we now know this factor to be interleukin 1. Polymorphonuclear granulocytes can be primed by MDP for an oxidative burst triggered by phorbol myristic acetate with the concomitant production of Il-1. MDP and derivatives of MDP have also been shown to stimulate macrophages as well as human endothelial cells to release colony stimulating factors.

Parenteral administration of MDP affords protection against a number of extracellular infections. Oral application at ten times the parenteral doses are also effective. MDP enhances the activity of the mononuclear-phagocytic system at doses as low as 5–10 mg per kg subcutaneously, as can be ascertained from the increase in the rate at which i.v. injected carbon particles are eliminated from the bloodstream (carbon clearance rate). Between five and ten times as much substance is sometimes required for protection against infection with lethal doses of infectious pathogens. It is, however, typical of the protective effects against gram-positive cocci, gram-negative rods and even *Candida albicans* that MDP or an effective MDP derivative is most effective when it has been administered 24 hours before experimental induction of the infection. In combination with antibiotic treatment, however, a clear therapeutic effect, which is additive to that of the antimicrobial therapy can still be observed four to six hours after experimental induction of the infection.

The dosage form of an MDP derivative also appears to play an important role for its therapeutic properties. Encapsulation of the N-acetyl-muramyl-L-aminobutyryl-D-isoglutamine in multilamellar liposomes leads to a reduction of the ED_{50} from 80 mg per kg to 5.5 mg per kg bodyweight in experimental infection in mice.

It has been shown that the encapsulation of MDP or MDP derivatives into multilamellar liposomes increases the uptake and the retention of the immune modulator by human monocytes and thus increases the specificity of drug action. When introduced in this form into experimental animals, MDP loses much of its typical toxicity which is characterized by fever, vasculitis and granulomatous reactions. The reason for this improved tolerability may relate to the fact that MDP when encapsulated into liposomes does not induce the formation of Il-1 in macrophages and endothelial cells. This very pronounced effect has been held responsible for the toxicity of the non-encapsulated material.

With such experimental results the outlook for the clinical use of MDP and its derivatives has become more promising. Earlier experiments had already suggested that at least the pyrogenic and the immunostimulating effects were not inseparable: MDP-induced fever was suppressed by indomethacin without any apparent modification of the adjuvant effect or the increase in resistance. Extensive efforts to create derivatives of MDP subsequently yielded products whose pyrogenic effects were clearly surpassed by the other two properties. The most interesting substance in this respect is the N-alanyl-D-glutaminyl-n-butyl ester derivative, which is on a par with MDP as an adjuvant in triggering humoral im-

Table 6.5. Adjuvant activity of MDP (Glu)-On-Bu in the immune response of 6–7-week-old mice to bovine serum albumin (RSA).

Immunization	Primary response (21 days)	Secondary response (day 36)
Controls	1.64	3.01
MDP	4.52	8.45
MDP (Glu)-On-Bu	4.2	8.43

mune responses *(Table 6.5)*. The non-pyrogenic derivative was also as effective as MDP in the protection it afforded against a number of bacterial infections, including *Klebsiella pneumoniae* in young mice (seven days old) or in splenectomized animals.

While MDP-treated rabbits responded to doses as low as 30 μg MDP per kg with a marked rise in temperature, the butyl ester itself was not pyrogenic even in doses of 10 mg per kg i.v. Plasma from animals given the n-butyl ester proved to be non-pyrogenic on transplantation to untreated rabbits, in contrast to plasma from MDP-treated animals. Like other exogenous pyrogenic substances (e.g. LPS), MDP immediately causes a sudden fall in granulocytes, lymphocytes and monocytes which lasts for five hours in granulocytes and up to 24 hours in lymphocytes and monocytes. Although n-butyl-MDP does not release endogenous pyrogen from mononuclear cells in vitro, supernatants of macrophages which have been incubated with the derivative nevertheless cause activation of lymphocytes. This would mean that, besides endogenous pyrogen, there is a non-pyrogenic lymphocyte-activating factor whose synthesis and release is selectively stimulated by MDP (Glu)-On-Bu.

It has recently been shown by several authors that MDP can act synergistically with interferon γ in making human monocytes tumoricidal. Fresh human monocytes, when exposed to γ-interferon (1,000 U/ml) or to 1 mg of MDP per ml did not become tumoricidal. However, when monocytes were exposed to much lower concentrations of both agents together they became cytolytic against a large variety of allogeneic tumour targets but do not kill normal cells. Analogous effects were also observed with MDP derivatives encapsulated into liposomes. The best activation an be observed if γ-interferon is introduced first, followed by the addition of the liposome-MTP-PE complex (muramyltripeptide phosphatidylethanolamine incorportated into liposomes). This observation could open up an interesting therapeutic possibility for the combined use of interferon γ and MDP derivatives in patients with metastasizing tumours.

6.3.4 Beta 1,3-D-glucan

These substances occur in bacteria, fungi, yeasts and higher plants. Although a number of different glucans have been investigated, the bulk of the experience has been gained with those derived from yeasts. Glucans may be found in highly polymeric form which is water-insoluble and has a very pronounced effect on macrophages, activating them to the point of cytotoxicity, secretion of colony-stimulating factors from activated macrophages and, on repeated dosing, to the formation of granulomas. But beta 1,3-D-glucan is still effective in less highly polymeric and in water-soluble form. The minimum chain length with which anything like full efficacy can still be achieved is approximately 16 D-glucose residues. Even single injections of beta 1,3-D-glucan protect experimental animals against a large number of otherwise lethal bacterial infections. The effective doses are in the region of 1–10 mg per kg. In the presence of beta 1,3-D-glucan serum lysozyme concentrations rise to five or six times the normal levels. The glucan-induced enhancement of *in vivo* phagocytosis by macrophages can be measured by the substantially increased clearance rate for colloidal carbon particles. Glucan-activated macrophages become cytotoxic for a number of tumour cells, though glucans are less effective in this respect than BCG or *C. parvum.* A number of other glucans have attracted more interest than the linear beta 1,3-D-glucan from *Saccharomyces cerevisiae* for their efficacy against syngeneic or allogeneic experimental tumours. These include lentinan, a beta 1,3-D-glucan from a fungus, Pachyman (beta 1,3-linked) D-glucan with beta (1,6-linked) branches and a peptidoglucan from *Coriolus versicolor,* which has become known in Japan under the designation *"Krestin"*. This substance also consists of a beta 1,3-D-glucan with beta 1,6 branches and, additionally, contains peptide residues which are covalently bound to the glucan. It has been reported that these fungal glucans do not have a direct effect on macrophages. In studies on thymectomized mice or in mice treated with antilymphocytic serum, lentinan proved unsuitable for induction of macrophage toxicity. This effect was achieved only in intact mice. In the light of these findings it can be concluded that the overall effect of these glucans depends on their effect on T-helper cells.

6.3.5 Coenzyme Q (ubiquinones)

Various forms of coenzyme Q were already being associated with pharmacological effects some decades ago. In particular, reference to a positively inotropic effect of coenzyme Q_{10} attracted considerable interest. More recently a number of ubiquinone derivatives have been investigated for immunostimulating effects. It turned out that coenzymes Q_7 and Q_8 stimulate murine macrophages *in vitro* and *in vivo*. Ubiquinones or coenzyme Q are lipid-soluble benzoquinones which are involved in almost all aerobic microorganisms in electron transport within the respiratory chain, for instance for the oxidation of succinate or NADH. Chemically, the ubiquinones consist of a 2,3-dimethoxy-5-methyl-benzoquinone, which has a varying number of isoprene residues at position 6. Depending on the number of isoprenes, the designation coenzyme Q_n ($n = 1$–10) or ubiquinone (X) is used, with X indicating the number of carbon atoms in the side chain.

Coenzyme Q_7 speeds up carbon clearance *in vivo,* and *in vitro* it enhances antibody-mediated phagocytosis of sheep erythrocytes and of bacteria by macrophages. These effects are accompanied by characteristic changes in electron micrographs of macrophages. In addition, when administered in doses of 10–50 mg per kg parenterally (i.v. or i.p.) coenzyme Q_7 protects mice against a number of experimental infections, though the protective effect of this substance, too, depends on its being administered early, i.e. 12–24 hours before induction of infection. The effect of coenzymes Q_7 and Q_8 is particularly striking in granulocytopenic mice – a condition that can be obtained by whole-body irradiation or by a single dose (200 mg per kg) of cyclophosphamide.

During the granulocytopenic phase, which lasts about three days, the mice are particularly sensitive to experimentally induced infections: the bacterial inocula required to produce lethal infections are many times lower than those required in healthy mice. It was first supposed that the ability of coenzyme Q_7 or Q_8 to enhance phagocytosis was solely responsible for the curative effects of these substances in experimental infections, but this is not the case. Like coenzyme Q_7, synthetic ubiquinone analogues stimulate phagocytosis *in vivo* and *in vitro,* but are ineffective in treatment of experimental infections in granulocytopenic mice. Analysis of this discrepancy revealed that a complete curative effect was exerted only by ubiquinones which stimulated the synthesis and secretion of colony stimulating factors in macrophages. This stimulation can be observed *in vitro* and *in vivo*. *In vivo* it causes a more rapid mobilization of granulocytes from the bone marrow. This effect seems to be essential for the curative properties of the ubiquinones.

6.3.6 Bestatin

Attempts had already been made in the 1970s to discover and isolate from microorganisms low-molecular-weight substances with immunostimulating effects. The methods used, however, were very indirect. They were partly based on the fact that certain enzymes such as aminopeptidases, alkaline phosphatases and esterases are located not only inside the cell but also on its surface. This applies to the surface of immune cells as well, hence to lymphocytes and macrophages. Inhibitors of these enzymes could therefore be expected to become attached to the surface of the cells. While searching for protease inhibitors, Umezawa and his colleagues found in 1976 a number of low-molecular-weight substances that inhibited leucine aminopeptidase, aminopeptidase B, esterases and an alkaline phosphatase. Bestatin, which inhibits leucine aminopeptidase and aminopeptidase B, proved to be the most interesting of these substances because it has – at least in part – the desired immunostimulant properties. Bestatin is a dipeptide (2-hydroxyphenyl-butyryl-leucine) with three asymmetric carbon atoms.

Bestatin has an effect of macrophages and possibly also on T-lymphocytes. When murine spleen cells are incubated with [^{3}H]-thymidine, the DNA synthesis activity of these cells can be measured by incorporation of [^{3}H]-thymidine into acid-stable material. This reaction is enhanced by bestatin, although only as long as both macrophages and T-cells are in the incubation mixture. Bestatin added to bone-marrow cultures at concentrations between 0.001 and 0.1 μg/ml enhanced the effect of a colony stimulating factor on the formation of colonies in soft agar by about one third of the values observed in control experiments. Daily doses of 0.05–5 mg per kg promote delayed-type hypersensitivity in mice. Bestatin can also inhibit growth of slow-growing tumours in mice.

Immunological and allegedly therapeutic effects have been observed at a clinical level as well: daily doses of between 10 and 100 mg brought the numbers of cytotoxic T-cells and NK-cells in patients with malignant tumours back to normal. Likewise, negative skin reactions to tuberculin and PPD (purified protein derivative) became positive under treatment with bestatin. These findings have been corroborated in more recent studies in which it could also be shown that bestatin given orally has the capacity to normalize impaired immune parameters in cancer patients after irradiation. Lymphocyte responses to PHA and pokeweed mitogen were improved as was the ability of B-cells to secrete IgM. It remains, however, doubtful whether any of these effects translate into clinical benefits.

Orally administered bestatin is well tolerated. 85% is eliminated with the urine. A serum level of 1–2 μg per ml is reached 1–2 hours after administration of a daily dose of 30 mg. Concentrations of more than 0.2–0.5 μg per ml are maintained for over three hours. About 10–15% of bestatin is oxidized to parahydroxybestatin. The plasma concentration of this molecule is 0.005–0.5 μg per ml. It is between five and ten times more active than bestatin.

6.4 Synthetic substances

6.4.1 *Levamisole*

Tetramisole, the racemate from 2,3,5,6-tetrahydro-6-phenylimidazo(2,1-b)-thiazole, was first used in treatment in 1966 as a broad-spectrum anthelmintic. Tetramisole and, more recently, the levorotatory isomer levamisole have been widely and successfully used in both human and veterinary medicine. Renoux and Renoux discovered in 1971 that tetramisole enhanced the protective effect of a Brucella vaccine in mice, a finding that sparked a large number of experimental and, ultimately, clinical studies of the immunomodulating activities of tetramisole and, more particularly, of levamisole.

Levamisole (molecular weight 240.75 daltons) is a stable, white, crystalline powder *(Fig. 6.15)*. The hydrochloride is readily soluble in most organic solvents. The substance undergoes hydrolysis in aqueous solutions and in an alkaline pH. Levamisole is, however, stable in a neutral or slightly acid pH and at low temperatures.

6.4.1.1 Pharmacokinetics

Levamisole is readily absorbed in most animal species after oral, subcutaneous and intramuscular administration. The plasma half-life of the unchanged substance is between one and four hours. The volume of distribution is high, and the substance can be detected in almost all tissues and fluids. The peak concentrations are found in the liver and kidneys, the organs in which levamisole is metabolized. In rats, less than 1% of a radioactive dose is found in the body after eight days, while 46% of the radioactive dose is eliminated in the urine and 40% in the feces within 48 hours. The eight metabolites found are less toxic than levamisole and have no anthelmintic effects.

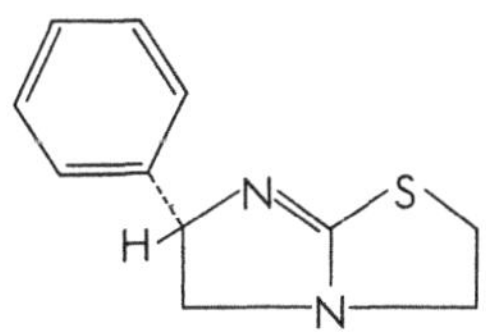

Figure 6.15. Molecular structure of levamisole.

In man, peak plasma levels of 0.5 ± 0.05 μg/ml are found two hours after oral intake of 150 mg [^{3}H]-levamisole. This is the concentration required for *in vitro* restoration of reduced macrophage and T-lymphocyte function. The plasma half-life of levamisole in man is four hours, and only very slight interindividual differences are found in the plasma levels. The substance therefore seems to be well absorbed in man. About 60% is eliminated with the urine within 24 hours. In the same period, about 4% of the radioactive material is found in the feces. The drug is extensively metabolized: only 6% of the radioactive material found in the urine and 4% of that in the stools represent the unchanged substance.

6.4.1.2 Mechanism of action

The anthelmintic properties of levamisole are the result of stimulation of autonomic ganglia in the parasites. Levamisole also stimulates heart rate and the intensity of cardiac contractions (positive inotropic effect). It has no effect on bacteria, viruses or fungi.

The molecule has an imidazole ring and its action may be similar to that of the imidazoles by influencing enzymes responsible for the synthesis and breakdown of cyclic nucleotides. The net effect of imidazole and levamisole on lymphocytes is enhancement of the intracellular concentrations of cyclic GMP (cGMP). Neither levamisole nor imidazole are mitogenic.

6.4.1.3 Immunopharmacological effects

In vitro systems: levamisole has been described as an immunorestorative substance, i.e. it does not affect, or scarcely affects, normally functioning immune cells but has the ability to restore normal function to damaged or hypofunctional immune cells. These restorative functions have been found in *in vitro* incubation of immune cells with levamisole and in *ex vivo* studies involving *in vivo* administration of the substance and *in vitro* investigations of the cells.

Levamisole can stimulate phagocytosis of human or animal polymorphonuclear leucocytes or macrophages. The ability of the compound to restore the chemotactic reaction of polymorphonuclear leucocytes and monocytes in patients whose leucocytes display abnormally low motility ("lazy leucocyte syndrome") has also been described. Levamisole enhances activation of lymphocytes by lymphokines (Il-2, interferon γ) or lymphokine production, particularly when the antigenic stimulus triggering these phenomena *in vitro* is suboptimal or when the cells are derived from anergic patients or mice. Levamisole stimulates protein and nucleic acid synthesis in resting lymphocytes and in mitogen- and antigen-stimulating cells. T-lymphocytes stimulated by contact with allogeneic cells also exhibit an acceleration of their protein and nucleic acid synthesis under the influence of levamisole. However, the compound does not seem to have any notable effect on B-cell function. The mechanism by which T-lymphocyte function is impaired (irradiation, cytotoxic substances, immunosuppression) does not seem to have any particular bearing on the restorative effect of levamisole. The toxicity of cytotoxic lymphocytes on allogeneic cells is enhanced by levamisole, and the effect of the substance, administered either before or during the sensitization phase, leads to an increase in the number of allogeneic cells killed by each lymphocyte. In patients with a diminished number of circulating T-cells levamisole was shown to restore the number of T-cells to normal. There is little change in the total number of lymphocytes.

In vivo test systems: levamisole restores delayed-type hypersensitivity reactions to various antigens in anergic patients. The suppression of DTH observed in elderly patients following influenza vaccination can be inhibited by levamisole. The same is true of cortisone-induced inhibition of DTH in rabbits. Clearance of colloidal particles from the blood can be enhanced in elderly or chronically ill patients, which is tantamout to normalization of this parameter. Analogous effects can be seen in animals whose phagocytic response had been suppressed by cortisone. Levamisole has an aggravating effect on a number of experimental autoimmune diseases: adjuvant arthritis in the rat is intensified by levamisole, as is experimentally induced allergic encephalomyelitis. In contrast, nephritis in the NZB/NZW mouse, a condition similar to lupus erythematosus, tends to be improved by levamisole. At all events, proteinuria and antinuclear antibodies develop more slowly under levamisole than in untreated control animals.

Antitumour effects in experimental animals: administered on its own, levamisole does not have any effect on the growth of primary or transplantable tumours. Within narrow methodological limits, however, levamisole can achieve an additional therapeutic effect if it is associated with cytoreductive treatment. The methodological limits refer to the dose of levamisole, which should not be higher than 5 mg per kg, and to timing of the treatment sequence in that the levamisole must be given several days after the cytoreductive therapy. This approach has beneficial effects in the treatment of experimental leukemia, in "Lewis lung" adenocarcinoma and in other tumours: survival time is prolonged, primary tumour weights are reduced, and the number of metastases (in Lewis lung adenocarcinoma) is reduced in such cases.

Positive effects have been achieved with levamisole in 77 of 382 experiments on rapidly growing tumours and in 59 of 200 experiments with slow-growth tumours.

Even within the above methodological limits, however, the course of *primary* malignant tumours in mice is scarcely affected. Positive results have been reported in only 14 of 78 experiments.

6.4.1.4 Clinical use

Levamisole has been tested in well over 1,000 patients with malignant disease. The results, however, are highly contradictory. Besides positive findings such as prolonged postsurgery survival in patients with stage one bronchial carcinoma, there are numerous reports which provide no evidence of improved survival for patients treated with levamisole. A negative tone is even taken in one large-scale study which comprised 720 mastectomized patients with positive lymph-node findings but no remote metastases and which compared the effects of 2.5 mg levamisole per kg, administered as an adjuvant to radiotherapy on two successive days for a period of 48 weeks, with those of radiotherapy on its own. After one year, the patients treated with levamisole for more than 24 weeks had a much higher recurrence rate than the controls or the patients in whom levamisole had to be withdrawn prematurely on account of side effects.

In all thoroughly documented, controlled studies of patients with rheumatoid arthritis the positive effect of levamisole compared with that of placebo is confirmed by a large number of clinical parameters. No explanation is as yet available for the positive effect of levamisole, but it could be due to a number of different mechanism: correction of disturbed function of the T-suppressor cells which normally prevent reactions to autoantigens, or, for that matter, the possibility that, as in NZB/NZW mice, levamisole brings about more effective elimination of immune complexes by the mononuclear-phagocytic system. It should be borne in mind that the negative feedback effect of prostaglandins which are released by inflammatory cells, i.e. by polymorphonuclear leucocytes and macrophages, in the inflamed joints, is restored or even enhanced by levamisole. Prostaglandins (PGE_2) normally inhibit macrophage and T-lymphocyte function. In-T lymphocytes this inhibition results in reduced secretion of lymphokines.

Levamisole has no effect on the concentration of circulating immunoglobulins or on antibody formation. A drop in circulating immune complexes can be observed in rheumatoid arthritis patients treated with levamisole. This finding has been interpreted as reflecting a drug-induced enhancement of previously reduced phagocytic activity in mononuclear cells. Elevated C-reactive protein in RA patients is restored to normal levels under levamisole. It has also been reported that the substance induces the formation of interferon in normal human lymphocytes. But *in vivo* studies have not revealed any antiviral effect that would suggest levamisole-mediated interferon formation.

In children suffering from repeated upper respiratory tract infections during the winter months, low doses of levamisole (1.25 mg per kg) significantly reduced the frequency and duration of infections. In patients with freshly diagnosed active tuberculosis and also in those with lepromatous leprosy, treatment with 150 mg levamisole, administered every week on two successive days in addition to chemotherapy, restored cutaneous reactions to tuberculin and lepromin. However, the additional treatment with levamisole did not noticeably speed up the recovery process.

To sum up: though levamisole is of proven therapeutic value in the treatment of rheumatoid arthritis, it has not yet acquired a regular place in the treatment of human tumours and infections, despite its confirmed immunopharmacological efficacy.

Most recently the enthusiasm for using levamisole as an immunostimulant agent appears to have subsided. The rather impressive stream of publications on the immunomodulatory function of levamisole which appeared during the first half of the eighties has degenerated into a modest trickle. No new indications have been reported. The "restoration" of impaired immune parameters in immunologically compromised patients has been repeatedly confirmed. As with many other drugs the clinical significance of these changes is not at all clear.

6.4.1.5 Side effects

As already mentioned, levamisole has been used clinically as an anthelmintic without any major adverse reactions being observed. The prolonged treatment periods in rheumatoid arthritis and in tumours, and possibly also the particular sensitivity of patients with rheumatic diseases, however, clearly revealed the substance's toxic profile, in particular the occurrence of agranulocytosis, which was observed in about 5% of all rheumatic patients, 2% of patients with malignant tumours, and only 0.2% of those with infectious diseases. Rheumatic patients also react relatively frequently to prolonged treatment with levamisole by developing urticaria and fever (7 and 1.5% respectively). These reactions often regress spontaneously in the course of treatment, however, and withdrawal of the substance is necessary only if they are accompanied by leucopenia or agranulocytosis. Sensory disturbances such as insomnia, excitation or impaired sense of taste or smell are found in 4–6% of all patients. About the same proportion of patients experience mild gastrointestinal reactions such as nausea, loss of appetite and, occasionally, vomiting or diarrhea. Withdrawal of therapy on account of these side effects is usually unneccesary.

6.4.2 Cimetidine

Cimetidine is a cyanoguanidine derivative of imidazole *(Fig. 6.16)*. It is a reversible competitive antagonist of the effects of histamine on H_2 receptors. Its effect on these receptors is very selective: H_1 receptors are not influenced by cimetidine, nor has the substance any effects that are mediated by H_1 receptors. The most important effect of histamine that is mediated by the H_2 receptors is stimulation of gastric secretion, and the therapeutic significance of cimetidine is due to its ability to inhibit this process. Cimetidine is in clinical use today as an effective agent for the treatment of duodenal ulcer.

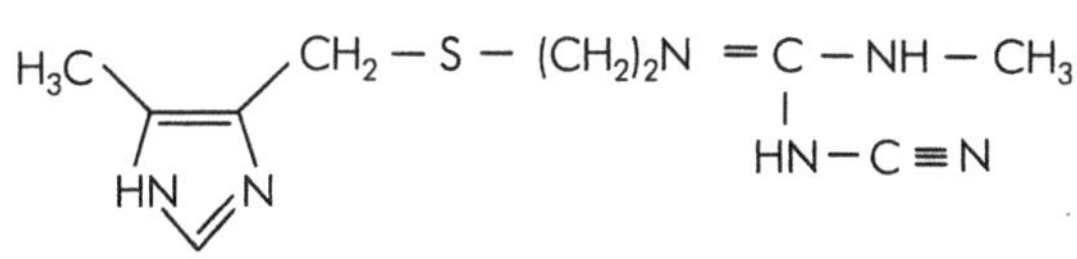

Figure 6.16. Molecular structure of cimetidine.

6.4.2.1 *Pharmacokinetics*

About 60% of cimetidine is absorbed on oral administration. Peak blood levels are reached after one to one and a half hours. A single oral dose is sufficient to obtain effective concentrations in the blood and at the site of action for about four hours. Most of an oral dose of cimetidine is eliminated unchanged in the urine within 24 hours. A small proportion enters the bile and, together with non-absorbed material, can be found in the feces. Cimetidine is distributed widely throughout almost all body tissues, an exception being the brain.

6.4.2.2 *Immunopharmacological effects*

Histamine exerts an activating effect on T-suppressor lymphocytes via H_2 receptors, thereby intensifying suppression of both the cell-mediated and the humoral immune response. Cimetidine antagonizes this effect. The histamine-triggered secretion of a suppressor factor by T-suppressor lymphocytes can be suppressed *in vitro* by cimetidine. *In vivo,* cimetidine prevents the induction of T-suppressor lymphocytes in mice carrying certain experimental tumours. Macrophages with suppressor activity, on the other hand, were not affected by cimetidine. In mice with Lewis lung carcinoma there seems to be a correlation between suppression of the induction of suppressor cells and prolongation of the mean survival time. Administered in doses of 0.2, 0.5 and 10 mg per kg, cimetidine inhibited T-cell suppressor activity, and there was a parallel increase in mean survival time. Similar effects have been observed in other animal models. An impressive prolongation of survival time was, for instance, obtained with doses of 15, 40 and 100 mg cimetidine per kg body weight in C57B1/6 mice which had been inoculated with a syngeneic lymphoma or syngeneic fibrosarcoma. 90–100% of mice inoculated with the experimental lymphoma died within 30 days. When cimetidine was given at a daily dose of 100 mg/kg body weight, 60–80% of the younger animals (two months old) survived for 30 days after inoculation. In the group of older animals (eight months) the corresponding survival rate was still 40–60%.

The ability of cimetidine to counteract T-suppressor cells may not be the only mechanism, perhaps not even the most important one, by which the drug exerts its immunostimulating effect. Several reports describe the induction of NK-cells in animals and the activation of these cells in human patients. The existence of a non-T-cell related mechanism is convincingly demonstrated by the finding that cimetidine significantly reduced the size of tumours, which were generated by inoculating nude mice with a human cell line derived from an ovarian carcinoma. In these experiments it was shown that spleen cells of cimetidine-treated but not of control animals acquired the ability to lyse the transplanted human tumour cell fourteen days after the institution of treatment (100 mg/kg/day orally).

6.4.2.3 Clinical findings

An immunopharmacological effect of cimetidine has also been observed in man: in patients taking cimetidine for duodenal ulcer, delayed-type allergic reactions to four antigens were tested on the skin before therapy and six weeks after it had been instituted. After the treatment eight patients showed a significant increase in erythema and induration at the site of injection. In eight control patients who had received either placebo or an antacid, skin reactions six weeks after the beginning of therapy were as weak as those observed before treatment had begun. Whether or not the suppressor-cell-inhibiting effect of cimetidine is also of benefit in the treatment of human tumours still remains to be seen. Although anecdotal reports indicate that this may be the case, solid evidence is lacking. In contrast, there is evidence that cimetidine may shorten the symptoms of herpes infections and bring about rapid disappearance of the skin lesions. A one-week course of treatment involving doses of 1,600 mg cimetidine on two days and 1,000 mg on the remaining days greatly speeded up the healing process in the skin lesions and appreciably shortened hyperalgesia states in 18 of 21 patients. Only in 3 patients did the healing process extend over several weeks. A four-week course of cimetidine (300 mg four times daily by mouth) in 4 patients with mucocutaneous candidiasis led to restoration of the cutaneous reaction to tuberculin, *Candida albicans* and streptokinase/streptodornase. In two of the patients the lymphocytes also produced MIF (migration inhibition factor) in the presence of *Candida* antigen after therapy. Four weeks after withdrawal of therapy all the cutaneous and leucocyte tests were again pathological. On resumption of therapy with cimetidine all 4 patients exhibited strongly positive skin tests to the above-mentioned antigens after a further four weeks. Their lymphocytes also produced MIF in the presence of *Candida* antigen. The candidiasis, however, was not influenced in any of the patients. Combined treatment with griseofulvin and cimetidine may also succed in eliminating *Candida* infection, which cannot be mananged with griseofulvin alone.

In 33 patients with AIDS-related complex (ARC) oral doses of cimetidine (1,200 mg/day) given for five months with an interruption of therapy for three weeks after the first three months of treatment, several parameters improved. At the end of the treatment period significant elevations of immunoglobulins (IgG, IgA) complement C4, B-lymphocytes and $CD4^+$ cells were observed. Moreover, the *in vitro* lymphoproliferation responses to plant mitogens were increased as compared with the values measured before treatment. The *in vivo* cell-mediated hypersensitivity reaction assessed by intradermal antigen application also improved significantly. These immunological changes correlated with clinical improvements, such as a reduction of febrile episodes, gain in body weight and performance status, although the clinical changes were not statistically significant. All immunological parameters were reversible after the first discontinuation of therapy and reimproved during the second two-month period of treatment.

A decrease in the CD4/CD8 cell ratio observed after surgery can apparently be diminished or even prevented by perioperative treatment with cimetidine but also with ibuprofen. These findings give indirect support to the negative influence that both histamine and prostaglandins have on the immune system after major operations.

The value of cimetidine as an immunostimulating agent cannot yet be reliably determined. Attemps to use the drug in combination with cytokines such as α-interferon are in progress but have not yet produced a sufficient number of data to allow any conclusive judgement.

6.4.2.4 *Side effects*

Cimetidine is generally well tolerated. Side effects are rare and usually not dangerous. Headache, dizziness, tiredness, muscle pain, constipation or diarrhea, and rash are among the reactions occasionally encountered. Plasma creatinine levels may be elevated and aminotransferase activity increased. Although, as already mentioned, very little cimetidine reaches the central nervous system, neurological symptoms have occasionally been described. Only elderly patients whose renal excretion is disturbed and who take cimetidine in large doses over a long period seem to be at risk. The symptoms observed in such cases included: confusion states, blurring of speech, hallucinations and apathy. Cimetidine has a slight antiandrogenic effect in rats and dogs. Gynecomastia has occasionally been observed in men and galactorrhea in women.

6.4.3 Isoprinosine

Isoprinosine (inosiplex, methisoprinol) is a complex containing inosine and the paracctaminobcnzoatc of N_1-N-dimethyl-amino-2-propanol in a molar ratio of 1:3. The efficacy of the complex is derived exclusively from inosine. The other components seem only to facilitate transport of inosine into the lymphocytes. After incubation of lymphocytes in the presence of the complex the intracellular concentrations of inosine found are three times as high as after incubation of the cells with an equimolar concentration of inosine alone. At concentrations of between 0.4 and 40 μg per ml, isoprinosine enhances blastogenesis triggered by phytohemagglutinin, concanavalin A or pokeweed mitogen. Not surprisingly, the stimulatory effect of isoprinosine on functional parameters of lymphocytes *in vitro* appears to be dependent on the media in which the cells are suspended. In Eagle's minimal essential medium, for instance, isoprinosine very distinctly enhances the proliferation responses of human mononuclear cells to phytohemagglutinin. However, when medium 199 (M-199) was used to culture the cells no such effect was observed. This difference was traced back to the presence of purines, specifically hypoxanthine and adenine, in M-199.

Lymphocytes from patients with systemic lupus erythematosus react particularly strongly to isoprinosine in the presence of mitogens while lymphocytes from patients with rheumatoid arthritis tend to exhibit a weaker reaction than that observed with normal lymphocytes. In the presence of PHA and isoprinosine, peripheral blood lymphocytes show enhanced ability to form Il-2. This effect, however, is seen only in the presence of a mitogen or antigen and is not elicited by isoprinosine alone.

In addition to its effects on T-cells, isoprinosine appears to have an effect on the function of antigen-stimulated B-cells. The number of plaque-forming cells in the Mishell-Dutton test is likewise enhanced by the presence of isoprinosine during antigenic stimulation.

Viral infections frequently impair the reactivity of human peripheral blood lymphocytes to mitogens and viral antigens. In many cases this transient form of immunosuppression is corrected by treatment with isoprinosine.

6.4.3.1 Pharmacokinetics

Isoprinosine is rapidly metabolized after oral or intravenous administration. The half-life of the inosine component is 50 minutes after an oral dose and only three minutes after i.v. administration. In animal experiments more than 90% of the inosine is excreted as allantoin and uric acid, and the remainder as hypoxanthine and adenine. The main elimination product is uric acid. The other components of the complex are oxidized and glucuronized and eliminated with the urine.

6.4.3.2 Clinical uses

A number of clinical studies have shown that a prolonged application of 1 to 3 g of isoprinosine per day restores depressed immune parameters back to normal values. Specifically, this could be demonstrated for the number and for the *in vitro* function of NK-cells and T-helper-cells. These effects were seen in elderly individuals, in immunosuppressed HIV-positive homosexuals with lymphadenopathy, in children with recurrent upper respiratory tract infections, in burned patients, uremic individuals, cancer patients and in patients after surgery. However, up to this day convincing evidence that these immunorestorative effects translate into therapeutic benefits is still lacking. However, since normalization of depressed immune parameters seems desirable and the compound is virtually non-toxic, its probational clinical use in immunosuppressed patients may be justified.

A number of clinical studies which suggested some clinical efficacy of isoprinosine will therefore be briefly described.

In a randomized double-blind study performed by French clinicians in Dakar, the effects of a five-day course of treatment with 50 mg isoprinosine per day on the course of acute measles in 59 children at high general risk were investigated. 55 of the children were less than three years of age. In the group of 30 children treated with isoprinosine there was one death as against four in the 29 children comprising the control group. The fact that in the isoprinosine group only 6 serious clinical complications of measles were observed as against 11 in the control group also suggests that isoprinosine was effective in this particular clinical setting.

Moreover, there is evidence to suggest that isoprinosine is therapeutically effective in subacute sclerosing panencephalitis (SSPE). A report was published in 1982 on a multicentre study in which 98 patients in the USA and Canada were treated for up to 9.5 years with isoprinosine. The survival times of these 98 patients were compared with those registered for three groups of SSPE patients in Israel, the Lebanon and USA who had contracted the disease at about the same time as the first group of patients but had been given different treatment or no treatment at all. In the isoprinosine patients the statistical probability of survival after two, four, six and eight years from onset of SSPE was 78%, 69%, 65% and 61% respectively, compared with 38%, 20%, 14% and 8% in the control group comprising the three populations already mentioned. There are, of course, weaknesses in this study. Apart from other minor criticisms, the control group was based on historical evidence, and no proper randomization was carried out. The study does, however, suggest that isoprinosine may prolong the life of patients with SSPE. Dyken and his colleagues arrived at a similar conclusion in their smaller-scale study published in 1982 in which they compared the degree of neurological dysfunction in 12 patients receiving isoprinosine with the same parameters in an historical control group of 15 untreated patients. During the first twelve months from onset of SSPE the two groups did not differ as regards the neurological parameters. From years two to five the group treated with isoprinosine exhibited a much lower degree of neurological dysfunction than the untreated group. This improvement seemed to be concentrated mainly on patients whose disease had developed more slowly between years two and five. Besides these examples of meticulously performed though by no means faultless studies, numerous reports have been published on the effectiveness of isoprinosine in a number of viral diseases such as viral encephalitis, aphthous stomatitis, hepatitis triggered by cytomegalovirus or herpes zoster. These reports are, however, anecdotal and could, at the most, spark more rigorous investigations.

6.4.3.3 Mechanism of action

Isoprinosine stimulates RNA synthesis in activated lymphocytes. As already mentioned, the effect appears to be derived solely from the presence of inosine. Lymphocytes seem to depend very much on the "salvage pathway" in purine biosynthesis. This is the metabolic pathway by which already synthesized purine reaches the cell interior, where it is then phosphorylated. Adenosine deaminase and nucleoside phosphorylase are enzymatic constituents of this pathway. Congenital dysfunction of these two enzymes is manifested clinically as immune deficiency. It can be accepted as a working hypothesis that in certain settings stimulated lymphocytes are not able to cover their purine needs by *de novo* synthesis but are dependent on the "import" of purines. In that case, the function of isoprinosine would simply be that of a rapidly utilizable purine building block for RNA and DNA synthesis. This hypothesis is substantiated by the observation reported in all pharmacological and clinical investigations that isoprinosine enhances events that are triggered by other factors (mitogens, antigens).

Two other purines, the hypoxanthine derivatives NPT 15392 and NPT 16416, should be mentioned in this context: as immunostimulants with a mechanism of action similar to that of isoprinosine, they have received considerable attention. However, lack of available data rules out any assessment of their clinical activity for the time being.

6.4.3.4 Side effects

Isoprinosine is virtually non-toxic. The LD_{50} in animal experiments is between 5 and 10 g per kg. Nausea is occasionally observed after prolonged treatment with high doses. Blood chemistry changes are confined to elevation of uric acid in the blood and urine.

6.4.4 Other synthetic immunostimulants

None of the following substances have so far received much clinical attention. They nevertheless constitute new chemical or biological approaches and therefore deserve brief mention. The immunostimulating effects of *diethyldithiocarbamate* (DTC) on laboratory animals may be summarized as follows: administered over a wide dosage range DTC brings about an increase in the number of spleen cells forming IgG against sheep erythrocytes. It enhances the reaction of peripheral blood lymphocytes to PHA and concanavalin A and also increases the DTH to sheep erythrocytes. In addition, DTC can compensate for the immunosuppression caused by cytoreductive treatment. Clinically, the substance seems to be well tolerated after a single dose. The reactivity of peripheral blood lymphocytes to T-cell antigens seems to stay enhanced for a week following a single dose. DTC has no effect on B-lymphocytes.

The substance is ineffective *in vitro* and does not appear to exert a direct action on lymphocytes *in vivo*. The effects of DTC on the development, mobilization and activation of T lymphocytes are more probably due to the fact that DTC induces hormone-like factors which do not stem from the thymus and which speed up T-cell maturation and activation.

Because of its chelating properties DTC has been used in treatment of metal intoxications. Daily doses of 30–50 mg per kg body weight over a period of weeks have not proved toxic. On slow intravenous injection even single doses of 5 mg per kg are well tolerated.

Azimexone is 2-[2-cyanaziridinyl-(1)]-2[2-carbomoylaziridinyl-(1)]-propane. This substance is still in clinical development. Azimexone administered in doses between 0.001 and 0.01 μg per ml has been reported to speed up the PHA-induced proliferation of lymphocytes and, above all, lymphokine-induced proliferation of macrophages. Both reactions are inhibited at higher concentrations, possibly as a result of induction of T-suppressor cells. The following immunological effects have been observed *in vivo:* enhancement of the DTH to oxazolone, increased intracellular destruction of bacteria by macrophages, increased NK-activity, accelerated granulopoiesis. In rats in which the natural defenses had been compromised by treatment with cyclophosphamide, azimexone increased survival rate from 60% to 100% in experimentally induced *Candida* infections. In animals given cyclophosphamide, azimexone also proved effective in the treatment of bacterial infections with various organisms, even with *P. aeruginosa.* Quantitatively, however, these results are less impressive than similar effects observed for glucans or, for that matter, ubiquinones.

The substance is well tolerated on intravenous administration of between 200 and 400 mg per day one to three times a week. Positive changes are observed in clinical immunological parameters such as the number of circulating lymphocytes, the activation rate of peripheral lymphocytes by PHA and concanavalin A, and cutaneous reactivity to dinitrochlorobenzene. However, the data available are insufficient to clearly define this substance in relation to the purine derivatives (isoprinosine, NPT 15392) or levamisole. Administered in high doses, it may cause toxic hemolytic anemia in experimental animals and in man. The therapeutic value of azimexone has still to be established.

7. Clinical Assessment and Perspectives

The most important methodological approaches to immunopharmacology have been described in the preceding chapters of this book. By way of conclusion, this final chapter will be devoted to an evaluation of current immunotherapeutic methods from the clinical viewpoint. On the one hand, such an evaluation must be based on past therapeutic needs which at the present time are not satisfied at all or only to a limited extent. In this context, one is tempted to make some tentative predictions on the further development of immunopharmacology and on the therapeutic options that this discipline will open. In order to restrict the amount of speculation inherent in such predictions, such extrapolations must be confined to a rather narrow time frame. In addition they must be based on known facts. Our predictions will be limited to approximately 10 years, which is the time span needed to find and to develop a new drug. Projects which are at present underway in the laboratories of major pharmaceutical manufacturers, biotechnology companies and some university laboratories will be the starting points for our future projections. Anything which is not recognizable today in at least rough outline will hardly have matured into a therapeutic drug by the end of this century.

It would, of course, be presumptuous to attempt a survey of all scientific activity currently under way in the immunopharmacological or immunotherapeutic field. Much will be overlooked by the individual observer, and what has gone unperceived today could be a source of surprising developments. As in the preceding chapters, therefore, no claim to completeness is made. Many experimental efforts, however, are taking shape. Above all, research projects can be perceived which are being pursued in several locations or which are heavily funded. The intensity with which certain problems are investigated hinges on two factors: technical feasibility and therapeutic needs. Therapeutic research must find its proper orientation between these two coordinates. Those projects which are built on existing scientific techniques and paradigms and which at the same time are driven by strongly perceived therapeutic needs are most likely to succeed *(Fig. 7.1)*. An attempt will be made on the following pages to identify some of these projects.

7.1 Immunosubstitution – antibodies

The value of substitution therapy with gamma-globulins in congenital hypo- or agammaglobulinemia is confirmed. Likewise, as we have already seen, treatment with intravenous gamma-globulin in immunohemolytic thrombocytopenic purpura and prophylaxis against Rhesus sensitization of Rh-negative mothers with antirhesus (D) gamma-globulins must be viewed as effective and well tolerated clinical measures. There is also no doubt about the effectiveness of

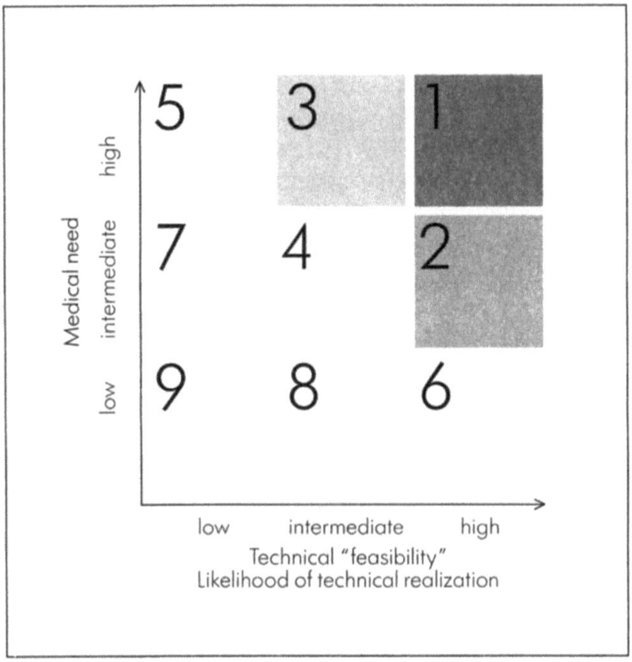

Figure 7.1. Therapeutic need and technical feasibility. The figures represent the likelihood of realization as calculated on the basis of selected criteria.

prophylaxis with hyperimmunoglobulins against hepatitis A and B, tetanus, rabies and measles. This is already an impressive list of prophylactic and therapeutic indications. Thus, the principle of "passive immunization" has established itself in medicine in a number of ways.

What direction will developments take in the next few years? Efforts are currently underway to find new indications for intravenous therapy with gamma-globulins. As we have already pointed out in Chapter 3, it will be difficult to demonstrate the effectiveness of treatment of severe bacterial infections with gamma-globulins as an adjunct to antibiotics. Any such studies will have to be large in scale in order to provide statistical confirmation of small differences in mortality rates or disease progression (duration). Recent studies have shown which infections are suitable for treatment with gamma-globulins and for clinical experimental investigation. The question whether there is any advantage in administering intravenous gamma-globulins as well as antimicrobial treatment in severe bacterial infections cannot be answered with a simple yes or no. The value of any such therapy is much more likely to be demonstrated in a specific clinical model; a positive result in a representative situation would then be generalized and extrapolated to similar situations. Diffuse fibrinous purulent peritonitis, such as occurs after perforation of the gastrointestinal tract, is a clinical model which might shed light on the efficacy of gamma-globulin therapy. A multicentre study based on a rather sophisticated trial protocol is currently in progress at various surgical centres in the Federal Republic of Germany. The aim of this prospective randomized study is to determine the effectiveness of intravenous therapy with gamma-globulins instituted no later than three hours after surgery in patients with fibrinous purulent peritonitis. Administered in addition to antibiotics, this treatment consists of a total of 40 g of human gamma-globulin and 2000 ml of IgM-enriched plasma over a period of five days following surgery. The aim of the assessment is to determine the mortality rate during the hospital stay. The results obtained with this type of clinical investigation will have a considerable bearing on the use of immunoglobulins in bacterial infections in the course of the next 10 years. If the results are favourable, the implications will not be restricted to diffuse fibrinous purulent peritonitis, but will extend to other bacterial infections.

A number of clinical investigations attest to the interest being shown in improving therapy of bacterial infections. Neonatal group-B streptococcal infection is an important cause of neonatal sepsis and meningitis. Group-B streptococci are encapsulated bacteria which are effectively eliminated from the body by phagocytes only if they have been previously osponized with antibodies. Newborn infants often do not possess specific antibodies against group-B streptococci and are therefore sensitive to these microorganisms. It has recently been shown that neonates can be provided with the necessary specific antibodies against group-B streptococci by administering a single intravenous dose of 500 mg IgG per kg bodyweight. Should the titres achieved prove to be effective, IgG prophylaxis in newborn infants with infections due to Streptococcus B will probably become a routine measure.

Attempts have been made for some time to develop intravenous hyperimmunoglobulins against Pseudomonas or gram-negative cell-wall antigens ("common core antigens") in patients with extensive burns or gram-negative sepsis. Although there is evidence that such preparations are effective, it is questionable whether this approach will be successful: in order to obtain hyperimmunoglobulins, vaccines have to be developed and volunteers have to be immunized with these vaccines before providing plasma from which gamma-globulins can be obtained. This is a complicated and extremely expensive procedure. A more likely approach would be to obtain equivalent effects with large doses of non-enriched, intravenously applied gamma-globulins. The good tolerance of some of the more recent preparations suggests that this approach could be successful. There is therefore a good chance that intravenous treatment with polyvalent gamma-globulins will find new applications in the field of bacterial infection.

A recent randomized, prospective, placebo-controlled study showed that standard gamma-globulin (SGG), administered at intervals of several days over a period of weeks, can greatly reduce the symptoms of pollen-induced allergy (rhinitis, asthma, conjunctivitis). There are two possible explanations for this surprising result. The administration of IgG-antibodies may have resulted in passive desensitization: this means that specific IgG-antibodies bind (block) pollen antigen, thereby "withdrawing" them from the reaction with IgE antibodies. This explanation is unlikely because such an effect would require relatively large amounts of the specific antipollen IgG-antibody. It is questionable whether the required amount of antibody can be supplied in several injections of 5 ml SGG. The second – and equally unsatisfactory – explanation concerns the occupancy of Fc receptors on mast cells by IgG-molecules. This explanation is also questionable, firstly on account of the relatively low amounts of IgG which were administered and, secondly, because of the low affinity of Fc-receptors for IgG-molecules! It must, however, be borne in mind that the biological half-life of IgG (approximately 21 days) is much longer than that of class E immunoglobulins and that for various reasons it is very difficult to estimate the effect of administering exogenous gamma-globulins on the "occupancy" of Fc receptors on mast cells. The treatment of allergic disorders by means of polyvalent gamma-globulins seems, however, to be an interesting therapeutic approach which could effectively supplement the range of already tried and tested methods such as desensitization of administration of antihistamines, antianaphylactics and corticosteroids.

Monoclonal antibodies are already being used in diagnosis. They are playing an increasingly important role in tumour diagnosis and in the clinical-pathological classification of tumours. The sensitivity and precision of tumour diagnosis, particularly with regard to monitoring the progression of tumours, will definitely increase, and better use will be made of therapeutic measures based on improved diagnostics than is today the case. It will probably become possible to carry out quantitative or semiquantitative fluorescence microscopy and radioautographic assays of the products of cellular and viral oncogenes using monoclonal antibodies to these proteins in human tumour cells, and the results of these determinations will be used to classify various human tumours. It is equally likely that classification of human tumours on the basis of the expression of different oncogenes will, in the course of time, assume increasing prognostic and therapeutic importance.

The therapeutic use of monoclonal antibodies has so far been hampered by the fact that only murine monoclonals were available. Of course, such antibodies induce vigorous immune responses in the human recipient which severely limit the time during which they can be administered. But even within the existing limitations, some clinical uses for monoclonal antibodies appear to be in principle feasible. The use of antibodies against the CD3 T-cell antigen is of proven value in the treatment of rejection episodes after allogeneic kidney and liver transplantations. Certain antibodies directed at other T-cell antigens such as CD4, CD8 or CD11 may have similar clinical applicability. Several antibodies appear to have some therapeutic potential in the treatment of human cancer, especially colorectal cancer, breast carcinoma, melanoma and malignant diseases of the lymphatic system. Similarly, antibiotics against herpes viruses and against common antigens on bacteria could become valuable therapeutic tools. All of these potential therapeutic uses will benefit from the availability of monoclonal antibodies in which most of the murine sequences have been replaced by human sequences. The technique of "humanizing" mouse monoclonal antibodies has progressed to the point where virtually all murine monoclonal antibodies can be transformed into weakly immunogenic or non-immunogenic proteins, in which all amino acid sequences except those which determine complementarity with a particular antigen (CDR = complementarity determining region) have been exchanged for sequences from human antibodies.

The artificial recombination of human heavy and light chain cDNAs with other cDNAs can, of course, also be applied to molecules other than antibodies, for instance to receptors. Hybrid molecules, containing the constant regions of human IgG or IgM heavy chains coupled to the first two domains of the CD4 receptor have recently been described. In these constructs, the CD4 domains take the place of the variable region of the human heavy chain. On account of the V1 and V2 domains of CD4, such hybrid molecules can bind the envelope protein (gp120) of the AIDS virus and prevent the infection of CD4 cells. In addition, however, these constructs can bind to Fc receptors through their human constant regions. By the same token they should be able to serve as antibody-like molecules in ADCC reactions against HIV-infected lymphocytes which carry gp120 on their surface. Moreover, some of the IgG-CD4 constructs have been shown to activate complement, which adds another element to their potential therapeutic value.

Tumour therapy with "humanized" monoclonal antibodies will be carried out with unchanged antibodies which initiate an antibody-mediated cytotoxic reaction against tumour cells. As already mentioned, such tumour therapy will also be based upon procedures which include the binding of organic metal compounds (and radioactive metals) or of toxins to antibodies.

7.2 Immunosuppression

A "humanized" anti-tac antibody, i.e., an antibody which binds to the smaller subunit of the Il-2 receptor with a dissociation constant (kd) of approximately 10^{-9} M, is currently in development. This agent is expected to be useful in the treatment of rejection episodes after organ transplantation and in the management of acute episodes in autoimmune diseases. Whether the antibody will also be used on a more protracted basis will largely depend on its immunogenicity. Antibodies with other specificities but serving a similar purpose are likely to appear in clinical development and perhaps, towards the end of the period under consideration, on the shelves of hospital pharmacies.

The status of drug-induced immunosuppression is still unsatisfactory despite cyclosporin A. Less nephrotoxic substances are urgently required, and some are being developed, but it is a moot point whether these new cyclosporins will lead to further therapeutic advances. Even if this should not be the case, cyclosporin A has – apart from its own intrinsic therapeutic value – pointed the way to new approaches to drug-induced immunosuppression, which should make further advances possible. One such approach stems for the insight that certain microorganisms elaborate immunosuppressive substances – just as they produce effective antibiotic and cytostatic substances. In addition, thanks to cyclosporin research and to the progress made in immunology and cell biology, we also know which methods have to be used to find metabolites of this kind in fermentation broths. Some interesting substances have already been detected by using established methods. The research work carried out in this field will probably lead to clinically exploitable results within the next ten years. The second approach which should facilitate the discovery of new immunosuppressive drugs is derived from studies on the mechanism of action of cyclosporin A. The molecular characteristics of cyclophilin, the cytoplasmic receptor molecule for cyclosporin A, have now been elucidated in some detail. In contrast to earlier findings, which seemed to indicate that cyclophilin is a protein kinase, several groups have now reported that this protein corresponds to an enzyme which causes *cis,trans* isomerization of peptidyl-prolyl bonds in proteins. An enzyme of this type would be expected to induce conformational changes in other proteins. A hypothesis tying the new findings into a unified concept assumes that upon the activation of a T-lymphocyte cyclophilin would also be activated and subsequently change the conformation of proteins which in turn regulate the synthesis of Il-2 and other lymphokines at the transcriptional level. This conformational change would then allow for the synthesis of Il-2. Cyclosporin has been shown to be a potent inhibitor of the peptidyl-prolin-*cis,trans* isomerase. Since the 3-dimensional structure of cyclophilin will soon be known, a rational synthesis of new compounds, acting at this site but perhaps avoiding some of cyclosporin's disadvantages should become possible in the not too distant future.

The characterization of immunosuppressive lymphokines is still in its infancy. Some findings suggest the existence of a lymphokine that is released by alloantigen-stimulated T-lymphocytes and induces other T-cells to differentiate into T-suppressor cells. The possible therapeutic exploitation of this discovery is likely to take longer than the ten years selected for this overview.

A rather promising, though still somewhat speculative, approach to finding more antigen-specific drugs against autoimmune diseases rests on the following rationale: antigens, consequently also self-antigens, are presented by HLA class-I or class-II molecules. There is a striking association between the occurrence of certain autoimmune diseases and the presence of specific HLA alleles. Almost 50% of all patients with rheumatoid arthritis carry particular subtypes of DR4 (Dw4 and Dw14). DR1 is also "overrepresented" in RA patients. At least one of these three alleles is found in 85% of all cases with rheumatoid arthritis. Other HLA molecules are associated with different autoimmune diseases: insulin-dependent juvenile diabetes with DQ 3.2, multiple sclerosis with DR2, myasthenia gravis with DR3 and celiac diseases with DQw2.

Obviously, the self-antigens which initiate the autoimmune response in all these diseases are presented by a limited number of well-defined HLA alleles. If these "receptors" could be blocked, one could perhaps prevent certain autoimmune responses leading to disease. The oligopeptides presented by class-II molecules bind with a dissociation constant (kd) of 10^{-6} to 10^{-7} M. It has already been possible to identify peptides which can associate with certain HLA molecules with affinities that are one to two orders of magnitude higher than those of the "natural" peptides: It has also been shown that the blockade of defined HLA or MHC molecules by tightly binding peptides can abrogate immune responses which are mediated by these antigen-presenting molecules. In pharmacological terms, one would have to look for receptor antagonists for DR1, DR4 and other MHC molecules. Such antagonists could either be very selective or somewhat "promiscuous" with respect to the total number of HLA molecules. At first one would look for peptides; subsequently non-peptidic molecules might serve the same purpose.

7.3 Antiallergic substances – suppression of the acute-type hypersensitivity reaction

Besides the clinical-empirical desensitization measures, histamine H_1-antagonists, disodium chromoglycate and glucocorticosteroids are the pillars of antiallergic treatment. Despite appropriate experimental and clinical evidence, there is no confirmation that substances such as ketotifene and oxatomide represent a different approach to treatment from the classic antihistamines. A continuation of the search for new antihistamines does not seem to hold out much prospect of success. Disodium chromoglycate is valuable in prevention of asthma. Its great drawback is its poor oral absorption, which rules out administration by mouth. The search for an orally absorbable analog has so far been unsuccessful, but will be continued. Recent results suggest, however, that this target might be within reach. An orally utilizable drug of the disodium chromoglycate type would not represent a theoretical advance in the prevention of asthma but would nevertheless be highly welcome in practical terms.

Pathophysiological theories on the development of bronchial asthma have increasingly spotlighted three substances in recent years. These are the leukotrienes C4, D4 and E4 (formerly known as SRS-A), prostaglandin D2, and platelet-activating factor (PAF). Antagonists for these physiological mediators are being sought in many laboratories. Since antagonists that are effective in animal experiments have already been described – thereby furnishing the chemical basis – it is probable that at least some of these projects will be successful. This applies particularly to leukotriene antagonists and to inhibitors of PAF activity. However, very few of the substances that have been described to date exhibit adequate oral activity.

The key enzyme for the development of leukotrienes is Δ^5-lipoxygenase. Inhibitors of this enzyme from various structural classes have been described: flavonoids, catechols, aminophenols, phenidones and hydroxyphenols. Some substances inhibit the enzyme both *in vitro* and – after intravenous administration – *in vivo*. However, no orally effective substances have been identified in this context either. What is more, the duration of action proved to be too short for potentially beneficial therapeutic use.

A solid body of evidence points to the importance of eosinophils in the generation of tissue damage in bronchial asthma. Il-5 has been shown to be the major hematopoietic factor supporting the differentiation of eosinophils and also activating these cells. An Il-5 receptor antagonist which would inhibit the proliferation and differentiation induction afforded by Il-5 might therefore represent a rather fundamental approach towards treating this disease. The receptor for Il-5 is the target of very intensive investigations. Once this structure is cloned, one can look for low molecular weight antagonists by screening for the inhibition of Il-5 binding to the receptor. After the three-dimensional structure of this receptor has become available, a more rational approach towards the design of receptor antagonists will be possible.

7.4 Antiinflammatory substances

The treatment of chronic inflammation with nonsteroidal antiinflammatory drugs has reached its limits. Substances such as indomethacin, mefenamine and ibuprofen inhibit cyclooxygenase and thereby suppress or at least reduce prostaglandin synthesis. This intervention partially or completely relieves the symptoms of inflammation, e.g. swelling, erythema, pain and dysfunction. At least in the case of rheumatoid arthritis, however, this symptomatic therapy does not mean that the process of tissue destruction associated with, or even triggered by, the inflammation, is halted. On the contrary: prostaglandin E2, one of the most important products of the cyclooxygenase pathway, has very important immunoregulatory functions which are all aimed at slowing down inflammatory processes. PGE_2 inhibits the synthesis of lymphokines in activated B- and T-cells, it reduces the generation of oxygen radicals, of Il-1 and of plasminogen activator in macrophages, it prevents or delays the degranulation of mast cells, antagonizes many of the actions of Il-4, in short: it generally down-modulates the mechanisms which contribute to the inflammatory process.

The secretion of Il-1 by activated macrophages is of particular pathophysiological significance. Inhibitors of prostaglandin synthesis would therefore suppress the symptoms of the inflammation which are directly caused by the prostaglandins. However, this symptomatic improvement in inflammation would be at the cost of losing an important regulatory element, PGE_2. *Fig. 7.2* illustrates these interconnections. The starting point of the pathophysiological process is the activated lymphocyte. These lymphocytes activate macrophages, which secrete Il-1 plasminogen activator and many other products and enhance their phagocytosis. PGE_2, which exerts a negative feedback effect both on the macrophages and on the activated lymphocytes, is also generated in the activated macrophages. Thus PGE_2 has a "calming" effect on the functional cycle outlined here. Cyclooxygenase inhibitors such as indomethacin enhance macrophage activation! It would, therefore, be logical to try to imitate the effect of this PGE_2: for example, by means of more stable analogues. Such attempts have already been made. The hydantoin derivatives of PGE_2 and the prostacycline derivative carbacycline are chemically stable in comparison with their natural analogues. Marked inhibition of lymphocyte stimulation by mitogens can be obtained with these analogues in concentrations ranging from 10^{-9} and 10^{-5} M. Whether these findings are sufficient to label these substances as potential antiinflammatory agents is still an open question. Imitation of the physiological role of PGE_2 nevertheless seems to be an approach that produces results.

After what has been said on the central role of Il-1 in the immune response and inflammatory processes, the wide-spread interest in finding and developing an Il-1 receptor antagonist appears to be a logical strategy. This is particularly tempting since both variants of Il-1, Il-1α and Il-1β, bind to the same receptor and elicit almost identical responses. The prospects for a receptor antagonist have recently been greatly improved by the discovery of a naturally occuring Il-1 inhibitor. The cDNA specifying synthesis of this protein was recovered from a cDNA gene bank. The complete protein contains 152 amino acids, 25 of which represent a leader sequence. The mature protein comprises 137 amino acids. It has a 26%

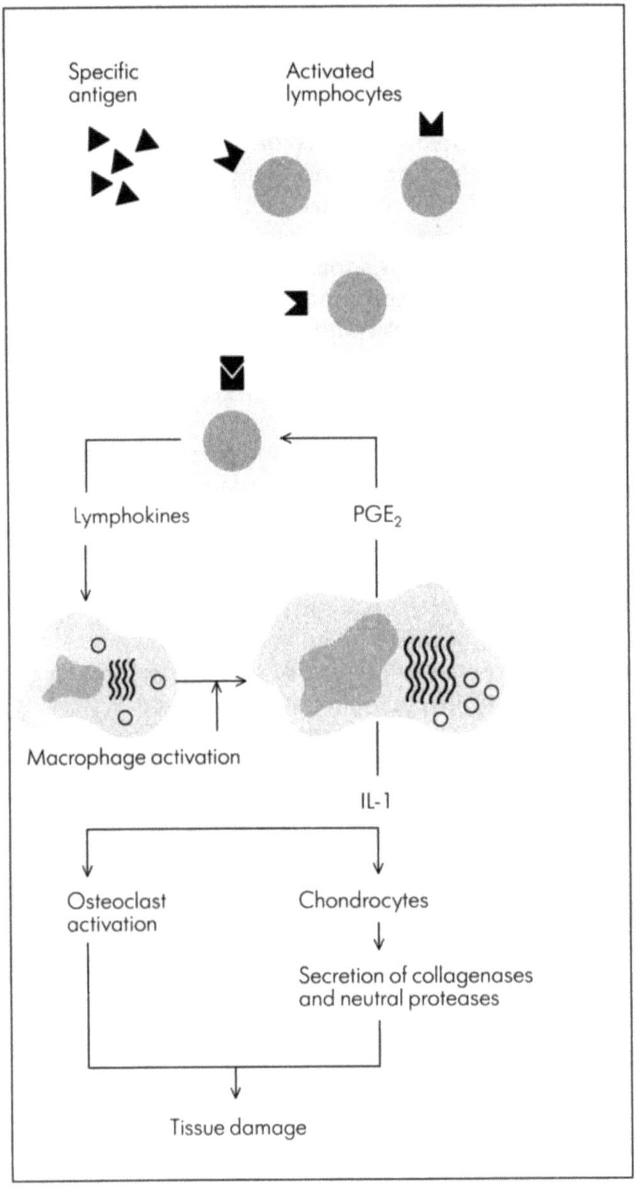

Figure 7.2. Connections between macrophage activation and tissue damage. For details see text.

amino acid sequence homology with Il-1α and a somewhat smaller homology with Il-1β. The three-dimensional structure of this protein is very similar to the corresponding structures of Il-1α and β, which have also recently been elucidated. The Il-1 inhibitor binds to the Il-1 receptor on EL-4 cells with an affinity which is intermediate between those for Il-1, α and β. It behaves entirely like a receptor antagonist without any agonistic efficacy of its own. The protein has already been shown to actively antagonize typical Il-1 effects. At a molar concentration ratio of 10 (Il-1 inhibitor / Il-1α or β), a 50% inhibition of the PGE2 release induced by I1-1 can be observed; at a ratio of 100, this inhibition is complete. Similarly, Il-1i at concentrations between 100 and 1000 ng/ml inhibits the interactions between neutrophils and endothelium which can be induced by Il-1. Local inflammatory responses to Il-1 in the rabbit skin can be antagonized by the inhibitor injected locally; Il-1 induced shock can be prevented and cartilage degradation, a typical disease-relevant consequence of the action of Il-1, is also antagonized effectively. Moreover, initial data indicate that doses of Il-1i in the range between 5 and 10 μg can effectively slow down the development of type-II collagen arthritis in mice even when treatment is started 12 days after the induction of the disease. Il-1i seems to be well tolerated by experimental animals: apart from its receptor-blocking effects, it does not seem to have any effects of its own. Thus, this human protein, the physiological significance of which is still unclear, seems to be a very promising candidate for the development a novel antiinflammatory drug. Of course, the ultimate goal must be to find a low molecular, non-peptidic compound with similar pharmacological properties.

Interferon-γ receptor antagonists or TNF receptor antagonists would also appear to be of potential value in interrupting inflammatory cascades, possibly also in down-modulating immune responses in certain autoimmune conditions. It appears likely that the search for such compounds will have resulted in novel drugs by the end of the nineties.

7.5 Immunostimulation – biological response modifiers

This field is the least satisfactory in immunotherapy. In fact no reliable, consistent therapeutic approach has been developed in this field. It should, however, be added that immunostimulation is still a very recent therapeutic principle and that some new substances in this category, e.g. the interferons, have been available for a relatively short time only. The disappointment surrounding the clinical efficacy of interferons in tumour therapy is a direct consequence of uncritical, exaggerated expectations. More precisely, the disappointment is felt predominantly by those who have never understood the biochemical and cell-biological effects of interferons and other lymphokines. The interferons will gradually consolidate their position in tumour therapy; they will be incorporated into new treatment regimens and tested for their suitability for combination with other substances. Such developments take time. The use of α-interferon against lymphomas, melanomas and, recently (in combination with vinblastine), also against renal cell carcinomas marks the beginning of the development of new therapeutic approaches which will take many years to come to fruition.

Interesting data are available on the synergistic effects of α- and γ-interferon. Isobologram curves are obtained for the combination of these two substances against a large number of tumour cells investigated *in vitro*; their synergistic effects are just as typical as the combination of β-lactam antibiotics and aminoglycosides against many bacteria.

The best route of administration for interferons has not yet been established. Since the development and the effect of interferons are predominantly "local" in nature, it may seem contradictory to administer large amounts of these lymphokines intravenously. Administration by way of the lymphatic vessels would be at least worth considering in regional processes. We know that with any severe trauma, and hence also with major surgery, the immunological defences of the organism are temporarily reduced. Particularly in cancer surgery, however, a reduction in cellular immunity and 'nonspecific resistance' is highly undesirable because it may lead to increased risk of metastasis formation. At present, the relationship between trauma and reduced defences, and the related interconnection between reduced defences and immunosuppression on the one hand and the tendency of a tumour to metastasize, on the other, are only vaguely understood. These connections are – at least clinically – difficult to quantify. We do not know, for instance, the extent to which a tumour patient is additionally at risk by temporary functional impairment of nonspecific or even specific defences. Lymphokines such as γ-interferon or Il-2 which can stimulate NK cells and macrophages could conceivably help overcome the temporary suppression of cellular defences occurring after surgery. It might even be possible to enhance the activity of tumour-destroying cells beyond normal levels for a limited period of time.

Though the interferons will not constitute the kind of breakthrough that the antibiotics were, they will nevertheless assume an increasingly important place in the treatment of viral infections and cancer in the course of the next few years. Especially in combination with Il-2, α-interferon holds out considerable promise for the treatment of certain tumours, e.g. melanoma and renal cell cancer. Also combinations of 5-fluorouracil and α-interferon appear to be capable of inducing synergistic effects, at least in some malignancies. *The overall conclusion from these findings – at least for the time being – may be that α-interferon, although of considerable merit by itself in certain viral and oncological diseases, has a much greater therapeutic potential in combination with other cytokines or with cytostatics. It appears likely that further progress with α-interferon will have to be sought mainly along these lines.*

The same may be true of interleukin 2. The early optimism regarding this protein was based on large-scale animal experiments which were carried out with Il-2, on clinical ex-vivo studies and a number of clinical trials which are still of a provisional character. Human Il-2 can expand LAK-cells and cytotoxic lymphocytes directed against tumours in mice, and drastically reduce the extent of metastasis of experimental tumours, for example the B16-melanoma. These positive results have not been completely reproduced in humans. However, after several adaptations of the original protocols, LAK-therapy in connection with Il-2 is now a rather well established therapeutic procedure.

High expectations are attached to the ability of Il-2 to expand cytotoxic lymphocytes. In this way immunoreactive T-cells directed against tumour antigens can be reconstituted after chemotherapy. The conditions for producing this effect in man are now being established. What is true for α-interferon may well turn out to be the case for Il-2: the use of this agent in combination with other cytokines (interferons and others) as well as conventional cytostatic drugs has yet to be elucidated.

Work on interferons is already well advanced, while Il-2 is still at a relatively early stage of clinical development. A number of other lymphokines with interesting therapeutic possibilities have been cloned and have been expressed in bacteria or mammalian cells (Chinese hamster ovary cells). The substances can now be investigated pharmacologically and tested and developed clinically. They include the tumour necrosis factors (TNFα and β) and the colony stimulating factors. The genes for TNFα and β have recently been cloned. Their sequence homology at the amino acid level is about 28%. TNFα is produced by macrophages and TNFβ by cytotoxic T-lymphocytes. Both factors have very similar cytotoxic effects on tumour cells. They can destroy tumour cells *in vitro*, and their effect is potentiated by the presence of interferons, notably γ-interferon. *In vivo*, both factors cause hemorrhagic necrosis of solid tumours after intralesional application. In experimental L1210 leukemia in the mouse, intraperitoneal administration of these lymphokines brought about a marked increase in survival. TNFα, the monocyte factor which has been studied more intensively than lymphotoxin (TNFβ), has attracted a lot of interest as a potential antitumour agent. Its synergistic effects with γ-interferon, which can be observed *in vitro*, have sparked much optimism.

The issue of the therapeutic use of TNFα is, however, complicated by the toxic properties of the protein. Like Il-1, TNF is a mediator of inflammatory responses. It induces the formation of prostaglandins and thromboxanes and induces shock. TNF is identical to "cachectin", a protein purified from activated macrophages by Cerami and Beutler. Cachectin, which is induced by endotoxins, inhibits lipoprotein lipase and helps to mobilize lipid stores. It also induces muscle wasting.

The finding that many of these severe toxic effects of TNF could be prevented or ameliorated by inhibitors, by cyclooxygenase-like indomethacin or by inhibitors of cycloxygenase and 5-lipoxygenase-like ibuprofen indicates that the therapeutic potential of TNF could be improved upon. This impression was supported by the finding that indomethacin did not affect the cytotoxicity of TNF for Hela cells *in vitro*. These and similar findings were taken as evidence that certain antiinflammatory drugs which interfered with the arachidonic acid cascade were useful in reducing the toxic effects of TNF without affecting its antineoplastic actions.

Clinical studies have so far not entirely corroborated this assumption. As expected, TNF proved to be very toxic in humans. Doses as low as 1–15 $\mu g/m^2$ body surface induced fever in 100 of the patients tested when applied intramuscularly and in 96% of all patients when injected intravenously. Other frequent side effects were chills, headache, fatigue, hypotension, anorexia and nausea. Antiinflammatory drugs reduced the severity, frequency and duration of such side effects. However, these drugs also seemed to reduce the direct toxic effects of TNF on tumours. Apparently TNF acts by two mechanisms: directly as a cytotoxic agent and indirectly through activation of NK-cells and macrophages. At least the first effect is reduced by cyclooxygenase inhibitors or steroids. It is not yet clear whether the indirect effects are also inhibited. The clinical use of TNF, therefore, is still surrounded by a great deal of uncertainty.

The rationale for the therapeutic use of colony stimulating factors has been described. It appears likely that within the next 10 or 12 years Il-3 and M-CSF will also be developed and used clinically. As already indicated in the previous chapter, combined use of colony stimulating factors may hold certain advantages over the use of single agents. Since Il-3 stimulates earlier phases of blood cell development, this factor may be a suitable tool to increase the precursor pool on which class two factors like M-CSF and G-CSF can subsequently act. It would therefore appear conceivable that the sequential use of Il-3 and G- or M-CSF might have better effects than the use of any of these factors alone. Il-1 and Il-6 are currently being evaluated for their hematopoietic effects in rodents and in primates. It appears that both of these proteins may play a role in the very early stages of hematopoiesis, possibly in the replication of committed stem cells or even pluripotent stem cells. At the time of writing, it is, however, not clear whether Il-1 acts directly on early precursor cells or via its induction of other factors like Il-3, Il-6 or GM-CSF in endothelial or stromal cells. Although Il-1 is a protein with pleiotropic effects there seem to be dose ranges in animals (rodents and cynomolgus monkeys) in which hematopoietic effects are clearly evident, while fever, acute phase protein synthesis, or the induction of weight loss and tissue damage are not yet seen. Should these findings also be conformed in humans, this could mean a further enlargement of the hematopoietic armamentarium.

So far it has been demonstrated that G-CSF and GM-CSF can reduce the myelotoxic side effects of cytoreductive therapy, as measured by the number of days with neutropenia (>1000 cells/μl), the number of fever episodes and the ability of patients to go through several cycles of chemotherapy. It is conceivable that colony stimulating factors can provide a support for bone-marrow function which makes even more aggressive and more extensive schemes of cytoreductive therapy possible than those being used today. Similar considerations also apply to the bone-marrow toxicity of azidothymidine (AZT). These possibilities will have to be explored in detail.

Experimentally, it has repeatedly been shown that a transient rise in functional granulocytes is a powerful strategy for the treatment of bacterial infections. With small bacterial inocula, GM- or G-CSF or Il-1 treatment may suffice to bring about a complete cure. With higher numbers of the infectious agent in question, antibiotics are needed in addition to the colony stimulating factor but in much lower doses than in untreated animals *(Fig. 7.3)*. In other words; CSFs might be powerful and attractive agents to be combined with antibiotics in severe infections. It is likely that we will see the emergence of such combined treatment modalities over the next 10 years.

The availability of Il-2, interferons and other lymphokines will, of course, make it possible to search selectively for substances which will interact as agonists or – as already mentioned – antagonists with the receptors of these lymphokines. In our ten-year period, however, the results of this approach are not likely to come to fruition.

The question whether progress in immunostimulation can be expected from derivatives of microbial structures must be treated with some caution. Despite considerable chemical efforts, it has not so far been possible to separate the macrophage-activating effects of muramyl-dipeptide from its pyrogenic effects and

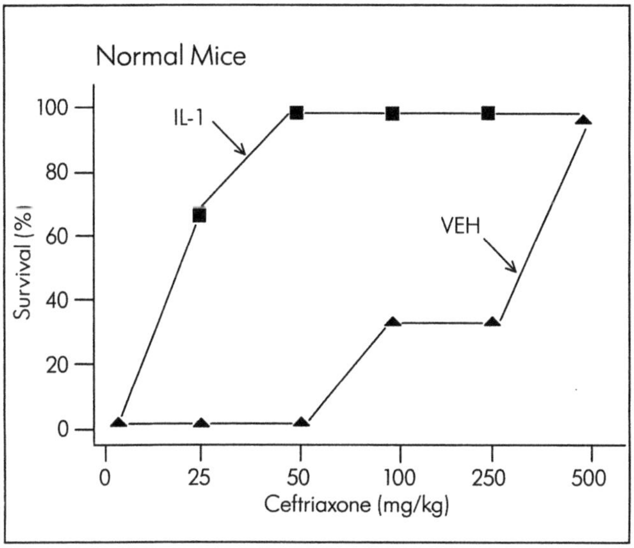

Figure 7.3. Effect of IL-1 on antibiotic therapy of Pseudomonas infection in normal mice. Mice were treated daily for 3 days with vehicle or IL-1 (25 μg/kg). Twenty-four hrs. after the last dose, mice were infected i.p. with 10^6 CFU (approx. 100 LD50 for normal mice) P. aeruginosa. At the time of infection, mice were also injected s.c. with various doses of Ceftriaxone (n = 6 mice per dose). Survival was recorded after 6 days.

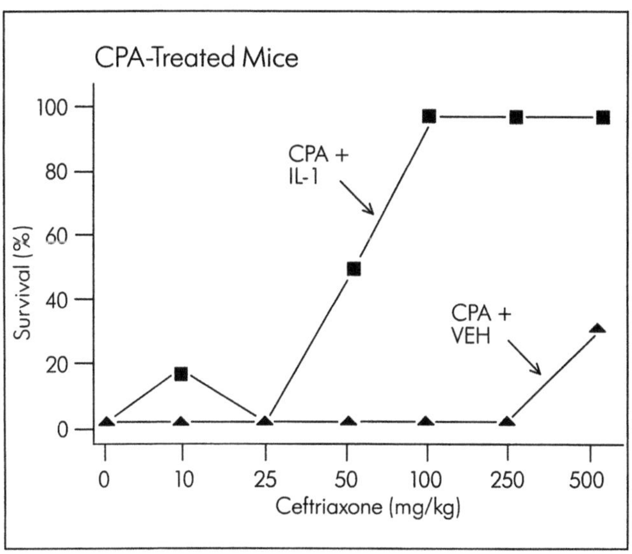

Effect of IL-1 on antibiotic therapy of Pseudomonas infection in bone marrow-suppressed mice. Mice were injected with CPA (150 mg/kg) and then were treated daily for 3 days with vehicle or 25 μg/kg IL-1. Twenty-four hrs. after the last dose, mice were infected i.p. with 10^6 CFU P. aeruginosa. At the time of infection, mice were injected s.c. with various doses of Ceftriaxone (6 mice per dose). Survival was recorded after 6 days.
CPA: cyclophosphamide

other undesirable actions in such a way that broad clinical use of such substances would seem to be feasible. It has already been mentioned that the incorporation of muramyl-dipeptide derivatives into multilamellar liposomes changes the toxicity profile of MDP quite dramatically. At least one such preparation which appears to be well tolerated and is at the same time effective in the activation of the mononuclear-phagocytic system is already in the early stages of clinical development and may be established as a clinically useful agent within the time period under "preview".

The development of microbial structures in connection with immunostimulation will, in the next few years, be increasingly displaced by genetic engineering and protein chemistry work on lymphokines and probably also by the search for low-molecular-weight, synthetic compounds with immunostimulating effects. In this last field, chance has played, and still plays, a prominent role. Levamisole, cimetidine and even isoprinosin were, after all, not synthesized as immunostimulants but were developed for quite different purposes.

General Literature

Chapter 1

Herberman RB (ed) (1980): Natural cell-mediated immunity against tumors. Academic Press, New York.
Herberman RB (ed) (1982): NK cells and other natural effector cells. Academic Press, New York.
Sirois P, Rola-Pleszczynski M (eds) (1983): Immunopharmacology. Elsevier Biomedical Press. Amsterdam, New York, Oxford (Research Monographs in Immunology, Vol 4.)
Wechter W, Longhman B (1984): Immunology in drug research. Progress in Drug Res Vol 28, 233–272. Birkhäuser, Basel.

Chapter 2

Bach F, Good RA (eds) (1980): Clinical immunology, Vol 4, Academic Press, New York, 1–198.
Gallin Jl, Fauci AS (eds) (1982): Phagocytic cells. Advances in Host Defense Mechanisms, Vol 1, Raven Press, New York.
Khan A, Hill NO (eds) (1982): Human lymphokines. Academic Press, New York, London, Paris, San Diego, San Francisco, São Paulo, Sydney, Tokyo, Toronto.
Litwin SD, Scott DW, Reisfeld RA, Flaherty L, Marcus DM (1989): Human immunogenetics. Basic principles and clinical relevance. Immunology Series, Vol 43, 319–328.
Nathan C, Yoshida R (1988): Cytokines: Interferon-γ. Inflammation: Basic principles and clinical correlates, Chapter 14, 229–251.
Roitt I (1988): Essential immunology. Blackwell Scientific Publication, 4. Auflage, Oxford, London, Edinburgh, Boston, Melbourne.
Sell S (ed) (1987): Immunology, immunopathology and immunity. Elsevier, New York, Amsterdam.

Chapter 3

Burton DR (1985): Immunoglobulin G: Functional sites. Molecular Immunology, Vol 22, No 3, 161–206.
Lattmann P (ed) (1982): Der klinische Einsatz von Immunglobulin (Gammaglobulin). Sandoz Produkte (Schweiz) AG, Basel.
Newland AC (1987): Idiopathic thrombocytopenic purpura and IgG: A review. Journal of Infection, Vol 15, Supplement 1, 41–49.
Nydegger UE (1981): Immunochemotherapy. Proceedings of a workshop on immunological and pathological aspects of i.v. immunglobulin prophylaxis and therapy. Academic Press, New York.

Chapter 4

AMA Council on Scientific Affairs (1986): Introduction to the management of immunosuppression. Connecticut Medicine, Vol 51, No 7, 447–452.
Borel JF (ed) (1986): Ciclosporin. Karger, Basel, München, Paris, London, New York, New Delhi, Singapore, Tokyo, Sydney.

Calabresi P, Parks RE (1980): Antiproliferative agents and drugs used for immunosuppression. In: The pharmacological basis of therapeutics (Goodman Gilman A, Goodman LS, Gilman A, eds). MacMillan Publishing Co, New York.
Cosimi AB (1987): Clinical development of orthclone OKT3 Transplantation Proceedings Vol 19, No 2, Suppl 1, 7–16.
Costanzo-Nordin MR et al (1987): Successful reversal of acute cardiac allograft rejection with OKT3 monoclonal antibody. Circulation, Vol 76 (Suppl. V), 71–80.
Hadden JW (1987): Immunopharmacology. Immunomodulation and immunotherapy, JAMA, Vol 258, No 20, 3005–3010.
Kahan BD (ed) (1984): Cyclosporine: Biological activity and clinical applications. Grune and Stratton, Orlando, Vol 1.
Kirkpatrick CH (1987): Transplantation immunology, JAMA, Vol 258, No 20, 2993–3000.
Padberg W, Schwemmle K, Dobroschke J, Kupiec-Weglinski JW, Tilney NL (1987): Immunosuppressive Therapie in der Transplantationschirurgie. Dtsch med Wschr, Vol 112, 1670–1674.
Vane J, Botting R (1987): Inflammation and the mechanism of action of anti-inflammatory drugs FASEBJ, Vol 1, 89–96.
White DJG (ed) (1981): Cyclosporin A. Elsevier Biomedical Press, Amsterdam, New York, Oxford.

Chapter 5

Goldberg ME (ed) (1981): Pharmacological and biochemical properties of drug substances, Vol 3, Published by: American Pharmaceutical Association, Academy of Pharmaceutical Sciences.
Ishizaka K (1988): IgE-binding factors and regulation of the IgE antibody response. Ann Rev Immunol, Vol 6, 513–534.
Morley J (1982): Bronchial hyperreactivity. Academic Press, London, New York, Paris, San Diego, San Francisco, São Paulo, Sydney, Tokyo, Toronto.
Oppenheim JJ, Rosenstreich DL, Potter M (eds) (1984): Cellular functions in immunity and inflammation. Elsevier/North Holland, New York, Amsterdam.
Parker W (1982): Allergic reactions in man. Pharmacological Reviews, Vol 34, No 1, 85–104.
Wilson JD (1983): Asthma and allergic diseases: A clinician's guide to diagnosis and management. ADIS Health Science Press, Sydney, Auckland, Bristol, Boston, Hong Kong, Tokyo.

Chapter 6

Adams DO, Hamilton TA (1984): The cell biology of macrophage activation. Ann Rev Immunol, Vol 2, 283–318.
Arrigoni-Martelli E (1981): Developments in drugs enhancing the immune responses. Meth and Find Exptl Clin Pharmacol, Vol 3 (4), 247–270.
Drews J (1984): Die Pharmakologie des Immunsystems: Klinische und experimentelle Perspektiven. In: Progress in Drug Research, Vol 28, 83–109. (E Jucker ed).
Drews J (1984): The experimental and clinical use of immune-modulating drugs in the prophylaxis and treatment of infections. Infection, Vol 12, 157–166.
Fidler IJ (1985): Macrophages and metastasis – A biological approach to cancer therapy: Presidential address. Cancer Research, Vol 45, 4714–4726.
Grob PJ, Fontana A (1982): Immunstimulantien und Infektionskrankheiten. Therap Umsch, Vol 39, No 9, 668–674.
Mertelsmann R, Welte K (1986): Human interleukin 2: Molecular biology, physiology and clinical possibilities. Immunobiol, Vol 172, 400–419.
Metcalf D (1985): The granulocyte-macrophage colony-stimulating factors. Science, Vol 229, 16–22.
Metcalf D (1988): Haemopoietic growth factors. Med J Austral, Vol 148, 516–519.

Mihich E (1986): Future perspectives for biological response modifiers: A viewpoint. Seminars in Oncology, Vol 13, No 2, 234–254.

Mihich E, Fefer A (eds) (1983): Biological response modifiers: Subcommittee Report. Subcommittee on Biological Response Modifiers. Board of Scientific Counselors, Division of Cancer Treatment. National Cancer Institute.

Nicola NA (1987): Why do hemopoietic growth factor receptors interact with each other? Immunology Today, Vol 8, No 5, 134–140.

Oettgen HF, Old LJ (1987): Tumor necrosis factor. Important Adv Oncol, Vol. 1987, 105–130.

Patterson R, Norman P (1982): Immunotherapy-Immunomodulation. JAMA, Vol 248, No 20, 2759–2772.

Smith KA (1988): Interleukin-2: Inception, impact, and implications. Science, Vol 240, 1169–1176.

Umezawa H (1980): Low-molecular-weight immunomodulators produced by microorganisms. Biotechnol Bioengineering, Vol XXII, Suppl 1, 99–110.

Werner GH, Floc F, Migliore-Samour D, Jollès P (1986): Immunomodulating peptides. Experientia, Vol 42, 521–531.

References

Chapter 1

Hibbs JB, Granger DL, Cook JL, Lewis AM (1983): Activated macrophage mediated cytotoxicity for transformed target cells. In: Mechanisms of cell-mediated cytotoxicity (Clark WR, Golstein P, eds), Plenum Press, New York and London, 315–335.

Key ME, Hoyer L, Bucana C, Hanna MG (1982): Mechanisms of macrophage-mediated tumor cytolysis. In: Mechanisms of cell-mediated cytotoxicity (Clark WR, Golstein P, eds). Plenum Press, New York and London, 265–310.

Kohler PF (1982): The autoimmune diseases. JAMA, Vol 248, No 20, 2646–2656.

Schultz RM, Chirigos MA (1980): Macrophage activation for nonspecific tumor cytotoxicity. Advances in Pharmacology and Chemotherapy, Vol 17, 157–193.

Chapter 2

Acuto O, Hussey RE, Fitzgerald KA, Protentis JP, Meuer SC, Schlossman SF, Reinherz EL (1983): The human T cell receptor: appearance in ontogeny and biochemical relationship of a and b subunits on IL-2 dependent clones and T cell tumors. Cell, Vol 34, 717–726.

Adams JM (1980): The organization and expression of immunoglobulin genes. Immunology Today, Vol 1, 10–17.

Allen PM (1987): Antigen processing at the molecular level. Immunology Today, Vol 8, No 9, 270–273.

Askenase PW, van Loveren H (1983): Delayed-type hypersensitivity: activation of mast cells by antigen-specific T-cell factors initiates the cascade of cellular interactions. Immunology Today, Vol 4, No 9, 259–264.

Babior BM (1984): The respiratory burst of phagocytes. J Clin Invest, Vol 73, 599–601.

Batchelor JR, McMichael AJ (1987): Progress in understanding HLA and disease associations. British Medical Bulletin, Vol 43, No 1, 156–183.

Bendtzen K (1988): Interleukin 1, interleukin 6 and tumor necrosis factor in infection, inflammation and immunity. Immunology Letters, Vol 19, 183–192.

Berger M, Wetzler EM, Wallis RS (1988): Tumor necrosis factor is the major monocyte product that increases complement receptor expression on mature human neutrophils. Blood, Vol 71, No 1, 151–158.

Bienenstock J, Tomioka M, Stead R, Ernst P, Jordana M, Gauldie J, Dolovich J, Denburg J (1987): Mast cell involvement in various inflammatory processes. Am Rev Respir Dis, Vol 135, 5–8.

Bjorkman PJ, Saper MA, Samraoui B, Bennett WS, Strominger JL, Wiley DC (1987): Structure of the human class I histocompatibility antigen, HLA-A2. Nature, Vol 329, 506–512.

Blüthmann H, Kisielow P, Uematsu Y, Malissen M, Krimpenfort P, Berns A, von Boehmer H, Steinmetz M (1988): T-cell specific deletion of T-cell receptor transgenes allows functional rearrangement of endogenous α and β-genes. Nature, Vol 334, 156–159.

Bjorkman PJ, Saper MA, Samraoui B, Bennett WS, Strominger JL, Wiley DC (1987): The foreign antigen binding site and T cell recognition regions of class I histocompatibility antigens. Nature, Vol 329, 512–539.

Bodmer WF (1987): The HLA system: structure and function. J Clin Pathol, Vol 40, 948–958.

Burgess AW, Metcalf D (1980): The nature and action of granulocyte-macrophage colony-stimulating factors. Blood, Vol 56, No 6, 947–958.

Buus S, Sette A, Colon SM, Miles C, Grey HM (1987): The relation between major histocompatibility complex (MHC) restriction and the capacity of Ia to bind immunogenic peptides. Science, Vol 235, 1353–1358.

Cambier JC, Ransom JT (1987): Molecular mechanisms of transmembrane signaling in B lymphocytes. Ann Rev Immunol, Vol 5, 175–199.

Campbell RD, Law SKA, Reid KBM, Sim RB (1988): Structure, organization, and regulation of the complement genes. Ann Rev Immunol, Vol 6, 161–195.

Dinarello CA (1989): Interleukin-1 and its related cytokines. Macrophage-Derived Cell Regulatory Factors. Cytokines, Vol 1, 105–154.

Dinarello CA, Clark BD, Puren AJ, Savage N, Rosoff PM (1989): The interleukin 1 receptor. Immunology Today, Vol 10, No 2, 49–51.

Dinarello CA (1986): Interleukin 1: Amino acid sequences, multiple biological activities and comparison with Tumor Necrosis Factor (Cachectin). The Year in Immunology, Vol 2, 68–89. Karger, Basel.

Edelman GM (1970): The structure and function of antibodies. Sci Am, Vol 223 (2), 34–42.

Farrar JJ, Benjamin WR, Hilfiker ML, Howard M, Farrar WL, Fuller-Farrar J (1982): The biochemistry, biology and role of interleukin 2 in the induction of cytotoxic T cell and antibody forming B cell responses. Immunological Rev, Vol 63, 129–166.

Fell PH, Tucker PW (1989): Immunoglobin genes. Human Immunogenetics: Basic principles and clinical relevance. Immunology Series, Vol 43, 181–202.

Germain RN (1986): Immunology. The ins and outs of antigen processing and presentation. Nature, Vol 322, 687–689.

Ghezzi P, Dinarello CA (1988): IL-1 induces IL-1. Specific inhibition of IL-1 production by IFN-γ. The Journal of Immunology, Vol 140, No 12, 4238–4244.

Gomperts BD, Cockcroft S, Howell TW, Nüsse O, Tatham PER (1987): The dual effector system for exocytosis in mast cells: Obligatory requirement for both Ca^{+2} and GTP. Bioscience Reports, Vol 7, No 5, 369–381.

Guyre, Munek (1989): In Schleimer RP, Claman HN, Oronsky AL (eds). Anti-inflammatory Steroid Actions. Basic and clinical aspects, Academic Press, 199–225.

Hadding U, Fassbender B (1988): Das Komplementsystem: Ein Funktionsträger für Infektabwehr und Immunregulation. Naturwissenschaften, Vol 75, 544–550.

Harriman GR, Strober W (1989): The immunobiology of interleukin-5. Cruse JM, Lewis RE Jr (eds): The year in immunology 1988. Immunoregulatory cytokines and cell growth. Year immunol Basel, Karger, Vol 5, 160–177.

Hedrick SM, Cohen DI, Nielsen EA, Davis MM (1984): Isolation of c-DNA clones encoding T-cell-specific membrane-associated proteins. Nature, Vol 308, 149–153.

Hedrick SM, Nielsen EA, Kavaler J, Cohen DI, Davis MM (1984): Sequence relationships between putative T-cell receptor polypeptides and immunoglobulins. Nature, Vol 308, 153–158.

Herberman RB (1986): Natural killer cells. Ann Rev Med, Vol 37, 347–352.

Hirano T, Taga T, Yamasaki K, Matsuda T, Tang B, Muraguchi A, Horii Y, Suematsu S, Hirata Y, Yawata H, Shimizu M, Kawano M, Kishimoto T (1989): A multifunctional cytokine (IL-6/BSF-2) and its receptor. Int Arch Allergy Appl Immunol, Vol 88, 29–33.

Kappes D, Strominger JL (1988): Human class II major histocompatibility complex genes and proteins. Ann Rev Biochem, Vol 57, 991–1028.

Kay NE (1986): Natural killer cells. Science, Vol 22, No. 4, 343–359.

Kennerly DA (1987): Preparation and characterization of mast cell cytoplasts. Journal of Immunological Methods, Vol 97, 173–183.

Kincade PW (1981): Formation of B lymphocytes in fetal and adult life. Advances in Immunology, Vol 31, 177–245.

Klein J, Juretic A, Constantin NB, Nagy ZA (1981): The traditional and a new version of the mouse H-2 complex. Nature, Vol 291, 455–460.

Knapp W, Rieber P, Dörken B, Schmidt RE, Stein H, vd Borne AEGKr (1989): Towards a better definition of human leucocyte surface molecules. Immunology Today, Vol 10, No 8, 253–258.

Lanzavecchia A (1987): Antigen uptake and accumulation in antigen-specific B cells. Immunological Rev, No 99, 40–51.

Larrick JW (1989): Native interleukin 1 inhibitors. Immunology Today, Vol 10, No 2, 61–65.

Leder P (1982): The genetics of antibody diversity. Sci Am, Vol 246 (5), 72–83.

Lopez AF, To LB, Yu-Chung Yang, Gamble JR, Shannon MF, Burns GF, Dyson PG, Juttner CA, Clark S, Vadas MA (1987): Stimulation of proliferation differentiation, and function of human cells by primate interleukin 3. Proc Natl Acad Sci USA, Vol 84, 2761–2765.

Lotzova E (1983/84): Natural immunity. Nat Immun Cell Growth Regul, Vol 3, 1–6.

Mace KF, Ehrke MJ, Hori K, Maccubbin DL, Mihich E (1988): Role of tumor necrosis factor in macrophage activation and tumoricidal activity. Cancer Research, Vol 48, 5427–5432.

Mach B, Gorski J, Rollini P, Berte C, Amaldi I, Berdoz J, Ucla C (1986): Polymorphism and regulation of HLA class II genes of the major histocompatibility complex. Cold Spring Harbor Symposia on Quantitative Biology, Vol LI, 67–74.

Malech HL, Gallin JI (1987): Current concepts: Immunology. Neutrophils in Human Diseases. New Engl J Med, Vol 317, No 11, 687–694.

Manser T, Wysocki LJ, Gridley T, Near Rl, Gefter ML (1985): The molecular evolution of the immune response. Immunology Today, Vol 6, No 3, 94–100.

Marrack P, Kappler J (1987): The T Cell receptor. Science, Vol 238, 1073–1079.

Marx JL (1987): Structure of MHC protein solved. Science, Vol 238, 613–614.

Matsushima K, Morishita K, Yoshimura T, Lavu S, Kobayashi Y, Lew W, Appella E, Kung HF, Leonard EJ, Oppenheim JJ (1988): Molecular cloning of a human monocyte-derived neutrophil chemotactic factor (MDNCF) and the induction of MDNCF mRNA by interleukin 1 and tumor necrosis factor. J Exp Med, Vol 167, 1883–1893.

Melchers F (1978): Introduction. Annual Report 1987, Basel Institute for Immunology, 8–22.

Milenkovic L, Rettori V, Snyder GD, Beutler B, McCann SM (1989): Cachectin alters anterior pituitary hormone release by a direct action in vitro. Proc Natl Acad Sci USA, Vol 86, 2418–2422.

Mills KHG (1986): Processing of viral antigens and presentation to class II-restricted T cells. Immunology Today, Vol 7, No 9, 260–263.

Mingari MC, Gerosa F, Carra G, Accolla RS, Moretta A, Zubler RH, Waldmann TA, Moretta L (1984): Human interleukin-2 promotes proliferation of activated B cells via surface receptors similar to those of activated T cells. Nature, Vol 312, 641–643.

Munker R, Koeffler HP (1987): Tumor Necrosis Factor: Recent advances. Klin Wschr, Vol 65, 345–352.

Nathan CF (1987): Secretory products of macrophages. J Clin Invest, Vol 79, 319–326.

Nicola NA, Vadas MA (1984): Hemopoietic colony-stimulating factors. Immunology Today, Vol 5, No 3, 76–80.

Ohara J-I (1989): Interleukin-4: Molecular structure and biochemical characteristics, biological function, and receptor expression. Cruse JM, Lewis RE Jr (eds): The year in immunology 1988. Immunoregulatory cytokines and cell growth. Year immunol. Basel, Karger, Vol 5, 126–159.

Osmond DG (1979): Generation of B lymphocytes in the bone marrow. In: Lymphocytes in the Immune Response (Cooper-Mosier-Scher-Vitetta, eds). Elsevier North Holland, Inc, 63–70.

Owen WF, Rothenberg ME, Petersen J, Weller PF, Silberstein D, Sheffer AL, Stevens RL, Soberman RJ, Austen KF (1989): Interleukin 5 and phenotypically altered eosinophils in the blood of patients with the idiopathic hypereosinophilic syndrome. J Exp Med, Vol 170, 343–348.

Pardoll DM, Kruisbeek AM, Fowlkes BJ, Coligan JE, Schwartz RH (1987): The unfolding story of T-cell receptor gamma. FASEBJ, Vol 1, 103–109.

Patton JS, Rice GC, Ranges GE, Palladino MA Jr (1989): Biology of the tumor necrosis factors. Macrophage-Derived Cell Regulatory Factors. Cytokines, Vol 1, 89–104.

Paul WE (1987): Interleukin 4/B cell stimulatory factor 1: one lymphokine, many functions. FASEBJ, Vol 1, No 6, 456–461.

Perlmutter DH, Colten HR (1989): Molecular basis of complement deficiencies. Immunodeficiency Reviews, Vol 1, 105–133.

Peters SP, Schleimer RP, Naclerio RM, MacGlashan DW Jr, Togias AG, Proud D, Freeland HS, Fox C, Adkinson NF Jr, Lichtenstein LM (1987): The pathophysiology of human mast cells. Am Rev Respir Dis, Vol 135, 1196–1200.

Ploegh HL, Orr HT, Strominger JL (1981): Major histocompatibility antigens: the human (HLA-A, -B, -C) and murine (H-2k, H-2D) class I molecules. Cell, Vol 24, 287–299.

Potter K, Leid RW (1986): A review of eosinophil chemotaxis and function in taenia taeniaeformis infections in the laboratory rat. Veterinary Parasitology, Vol 20, 103–116.

Rajewsky K, Förster I, Cumano A (1987): Evolutionary and Somatic Selection of the Antibody Repertoire in the Mouse. Science, Vol 238, 1088–1094.

Reid KB (1983): Proteins involved in the activation and control of the two pathways of human complement. Biochem Soc Trans, Vol 1, 1–12.

Reinherz EL, Acuto O, Fabbi M, Bensussan A, Milanese C, Royer HD, Meuer SC, Schlossman SF (1984): Clonotypic surface structure on human T-lymphocytes: Functional and biochemical analysis of the antigen receptor complex. Immunological Rev, Vol 81, 95–129.

Reinherz EL, Kung PC, Goldstein G, Levey R, Schlossman SF (1980): Discrete stages of human intrathymic differentiation: Analysis of normal thymocytes and leukemic lymphoblasts of T-cell lineage. Proc Natl Acad Sci USA, Vol 77, 1588–1592.

Sanderson CJ, Campbell HD, Young IG (1988): Molecular and cellular biology of eosinophil differentiation factor (interleukin-5) and its effects on human and mouse B cells. Immunological Rev, No 102, 29–50.

Schwartz LB, Bradford TR, Irani A-MA, Deblois G, Craig SS (1987): The major enzymes of human mast cell secretory granules. Am Rev Respir Dis, Vol 135, 1186–1189.

Scollay R, Bartlett P, Shortman K (1984): T-cell development in the adult murine thymus: Changes in the expression of the surface antigens Ly2, L3T4 and B2A2 during development from early precursor cells to emigrants. Immunological Rev, No 82, 79–103.

Shaw S (1987): Characterization of human leukocyte differentiation antigens. Immunology Today, Vol 8, 1, 1–3.

Siegel JP, Sharon M, Smith PL, Leonard WJ (1987): The IL-2 receptor β chain (p70): Role in mediating signals for LAK, NK, and proliferative activities. Science, Vol 238, 75–78.

Silverton EW, Navia MA, Davies DR (1977): Three-dimensional structure of an intact human immunoglobulin. Proc Natl Acad Sci USA, Vol 74, 5140–5144.

Sprent J, Lo D, Gao E-K, Ron Y (1988): T cell selection in the thymus. Immunological Rev, No 101, 173–190.

Stasny P, Ball EJ, Dry PJ, Nunez G (1983): The human immune response region (HLA-D) and disease susceptibility. Immunological Rev, Vol 70, 113–153.

Stites DP, Pavia CS (1979): Ontogeny of human T cells. Pediatrics, Vol 64/Suppl, 795–802.

Sudo T, Ito M, Ogawa Y, Iizuka M, Kodama H, Kunisada T, Hayashi S-I, Ogawa M, Sakai K, Nishikawa S, Nishikawa S-I (1989): Interleukin 7 production and function in stromal cell-dependent B cell development. J Exp Med, Vol 170, 333–338.

Sugamura K, Fujii M, Kobayashi N, Sakitani M, Hatanaka M, Hinuma Y (1984): Retrovirus-induced expression of interleukin 2 receptors on cells of human B-cell lineage. Proc Natl Acad Sci USA, Vol 81, 7441–7445.

Sullivan KE, Calman AF, Nakanishi M, Tsang SY, Wang Y, Peterlin BM (1987): A model for the transcriptional regulation of MHC class II genes. Immunology Today, Vol 8, No 10, 289–293.

Timonen T, Ortaldo JR, Herberman RB (1981): Characteristics of human large granular lymphocytes and relationship to natural killer and K cells. J Exp Med, Vol 153, 569–582.

Todd RF, Liu DY (1986): Mononuclear phagocyte activation: Activation-associated antigens. Federation Proceedings, Vol 45, No 12, 2829–2836.

Toivanen P, Uksila J, Leino A, Lassila O, Hirvonen T, Ruuskanen O (1981): Development of mitogen responding T cells and natural killer cells in the human fetus. Immunological Rev, Vol 57, 89–105.

Tonegawa S (1983): Somatic generation of antibody diversity. Nature, Vol 302, 575–581.

Tonegawa S et al (1981): Somatic reorganization of immunoglobulin genes during lymphocyte differentiation. Cold Spring Harbor Symp Quant Biol, Vol 45, 839–858.

Tsoukas CD, Valentine M, Lotz M, Vaughan JH, Carson DA (1984): The role of the T3 molecular complex in antigen recognition and subsequent activation events. Immunology Today, Vol 5, No 11, 311–313.

Vadas MA, Lopez AF (1984): Regulation of granulocyte function by colony-stimulating factors. Lymphokine Research, Vol 3, 45–50.

Volpé R (1986): Autoimmune Thyroid Disease. A Perspective. Mol Biol Med, Vol 3, 25–51.

Weissmann C, Weber H (1986): The interferon genes. Progress in Nucleic Acid Research and Molecular Biology, Vol 33, 251–301.

Westwick J, Li SW, Camp RD (1989): Novel neutrophil-stimulating peptides. Immunology Today, Vol 10, No 5, 146–147.

Williams AF (1987): A year in the life of the immunoglobulin superfamily. Immunology Today, Vol 8, No 10, 298–303.

Williams LW, Burks W, Steele RW (1988): Complement: Function and clinical relevance. Annals of Allergy, Vol 60, 293–301.

Woodruff MFA (1986): The cytolytic and regulatory role of natural killer cells in experimental neoplasia. Biochimica et Biophysica Acta, Vol 865, 43–57.

Yanagi Y, Yoshikai Y, Leggett K, Clark StP, Aleksander I, Mak TW (1984): A human T cell-specific cDNA clone encodes a protein having extensive homology to immunoglobulin chains. Nature, Vol 308, 145–149.

Zinkernagel RM (1978): Major transplantation antigens in host responses to infection. Hosp Pract, Vol 13 (7), 83–92.

Zinkernagel RM, Doherty PC (1974): Restriction of in vitro T cell-mediated cytotoxicity in lymphocytic choriomeningitis within a syngeneic or semiallogeneic system. Nature, Vol 248, 701–702.

Chapter 3

Abe T, Matsuda J, Kawasugi K, Yoshimura Y, Kinoshita T, Kazama M (1983): Clinical effect of intravenous immunoglobulin on chronic idiopathic thrombocytic purpura. Blut, Vol 47, 69–75.

Barandun S (1983): Passive Immunisierung mit Immunglobulinen. Therap Umsch, Band 40, Heft 3, 257–260.

Barandun S, Kistler P, Jeunet F, lsliker H (1962): Intravenous administration of human gammaglobulin. Vox Sang, Vol 7, 157.

Barandun S, Skvaril F, Morell A (1976): Prophylaxe und Therapie mit Gammaglobulin. Schweiz med Wschr, Vol 106, 533–580.

Böhm D (1987): Erfahrungen mit einem Pseudomonas-Immunglobulin bei beatmeten Patienten mit Pseudomonas-Pneumonie auf einer chirurgischen Intensivstation. Infection, Vol 15, Supplement 2, 64–66.

Brady LW, Woo DV, Heindel ND, Markoe AM, Koprowski H (1987): Therapeutic and diagnostic uses of modified monoclonal antibodies. Int J Radiation Oncology Biol Phys, Vol 13, No 10, 1535–1544.

Carroll RR, Noyes WD, Rosse WF, Kitchens CS (1984): Intravenous immunoglobulin administration in the treatment of severe chronic immune thrombocytopenic purpura. Amer J Med, March 30, Vol 76, 181–186.

Class I, Junginger W, Kloss T (1987): Use of pseudomonas immunoglobulin in ventilated patients at an interdisciplinary surgical intensive care station. Infection, Vol 15, Supplement 2, 67–70.

Conley ME, Delacroix DL (1987): Intravascular and mucosal immunoglobulin A: Two separate but related systems of immune defense? Ann Intern Med, Vol 106, No 6, 892–899.

Dalhoff A (1983): In vitro- und In vivo-Untersuchungen zur Wirkung von Acylureido-Penicillinen mit Immunglobulin G bei Problembakterien. Münch med Wschr, Vol 125, Suppl 2, 150–158.

Dawson DM, Carter JL, Hafler DA, Weiner HL (1987): Immunosuppression in progressive multiple sclerosis with high dose intravenous cyclophosphamide and monoclonal antibodies. Rivista di Neurologia, Vol 57, No 2, 88–91.

Dreesman G, Kennedy RC (1985): Antiidiotypic antibodies: Implication of image-based vaccines for infectious diseases. J Infect Dis, Vol 151, 761–765.

Dreikorn K, Doerr HW, Geursen RG, Braun R, Klingenfuss H, Fuchs M (1986): Immunglobulin-Prophylaxe von Cytomegalie-Virusinfektionen nach Nierentransplantation. Die gelben Hefte XXVI, 105–113.

Emanuel D, Gold J, Colacino J, Lopez C, Hammerling U (1984): A human monoclonal antibody to cytomegalovirus (CMV). The Journal of Immunology, Vol 133, No 4, 2202–2205.

Emmrich F (1987): Perspektiven der Anwendung monoklonaler Antikörper in der Therapie neoplastischer Erkrankungen. Onkologie, Vol 10, 121–124.

Erlich KS, Mills J (1986): Passive immunotherapy for encephalitis caused by Herpes Simplex virus. Reviews of Infectious Diseases, Vol 8, Supplement 4, 439–445.

Flood PM, Kripke ML, Rowley DA, Schreiber H (1980): Suppression of tumor rejection by autologous anti-idiotypic immunity. Proc Natl Acad Sci USA, Vol 77, No 3, 2209–2213.

Freda VJ, Gorman JG, Pollack W, Bowe E (1975): Prevention of Rh hemolytic disease – ten years' clinical experience with Rh immune globulin. New Engl J Med, Vol 292, 1014–1016.

Good RA (1982): Concluding remarks: Intravenous gamma globulin therapy. Journal of Clinical Immunology, Vol 2, No 2, 48S–49S.

Good RA (1982): Introductory comments. Intravenous gammaglobulin therapy. Journal of Clinical Immunology, Vol 2, No 2, 5S–6S.

Goodwin RA, Tuttle SE, Bucci DM, Jewell SD, Martin EW, Steplewski Z (1987): Tumor-associated antigen expression of primary and metastatic colon carcinomas detected by monoclonal antibody 17-1A. Brief Scientific Reports, Vol 88, No 4, 462–467.

Greisman SE, Johnston CA (1988): Failure of antisera to J5 and R595 rough mutants to reduce endotoxemic lethality. J Infect Dis, Vol 157, No 1, 54–64.

Hanson LA, Björkander J, Robbins JB, Schneerson R, Söderström R, Söderström T (1986): IgG subclass deficiencies. Vox Sang, Vol 51, Supplement 2, 50–56.

Heidl G, Davaris P, Zwadlo G, Jagoda MS, Düchting S, Bierhoff E, Grüter T, Krieg V, Sorg C (1987): Association of macrophages detected with monoclonal antibody 25 F 9 with progression and pathobiological classification of gastric carcinoma. Journal of Cancer Research Clinical Oncology, Vol 113, 567–572.

Herlyn M, Steplewski Z, Herlyn D, Koprowski H (1979): Colorectal carcinoma-specific antigen: Detection by means of monoclonal antibodies. Proc Natl Acad Sci USA, Vol 76, No 3, 1438–1442.

Hervé P (1987): Utilisation des anticorps monoclonaux pour la prévention de la réaction du greffon contre l'hôte et de l'hôte contre son greffon au cours des greffes de moelle osseuse allogénique. Néphrologie, Vol 8, 103–108.

Huser JH, Schwander D, Wegmann A, Chariatte N, Fässler MA (1986): Verträglichkeit und Verweildauer eines intravenösen Immunglobulinpräparates bei immunologisch gesunden Personen und Verträglichkeit bei Patienten mit Hypogammaglobulinämie infolge chronischer lymphatischer Leukämie. Schweiz med Wschr, Vol 116, No 5, 151–156.

Imbach P, Barandun S, Baumgartner C, Hirt A, Hofer F, Wagner HP (1981): High-dose intravenous gammaglobulin therapy of refractory in particular idiopathic thrombocytopenia in childhood. Helv paediat Acta, Vol 36, 81–86.

Imbach P, Barandun S, d'Apuzzo V, Baumgartner C, Hirt A, Morell A, Rossi E, Schöni M, Vest M, Wagner HP (1981): High-dose intravenous gammaglobulin for idiopathic thrombocytopenic purpura in childhood. Lancet 1, 1228–1230.

Imbach P, Jungi TW (1983): Possible mechanisms of intravenous immunoglobulin treatment in childhood idiopathic thrombocytopenic purpura (ITP). Blut, Vol 46, 117–124.

Just H-M, Metzger M, Vogel W, Pelka RB (1986): Einfluss einer adjuvanten Immunglobulintherapie auf Infektionen bei Patienten einer operativen Intensiv-Therapie-Station. Klin Wschr, Vol 64, 245–256.

Klingemann H-G (1987): Graft versus Host-Erkrankung: Prophylaxe und Therapie mit monoklonalen Antikörpern. Die gelben Hefte XXVII, 77–84.

Kohl S, Loo LS (1986): In vitro and in vivo antibody-dependent cellular cytotoxicity of intravenous immunoglobulin G preparations against Herpes Simplex virus. Reviews of Infectious Diseases, Vol 8, Supplement 4, 446–448.

Köhler G, Milstein C (1975): Continuous cultures of fused cells secreting antibody of predefined speciticity. Nature, Vol 256, 495–497.

Köhler H (1980): Idiotypic network interactions. Immunology Today, 18–21 (July 1980).

Koprowski H, Herlyn D, Lubeck M, DeFreitas E, Sears HF (1984): Human antiidiotype antibodies in cancer patients: Is the modulation of the immune response beneficial for the patients? Proc Natl Acad Sci USA, Vol 81, 216–219.

Kurata Y, Tsubakio T, Yonezawa T, Tarui S (1983): High-dose gammaglobulin therapy for idiopathic thrombocytopenic purpura in adults. Acta haemat, Vol 69, 391–397.

Lewis RB, Matzke DS, Albrecht TB, Pollard RB (1986): Assessment of the presence of cytomegalovirus-neutralizing antibody by a plaque-reduction assay. Reviews of Infectious Diseases, Vol 8, Supplement 4, 434–438.

Masuho Y, Matsumoto Y-I, Sugano T, Fujinaga S, Minamishima Y (1987): Human monoclonal antibodies neutralizing human cytomegalovirus. J gen Virol, Vol 68, 1457–1461.

Matzku S (1987): What's new in cancer monitoring? Path Res Pract, Vol 182, 699–703.

Michie SA, Spagnolo DV, Dunn KA, Warnke RA, Rouse RV (1987): A panel approach to the evaluation of the sensitivity and specificity of antibodies for the diagnosis of routinely processed histologically undifferentiated human neoplasms. Brief Scientific Reports, Vol 88, No 4, 457–462.

Miller R, Maloney D, Warnke R, Levy R (1982): Treatment of B-cell lymphoma with monoclonal anti-idiotype antibody. New Engl J Med, Vol 306, 517–522.

Miller RA, Levy R (1981): Response of cutaneous T cell lymphoma to therapy with hybridoma monoclonal antibody. Lancet 2, 226–230.

Morell A, Skvaril F (1980): Struktur und biologische Eigenschaften von Immunglobulinen und Gammaglobulin-Präparaten. II. Eigenschaften von Gammaglobulin-Präparaten. Schweiz med Wschr, Vol 110, 80–85.

Newland AC, Treleaven JG, Minchinton RM, Waters AH (1983): High-dose intravenous IgG in adults with autoimmune thrombocytopenia. Lancet, 84–87.

Newland AC, Boots MA, Patterson KG (1984): Intravenous IgG for autoimmune thrombocytopenia in pregnancy. New Engl J Med, Vol 310, 261–262.

Odermatt BF, Knecht H, Hagen MF, Fehr J, Rüttner JR (1987): Diagnostic and prognostic value of monoclonal antibodies in immunophenotyping of T cell lymphomas. Acta haemat, Vol 77, 72–77.

Oldham RK (1987): Monoclonal antibodies: Does sufficient selectivity to cancer cells exist for therapeutic application? Journal of Biological Response Modifiers, Vol 6, 227–234.

Oral A, Nusbacher J, Hill JB, Lewis JH (1984): Intravenous gamma globulin in the treatment of chronic idiopathic thrombocytopenic purpura in adults. Amer J Med, March 30, Vol 76, 187–192.

Pandolfi F, Cafaro A, Scarselli E (1987): Relevance of monoclonal antibody phenotyping and of genetic studies in the classification of T-cell leukemia/lymphoma. Onkologie, Vol 10, 134–136.

Pietersz GA, Kanellos J, Smyth MJ, Zalcberg J, McKenzie IFC (1987): The use of monoclonal antibody conjugates for the diagnosis and treatment of cancer. Immunology and Cell Biology, Vol 65 (Pt 2), 111–125.

Pirofsky B (1987): Clinical use of a new pH 4.25 intravenous immunoglobulin preparation (gamimune-N). Journal of Infection, Vol 15, Supplement 1, 29–37.

Pollack S, Cunningham-Rundles C, Smithwick EM, Barandun S, Good RA (1982): High-dose intravenous gamma globulin for autoimmune neutropenia. New Engl J Med, Vol 307, 253.

Price BJ (1987): Monoclonal antibodies: The coming revolution in diagnosis and treatment of human disease. Thirteenth Daniel C. Baker, Jr, Memorial Lecture. Ann Otol Rhinol Laryngol, Vol 96, 497–504.

Raventos A, DeNardo SJ, DeNardo G (1987): Prospects for radiolabeled monoclonal antibodies in metastatic disease. Journal of Thoracic Imaging, Vol 2, Issue 4, 44–49.

Report (1969): Prevention of primary Rh Immunization: First report of the Western Canadian trial, 1966–1968. The Canadian Medical Association Journal. Vol 100, No 22, 1021–1024.

Riesen W (1980): Struktur und biologische Eigenschaften von Immunglobulinen und Gammaglobulin-Präparaten. I. Struktur und Funktion von Immunglobulinen. Schweiz med Wschr, Vol 110, 74–79.

Römer J, Morgenthaler J-J, Scherz R, Skvaril F (1982): Characterization of various immunoglobulin preparations for intravenous application. I. Protein composition and antibody content. Vox Sang, Vol 42, No 2, 62–73.

Römer J, Späth PJ, Skvaril F, Nydegger UE (1982): Characterization of various immunoglobulin preparations for intravenous application. II. Complement activation and binding to staphylococcus protein A. Vox Sang, Vol 42, No 2, 74–80.

Rother K (1986): Antiinfektiöse Therapie mit Immunglobulinen. Die gelben Hefte XXVI, 97–104.

Schmidt RE, Budde U, Bröschen-Zywietz C, Schäfer G, Mueller-Eckhardt C (1984): High dose gammaglobulin therapy in adults with idiopathic thrombocytopenic purpura (ITP). Clinical Effects. Blut, Vol 48, 19–25.

Schulte-Wissermann H, Schofer O, Dinkel E (1982): Die Therapie mit Gammaglobulin. Struktur, Wirkungsweise und Einsatzmöglichkeiten intravenös applizierbarer Gammaglobulinpräparate. Immun Infekt, Vol 10, 98–109.

Schur PH (1987): IgG subclasses – a review. Annals of Allergy, Vol 58, 89–99.

Sickle-Santanello BJ, O'Dwyer PJ, Mojzisik C, Tuttle SE, Hinkle GH, Rousseau M, Schlom J, Colcher D, Thurston MO, Nieroda C, Sardi A, Farrar WB, Minton JP, Martin EW Jr (1987): Radioimmunoguided surgery using the monoclonal antibody B72.3 in colorectal tumors. Dis Col & Rect, Vol 30, 761–764.

Sidiropoulos D, Böhme U, Muralt G von, Morell A, Barandun S (1981): Immunglobulinsubstitution bei der Behandlung der neonatalen Sepsis. Schweiz med Wschr, Vol 111, 1649–1655.

Smith LH, Teng NNH (1987): Clinical applications of monoclonal antibodies in gynecologic oncology. Cancer, Vol 60, 2068–2074.

Soulillou JP, Le Mauff B, Olive D, Delaage M, Peyronnet P, Hourmant M, Mawas C, Hirn M, Jacques Y (1987): Prevention of rejection of kidney transplants by monoclonal antibody directed against interleukin 2. Lancet, 1339–1342.

Steiner E, Aigner F, Kathrein H, Huber C, Margreiter R (1984): Zum Wert prophylaktischer Immunglobulingabe bei Kadavernierentransplantation. Wien klin Wschr, Vol 96, Heft 7, 264–266.

Stephan W, Dichtelmüller H (1983): Intravenous immunoglobulin preparations. Lancet, May 14, 1111.

Stiller RC (1976): Clinical immunosuppression with antilymphocyte globulin. CMA Journal, Vol 115, 1190–1191.

Stuart FP, Scollard DM, McKeam TJ, Fitch FW (1976): Cellular and humoral immunity after allogeneic renal transplantation in the rat. V. Appearance of anti-idiotypic antibody and its relationship to cellular immunity after treatment with donor spleen cells and alloantibody. Transplantation, Vol 22, No 5, 455–466.

Stuttmann R, Petrovici V, Hartert M (1987): Prophylaxe mit einem Pseudomonas-Immunglobulin bei Brandverletzten. Infection, Vol 15, Supplement 2, 71–75.

Taylor HE, Ackman CF, Horowitz I (1976): Canadian clinical trial of antilymphocyte globulin in human cadaver renal transplantation. CMA Journal, December 18, 1976, Vol 115, 1205–1208.

Wain SL, Borowitz MJ (1987): Practical application of monoclonal antibodies to the diagnosis and classification of acute leukaemias. Clin Lab Haemat, Vol 9, 221–244.

Warrier I, Lusher JM (1984): Intravenous gamma globulin treatment for chronic idiopathic thrombocytopenic purpura in children. Amer J Med, March 30, Vol 76, 193–198.

Yap PL (1987): The use of intravenous immunoglobulin for the treatment of infection: An overview. Journal of Infection, Vol 15, Supplement 1, 21–28.

Chapter 4

Aarsman AJ, Mynbeck G, van den Bosch H, Rothhut B, Prieur B, Comera C, Jordan L, Russo-Marie F (1987): Lipocortin inhibition of extracellular and intracellular phospholipase A2 is substrate concentration dependent. FEBS letters. Elsevier Science publishers B.V. (Biomedical Division), Vol 219, No 1, 176–180.

Becker P, Gloss B, Schmid W, Strähle U, Schütz G (1986): In vivo protein-DNA interactions in a glucocorticoid response element require the presence of the hormone. Nature, Vol 324, 686–688.

Blackwell GJ, Camuccio R, Di Rosa M, Flower RJ, Parente L, Persico P (1980): Macrocortin: A polypeptide causing the antiphospholipase effect of glucocorticoids. Nature, Vol 287, 147–149.

Borel JF (1984): Animal experiments with Cyclosporin. Triangle 23, No 3/4, 153–158.

Broyer M, Gagnadoux MF, Guest G, Niaudet P (1987): Triple therapy including cyclosporine A versus conventional regimen. A randomized prospective study in pediatric kidney transplantation. Transplant Proceedings, Vol 19, 3582–3585.

Canafax D, Draxler C (1987): Monoclonal antilymphocyte antibody (OKT3). Treatment of acute renal allograft rejection. Pharmacotherapy, Vol 7 (4), 121–124.

Cantarovitch D, Le Mauff B, Hourmant M, Giral M, Denis M, Hirn M, Jacques Y, Soulillou JP (1989): Anti-interleukin 2 receptor monoclonal antibody in the treatment of ongoing acute rejection episodes of human kidney graft. A pilot study. Transplantation, Vol 47, 454–457.

Chirico G, Rondini G, Plebani A, Chiara A, Massa M, Ugazio AG (1987): Intravenous gammaglobulin therapy for prophylaxis of infection in high-risk neonates. The Journal of Pediatrics, Vol 110, No 3, 437–442.

Cohen JJ, Duke RC (1984): Glucocorticoid activation of a calcium-dependent endonuclease in thymocyte nuclei leads to cell death. The Journal of Immunology, Vol 132, No 1, 38–42.

Collier D, Calne R, Thiru S, Friend PJ, Lim S, White DJG, Kohno H, Levickis J (1988): FK 506 in experimental renal allografts in dogs and primates. Transplantation Proceedings, Vol 20, No 1, 226–228.

Colombani PM, Robb A, Hess AD (1985): Cyclosporin A binding to calmodulin: A possible site of action on T lymphocytes. Science, Vol 228, 337–339.

Cosimi AB (1987): Clinical development of orthoclone OKT3. Transplantation Proceedings, Vol 9, Suppl 1, No 2, 7–16.

Cupps TR, Fauci AS (1982): Corticosteroid-mediated immunoregulation in man. Immunological Rev, Vol 65, 134–155.

Davidson FF, Dennis EA, Powell M, Glenney JR (1987): Inhibition of Phospholipase A2 by "Lipocortins" and calpactins. An effect of binding to substrate phospholipids. The Journal of Biological Chemistry, Vol 262, No 4, 1698–1705.

Dupont E, Wybran J, Toussaint C (1984): Glucocorticosteroids and organ transplantation. Transplantation, Vol 37, No 4, 331–334.

Editorial (1983): Cyclosporin in autoimmune disease. Lancet, April 20, 909–911.

Gerrard TL, Cupps TR, Jurgensen CH, Fauci AS (1984): Hydrocortisone-mediated inhibition of monocyte antigen presentation: Dissociation of inhibitory effect and expression of DR antigens. Cellular Immunology, Vol 85, 330–339

Ghiara P, Meli R, Parente L, Persico P (1984): Distinct inhibition of membrane-bound and lysosomal phospholipase A_2, by glucocorticoid-induced proteins. Biochemical Pharmacology, Vol 33, No 9, 1445–1450.

Glass NR (1986): Immunosuppressive strategy for transplantation: Historical perspective and developing concepts. Seminars in Nephrology, Vol 6, No 3, 296–304.

Goldstein G (1987): Overview of the development of orthoclone OKT3. Monoclonal antibody for therapeutic use in transplantation. Transplantation Proceedings, Vol 19, No 2, Suppl 1, 1–6.

Griffin PJA, Ross WB, Ross WB , Williams JD, Salaman JR (1987): Low-dose cyclosporine monotherapy in renal transplantation. Transplantation Proceedings, Vol 19, No 5, 3685–3686.

Grundmann R, Wienand P, Hesse U (1987): Sequential conventional and cyclosporine therapy in cadaver renal transplantation. A prospective randomized trial. Transplantation Proceedings, Vol 19, No 5, 4033–4034.

Hiesse C, Fries D, Charpentier B, Neyrat N, Rieu P, Cantarovich M, Lantz O, Bellamy J, Benoît G (1987): Optimal results in cadaver-donor renal transplantation using prophylactic ALG, Cyclosporine, and Prednisone. Transplantation Proceedings, Vol 19, 3670–3671.

Homo-Delarche R (1984): Glucocorticoid receptors and steroid sensitivity in normal and neoplastic human lymphoid tissues: A review. Cancer Research, Vol 44, 431–437.

Huang KS, McGray P, Mattaliano RJ, Burne CE, Pingchang Chow E, Sinclair LK, Pepinsky RB (1987): Purification and characterization of proteolytic fragments of lipocortin I that inhibit Phospholipase A2. The Journal of Biological Chemistry, Vol 262, No 16, 7639–7645.

Imoto EM, Glanville AR, Baldwin JC, Theodore J (1987): Kidney function in heart-lung transplant recipients: The effect of low-dosage cyclosporine therapy. J Heart Transplant, Vol 6, No 4, 204–213.

Inamura N, Hashimoto M, Nakahara K, Aoki H, Yamaguchi I, Kohsaka M (1988): Immunosuppressive effect of FK506 on collagen-induced arthritis in rats. Clinical Immunology and Immunopathology, Vol 46, 82–90.

Jantzen H, Strähle U, Gloss B, Stewart F, Schmid W, Boshart M, Miksicek R, Schütz G (1987): Cooperativity of glucocorticoid response elements located far upstream of the tyrosine aminotransferase gene. Cell, Vol 49, 29–38.

Kahan B (1984): Cyclosporine: A powerful addition to the immunosuppressive armamentarium. Amer J Kidney Diseases, Vol 3, 444–455.

Kenmochi T, Asano T, Enomoto K, Goto T, Nakagori T, Sakamoto K, Horie H, Ochiai T, Isono K (1988): The effect of FK 506 on segmental pancreas allografts in mongrel dogs. Transplantation Proceedings, Vol 20, No 1, 223–225.

Keown PA, Stiller CR, Wallace AC (1987): Effect of cyclosporine on the kidney. The Journal of Pediatrics, Vol 111, No 6, part 2, 1029–1033.

Khan BD (1987): Immunosuppressive therapy with cyclosporine for cardiac transplantation. Circulation, Vol 75, No 75, 40–56.

Kino T, Hatanaka H, Susumu Miyata, Inamura N, Nishiyama M, Yajima T, Goto T, Okuhara M, Kohsaka M, Aoki Hatsuo, Ochiai T (1987): FK 506, a novel immunosuppressant isolated from a streptotimyces. II. Immunosuppressive effect of FK 506 in vitro. The Journal of Antibiotics, Vol 40, No 9, 1256–1265.

Klock G, Strähle U, Schütz G (1987): Oestrogen and glucocorticoid responsive elements are closely related but distinct. Nature, Vol 329, 734–736.

Krönke M, Leonard WJ, Depper JM, Arya SK, Wong-Staal F, Gallo RC, Waldmann TA, Greene WC (1984): Cyclosporin A inhibits T-cell growth factor gene expression at the level of mRNA transcription. Proc Natl Acad Sci USA, Vol 81, 5214–5218.

Lafferty KJ, Borel JF, Hodgkin P (1983): Cyclosporine-A: Models for the mechanism of action. In: Cyclosporine: Biological Properties and Clinical Applications. Grune and Stratton, Orlando 1983.

Lennard TWJ, Venning M, Donelly PK, Wilson RG, Parrott NR, Elliot RW, Proud G, Farndon JR, Ward MK, Wikinson R, Taylor RMR (1987): Conversion of immunosuppression in renal allograft recipients from Cyclosporine A to Azathioprine and Prednisolone 6 months after transplantation. Transplantation Proceedings, Vol 19, No 5, 3594–3596.

Lundgren JD, Hirata F, Marom Z, Logun C, Steel L, Kaliner M, Shelhamer J (1988): Dexamethasone inhibits respiratory glycoconjugate secretion from feline airways in vitro by the induction of lipocortin (Lipomodulin) synthesis. Am Rev Respir Dis, Vol 137, 353–357.

Merion RM, White DJ, Thiru S, Evans DB, Calne RY (1984): Cyclosporine: Five years' experience in cadaveric renal transplantation. New Engl J Med, Vol 310, No 3, 148–154.

Morris PJ (1987): Therapeutic strategies in immunosuppression after renal transplantation. The Journal of Pediatrics, Vol 111 (6, part 2), 1004–1007.

Mourad G, Legendre C, Argiles A, Bonardet A, Mion C (1987): Triple drug immunosuppression (cyclosporine, Azathiopine and low-dose prednisolone): A safe and effective regimen in first-cadaver kidney transplantation. Transplantation Proceedings, Vol 19, No 5, 3672–3673.

Myers BD, Ross J, Newton L, Luetscher J, Perlroth M (1984): Cyclosporine-associated chronic nephropathy. New Engl J Med, Vol 311, No 11, 699–705.

Najarian JS, Fryd DS, Strand M, Canafax DM, Ascher NL, Payne WD, Simmons RL, Sutherland DER (1985): A single institution, randomized, prospective trial of cyclosporine versus azathioprine-antilymphocyte globulin for immunosuppression in renal allograft recipients. Ann Surg, Vol 201, No 2, 141–157.

Norman DJ, Shield CF, III, Barry JM, Hennel K, Funnel MB, Lemon J (1987): Therapeutic use of OKT3 monoclonal antibody for acute renal allograft rejection. Nephron, Vol 46, Suppl 1, 41–47.

Ochiai T, Nakajima K, Nagata M, Asano T, Uematsu T, Goto T, Hori S, Kenmochi T, Nakagoori T, Isono K (1987): New immunosuppressive drugs. Drugs presumably affecting lymphocytes. Effect of a new immunosuppressive agent, FK 506, on heterotopic cardiac allotransplantation in the rat. Transplantation Proceedings, Vol 19, No 1, 1284–1286.

Ochiai T, Sakamoto K, Nagata M, Nakajima K, Goto T, Hori S, Kenmochi T, Nakagori T, Asano T, Isono K (1988): Studies on FK506 in experimental organ transplantation. Transplantation Proceedings, Vol 20, No 1, 209–214.

Oosterhuis B, Ten Berge I, Schellekens P, Van Boxtel C (1987): Concentration-dependent effects of prednisolone on lymphocyte subsets and mixed lymphocyte culture in humans. The Journal of Pharmacology and Experimental Therapeutics, Vol 243, No 2, 716–722.

Payvar F, DeFranco D, Firestone GL, Edgar B, Wrange Ö, Okret S, Gustafsson J-A, Yamamoto KR (1983): Sequence-specific binding of glucocorticoid receptor to MTV DNA at sites within and upstream of the transcribed region. Cell, Vol 35, 381–392.

Penn I (1983): Lymphomas complicating organ transplantation. In: Cyclosporine A: Biological Properties and Clinical Applications. (Kahan B., Borel JF, eds) Grune and Stratton, Orlando.

Prince H E, Ettenger RB, Dorey FJ, Fine RN, Fahey JL (1984): Azathioprine suppression of natural killer activity and antibody-dependent cellular cytotoxicity in renal transplant recipients. Journal of Clinical Immunology, Vol 4, No 4, 312–318.

Quesniaux V, Schreier M, Wenger R, Hiestand P, Hardling M, Van Regenmortel M (1987): Cyclophilin binds to the region of cyclosporine involved in its immunosuppressive activity. Eur J Immunol, Vol 17, 1359–1365.

Rapport FT (1984): Cyclosporine: Panacea or mirage? Amer J Kidney Diseases, Vol 3, No 6, 440–443.

Reis HJ, Hopt UT, Greger B, Schrareck WD, Bockhorn H (1987): Antirejection treatment in kidneys transplantation. Is there a proved rationale for the general use of monoclonal antibodies? Transplantation Proceedings, Vol 19, No 5, 3565–3569.

Rosman M, Bertino JR (1973): Azathioprine. Ann Intern Med, Vol 79, 694–700.

Rothhut B, Comera C, Prieur B, Errasfa M, Minassian G, Russo-Marie F (1987): Purification and characterization of a 32-kDa phospholipase A2 inhibitory protein (lipocortin) form human peripheral blood mononuclear cells. FEBS letters, Vol 219, No 1, 169–175.

Rothhut B, Russo-Marie F, Wood J, DiRosa M, Flower RJ (1983): Further characterization of the glucocorticoid-induced antiphospholipase protein "renocortin". Biochemical and Biophysical Research Communications. Vol 117, No 3, 878–884.

Sawada S, Suzuki G, Kawase Y, Takaru F (1987): Novel immunosuppressive agent, FK506. In vitro effects on the cloned T cell activation. The Journal of Immunology, Vol 139, 1797–1803.

Schlitt HJ, Christians U, Wonigeit K, Sewing KF, Pichlmayr R (1987): Immunosuppressive activity of cyclosporine metabolites in vitro. Transplantation Proceedings, Vol 19, 4248–4251.

Schütz G (1988): Control of the gene expression by steroid hormones. Biol Chem. Hoppe-Seyler, Vol. 369, 77–86.

Shield CF, Norman DJ, Marlett P, Fucello AJ, Goldstein G (1986): Comparison of antimouse and antihorse antibody production during the treatment of allograft rejection with OKT3 or antithymocyte globulin, Nephron, Vol 46, Suppl. 1, 48–51.

Sobh MA, Shebab Eldein AB, Moustafa FE, Ghoneim MA (1987): Elective conversion from cyclosporin to Azathioprine in living related donor kidney transplants. Nephrol Dial Transplant, Vol 2, 258–260.

Spreafico F, Tagliabue A, Vecchi A (1982): Chemical immunodepressants. In: Immunpharmacology (Sirois P, Rola-Pleszczynski M, eds) Elsevier Biomedical Press, Amsterdam, New York. Oxford.

Stiller CR, Dupré J, Gent M, Jenner MR, Keown PA, Laupacis A, Martell R, Rodger NW, Grafenried B V, Wolfe BMJ (1984): Effects of cyclosporine immunosuppression in insulin-dependent diabetes mellitus of recent onset. Science, Vol 223, 1362–1367.

Sutherland DR, Strand M, Fryd D, Ferguson RM, Simmons RL, Ascher NL, Najarian JS (1984): Comparison of azathioprine-antilymphocyte globulin versus cyclosporine in renal transplantation. Amer J Kidney Diseases, Vol 3, 456–461.

Szewczyck Z, Hruby Z, Uzar J, Skora K, Szydlowski Z, Witkiewicz W, Patrzalek D (1987): Dramatic reduction in sandimmune (CyA) dosage may be effective in reversal of severe hyperbilirubinemia and post-transplant acute kidney failure linked to CyA toxicity. Transplantation Proceedings, Vol 19, No 5, 4021–4024.

Todo S, Demetris AJ, Ueda Y, Imventarza K, Okuda K, Casavilla A, Cemaj S, Ghalab A, Mazzaferro V, Rhoe BS, Tonghua L, Makowka L, Starzl TE (1987): Canine kidney transplantation with FK-506 alone or in combination with cyclosporine and steroids. Transplantation Proceedings, Vol 19, Suppl 6, 57–61.

Todo S, Ueda Y, Demetris JA, Imventarza O, Nalesnik M, Venkataramanan R, Makowka L, Starzl TE: Immunosuppression of canine, monkey, and baboon allografts by FK 506: with special synergism with other drugs and to tolerance induction. Surgery, Vol 104, No 2, 239–249.

Van Vliet E, Melis M, van Ewijk W (1986): The influence of Dexamethasone treatment on the lymphoid and stromal composition of the mouse thymus: a flowcytometric and immunohistological analysis. Cellular Immunology, Vol 103, 229–240.

Vanrenterghem Y, Waer M, Roels L, Lerut T, Michielsen P (1987): Is cyclosporine-associated nephrotoxicity progressive? Transplantation Proceedings, Vol 19, 4031–4032.

Venkataramanan R, Warty VS, Zemaitis MA, Sanghvi AT, Burckart GJ, Seltman H, Todo S, Makowka L, Starzl TE (1987): Biopharmaceutical aspects of FK-506. Transplantation Proceedings, Vol 19, Suppl 6, 30–35.

Versluis DJ, Wenting GJ, Derx FHM, Schalekamp MADH, Jeekel J, Weimar W (1987): Who should be converted from cyclosporine to conventional immunosuppression in kidney transplantation, and why. Transplantation, Vol 44, No 3, 387–389.

Von der Ahe D, Janich S, Schneidereit C, Renkawitz R, Schütz G, Beato M (1985): Glucocorticoid and progesterone receptors bind to the same sites in two hormonally regulated promoters. Nature, Vol 313, 706–709.

Weiner LM (1987): Monoclonal antibody therapy. American Association of Occupational Health Nurses Journal, Vol 35, No 4, 175–178.

Zannier A, Mutin M, Touraine JL, Traeger J (1987): Differentiation of cyclosporin A: Induced nephrotoxicity from acute rejection in renal transplantation using fine-needle aspiration biopsies. Transplantation Proceedings, Vol 15, No 5, 3630–3632.

Zeevi A, Duquesnoy R, Eiras G, Rabinovitch H, Todo S, Makowka L, Starzl TE (1988): In vitro immunosuppressive effects of FK506 in combination with other drugs. Transplantation Proceedings, Vol 20, 220–222.

Chapter 5

Akasaki M, Jardieu P, Ishizaka K (1986): Immunosuppressive effects of glycosylation inhibiting factor on the IgE and IgG antibody response. The Journal of Immunology, Vol 136, No 9, 3172–3179.

Alm PE (1984): Modulation of mast cell cAMP levels. Int Arch Allergy Appl Immun, Vol 75, 375–378.

Alt FW, Blackwell TK, Yancopoulos GD (1987): Development of the primary antibody repertoire. Science, Vol 238, 1079–1087.

Askenase PW, Schwartz A, Siegel JN, Gershon RK (1981): Role of histamine in the regulation of cell mediated immunity. Int Arch Allergy Appl Immun, Vol 66 (Suppl 1), 225–233.

Azuma M, Hirano T, Miyajima H, Watanabe N, Yagita H, Enomoto S, Furusawa S, Ovary Z, Kinashi T, Honjo T, Okumura K (1987): Regulation of murine IgE production in SJA/9 and nude mice. Potentiation of IgE production by recombinant interleukin 4. The Journal of Immunology, Vol 139, No 8, 2538–2544.

Balch CM, Dougherty PA, Cloud GA, Tilden AB (1983): Prostaglandin E_2-mediated suppression of cellular immunity in colon cancer patients. Surgery, Vol 92, No 1, 72–77.

Batchelor JR, McMichael J (1987): Progress in understanding HLA and disease associations. British Medical Bulletin, Vol 43, No 1, 156–183.

Beaven MA, Moore JP, Smith GA, Hesketh TR, Metcalfe JC (1983): The calcium signal and phosphatidylinositol breakdown in 2H3 cells. The Journal of Biological Chemistry, Vol 259, 7137–7142.

Befus D (1987): The role of the mast cell in allergic bronchospasm. Can J Physiol Pharmacol, Vol 65, 435–441.

Bernstein IL (1981): Cromolyn sodium in the treatment of asthma: Changing concepts. J Allergy Clin Immunol, Vol 68, No 4, 247–253.

Berridge MJ, Irvine RF (1984): Inositol triphosphate, a novel second messenger in cellular signal transduction. Nature, Vol 312, 315–321.

Bonney RJ, Humes JL (1984): Physiological and pharmacological regulation of prostaglandin and leukotriene production by macrophages. Journal of Leukocyte Biology, Vol 35, 1–10.

Bottomly K (1988): A functional dichotomy in CD4 + T lymphocytes. Immunology Today, Vol 9, No 9, 268–274.

Bunting S, Moncada S, Vane JR (1983): The prostacyclin-thromboxane A_2 balance: pathophysiological and therapeutic implications. British Medical Bulletin, Vol 39, No 3, 271–276.

Craps LP (1985): Immunologic and therapeutic aspects of ketotifen. J Allergy Clin Immunol, Vol 76, 389–393.

Craps LP (1985): Ketotifen: Highlights in Asthmology. Springer, Heidelberg. Berlin, New York.

Craps LP, Greenwood C, Ney UM (1985): Ketotifen and asthma. In: Bronchial-Asthma-Mechanisms and Therapeutics, 2nd edition (Weiss EB, Segal MS, Stein M, eds). Little, Brown and Co, Boston, Mass, 734–740.

Craps LP, Ney UM (1984): Ketotifen: Current views on its mechanism of action and their therapeutic implications. Respiration, Vol 45, 411–421.

Davies RJ, Moodley I (1982): Antiallergic compounds. Pharmac Ther, Vol 17, 279–297.

Deguchi H, Suemura M, Ishizaka A, Ozaki Y, Kishimoto S, Yamamura Y, Kishimoto T (1983): Immunoglobulin E class specific suppressor T cells and factors in humans. The Journal of Immunology, Vol 131 (6), 2751–2756.

Delespesse G, Sarfati M, Hofstetter H (1989): Human IgE-binding factors. Immunology Today, Vol 10, No 5, 159–164.

Delespesse G, Sarfati M, Peleman R (1989): Influence of recombinant IL-4, IFN-α, and IFN-γ on the production of human IgE-binding factor (soluble CD23). The Journal of Immunology, Vol 142, No 1, 134–138.

Delespesse G, Sarfati M, Hofstetter H, Frost H, Kilchherr E, Suter U (1989): Human FcεR II and IgE-binding factors. Int Arch Allergy Appl Immun, Vol 88, 18–22.

Diamant B (1982): Histamine secretion: Research in retrospect. Agents and Actions. Vol 12, 1/2, 5–11.

Eiser NM (1982): Histamine antagonists and asthma. Pharmac Ther, Vol 17, 239–250.

Esser C, Radbruch A (1989): Rapid induction of transcription of unrearranged sγ 1 switch regions in activated murine B cells by interleukin 4. The EMBO Journal, Vol 8, No 2, 483–488.

Fernandez JM, Neher E, Gomperts BD (1984): Capacitance measurements reveal stepwise fusion events in degranulating mast cells. Nature, Vol 312, 29 November 1984, 453–454.

Finkelman FD, Katona IM, Mosmann TR, Coffman RL (1988): IFN-γ regulates the isotypes of Ig secreted during in vivo humoral immune responses. The Journal of Immunology, Vol 140, No 4, 1022–1027.

Finkelman FD, Katona IM, Urban JF Jr, Holmes J, Ohara J, Tung AS, Sample J, Paul WE (1988): IL-4 is required to generate and sustain in vivo IgE responses. The Journal of Immunology, Vol 141, No 7, 2335–2341.

Galizzi J-P, Cabrillat H, Rousset F, Ménétrier C, de Vries JE, Banchereau J (1988): IFN-γ and prostaglandin E_2 inhibit IL-4 induced expression of FcεR2/CD23 on B lymphocytes through different mechanisms without altering binding of IL-4 to its receptor. The Journal of Immunology, Vol 141, No 6, 1982–1988.

Geha RS (1988): Regulation of IgE synthesis in atopic disease. Hospital Practice, Vol 23, No 2, 91–102.

Gemsa D, Deimann W, Bärlin E, Seitz M, Leser H-G (1982): Die Rolle von Prostaglandinen aus Makrophagen bei Regulation und Suppression der Immunantwort. Allergologie, Jahrgang 5, Nr 4, 142–150.

Gigl G, Hartweg D, Sanchez-Delgado E, Metz G, Gietzen K (1987): Calmodulin antagonism: A pharmacological approach for the inhibition of mediator release from mast cells. Cell Calcium, Vol 8, 327–344.

Gleich JG, Adolphson CR (1986): The eosinophilic leukocyte: Structure and function. Advances in Immunology, Vol 39, 177–253.

Goetzl EJ, Payan DG, Goldman DW (1984): Immunopathogenetic roles of leukotrienes in human diseases. Journal of Clinical Immunology, Vol 4, No 2, 79–84.

Gomperts BD (1983): Involvement of guanine nucleotide-binding protein in the gating of Ca^{2+} by receptors. Nature, Vol 306, 3 November 1983, 64–66.

Goodwin JS, Ceuppens J (1983): Regulation of the immune response by prostaglandins. Journal of Clinical Immunology, Vol 3, No 4, 295–315.

Gordon J, Flores-Romo L, Cairns JA, Millsum MJ, Lane PJ, Johnson GD, MacLennan ICM (1989): CD23: a multi-functional receptor/lymphokine? Immunology Today, Vol 10, No 5, 153–157.

Hamann KJ, Barker RL, Loegering DA, Gleich GJ (1987): Comparative toxicity of purified human eosinophil granule proteins for newborn larvae of Trichinella spiralis. J Parasitol, Vol 73, No 3, 523–529.

Hansel TT (1987): Leucocyte typing – OKCD? Lancet Dec 12, 1382–1383.

Hansen BL (1986): Why do some individuals produce autoreactive antibodies against receptors and/or their ligands? A possible answer to the question. A review with implications. Scand J Immunol, Vol 24, 363–370.

Hanson JM, Rumjanek VM, Morley J (1982): Mediators of cellular immune reactions. Pharmac Ther, Vol 17, 165–198.

Hassner A, Saxon A (1984): Isotype specific human suppressor T cells for immunoglobulin E synthesis activated by immunoglobulin E antiimmunoglobulin E immune complexes. The Journal of Immunology, Vol 132 (6), 2844–2849.

Huff TF, Yodoi J, Uede T, Ishizaka K (1984): Presence of an antigenic determinant common to rat IgE-potentiating factor, IgE-suppressive factor, and Fc_{ε} receptors on T and B lymphocytes. The Journal of Immunology, Vol 132, No 1, 406–412.

Ishizaka K, Jardieu P, Akasaki M, Iwata M (1987): T cell factors involved in the regulation of the IgE synthesis. Int Arch Allergy Appl Immun, Vol 82, 383–388.

Ishizuka Y, Imai A, Nakashima S, Nozawa Y (1983): Evidence for de novo synthesis of phosphatidylinositol coupled with histamine release in activated rat mast cells. Biochemical and Biophysical Research Communications, Vol 111, No 2, 581–587.

Iwata M, Adachi M, Ishizaka K (1988): Antigen-specific T cells that form IgE-potentiating factor. IgG-potentiating factor, and antigen-specific glycosylation-enhancing factor on antigenic stimulation. The Journal of Immunology, Vol 140, No 8, 2534–2542.

Iwata M, Akasaki M, Ishizaka K (1984): Modulation of the biologic activities of IgE-binding factor. VI. The activation of phospholipase by glycosylation enhancing factor. The Journal of Immunology, Vol 133, No 3, 1505–1512.

Iwata M, Fukutomi Y, Hashimoto T, Sato Y, Sato H, Ishizaka K (1987): Augmentation of the antibody response by antigen-specific glycosylation-enhancing factor. The Journal of Immunology, Vol 138, No 8, 2561–2567.

Iwata M, Huff TF, Ishizaka K (1984): Modulation of the biologic activities of IgE-binding factor. V. The role of glycosylation-enhancing factor and glycosylation-inhibiting factor in determining the nature of IgE-binding factors. The Journal of Immunology, Vol 132, No 3, 1286–1293.

James MP, Kennedy AR, Eady RAJ (1982): A microscopic study of inflammatory reactions in human skin induced by histamine and compound 48/80. J Investig Dermatol, Vol 78, No 5, 406–413.

Jardieu P, Uede T, Ishizaka K (1984): IgE-binding factors from mouse T lymphocytes. III. Role of antigen-specific suppressor T-cells in the formation of IgE-suppressive factor. The Journal of Immunology, Vol 133, No 6, 3266–3273.

Joly F, Bessou G, Benveniste J, Ninio E (1987): Ketotifen inhibits paf-acether biosynthesis and β-hexosaminidase release in mouse mast cells stimulated with antigen. European Journal of Pharmacology, Vol 144, 133–139.

Kanowith-Klein S, Saxon A (1986): Regulation of ongoing IgE synthesis by human T-cell supernatants derived from atopic and nonatopic donors. Int Arch Allergy Appl Immun, Vol 80, 33–38.

Katz DH (1984): Regulation of the IgE system: Experimental and clinical aspects. Allergy, Vol 39, 81–106.

Katz DH, Chen S-S, Liu F-T, Bogowitz CA, Katz LR (1984): Biologically active molecules regulating the immunoglobulin E antibody system, biochemical and biological comparisons of suppressive factor of allergy and enhancing factor of allergy. J Mol Cell Immunol, Vol 1 (3), 157–166.

Kennerly DA (1987): Preparation and characterization of mast cell cytoplasts. J Immunol Meth, Vol 97, 173–183.

Kikutani H, Inui S, Sato R, Barsumian EL, Owaki H, Yamasaki K, Kaisho T, Uchibayashi N, Hardy RR, Hirano T, Tsunasawa S, Sakiyama F, Suemura M, Kishimoto T (1986): Molecular structure of human lymphocyte receptor for immunoglobulin E. Cell, Vol 47, 657–665.

König W, Pfeil P, Hofmann U, Bujanowski-Weber J, Knöller I (1987): Cellular requirements of IgE-antibody regulation. Path Biol, Vol 35, No 10, 1440–1445.

Kosaka Y, Kawabe H, Ishii A (1987): Oxatomide inhibits the release of bronchoconstrictor arachidonic acid metabolites (LTC_4 and PGD_2) from rat mast cells and guinea-pig lung. Agents and Actions, Vol 21, 32–37.

Kraemer MJ, Ochs HD, Furukawa CT, Wedgwood RJ (1982): In-vitro studies of the hyperimmunoglobulin-E disorders: Suppression of spontaneous immunoglobulin E synthesis by allogeneic suppressor T lymphocytes. Clin Immunol Immunopathol, Vol 25 (2), 157–164.

Kuriyama K, Hiyama Y, Nagatahira R, Okuda T, Saito K, Ito K (1986): An antiallergic activity of disodium cromoglycate unrelated to mast cell activation. Agents and Actions, Vol 18, 473–478.

Lagunoff D, Martin TW, Read G (1983): Agents that release histamine from mast cells. Ann Rev Pharmacol Toxicol, Vol 23, 331–351.

Leung DYM, Brozek C, Frankel R, Geha RS (1984): IgE-specific suppressor factors in normal human serum. Clin Immunol Immunopathol, Vol 32 (3), 339–350.

Leung DYM, Geha RS (1984): Regulation of IgE synthesis in man. Clinical Immunology Reviews, Vol 3 (1), 1–24.

Lim LK, Hunt NH, Eichner RD, Weidemann MJ (1983): Cyclic AMP and the regulation of prostaglandin production by macrophages. Biochemical and Biophysical Research Communications, Vol 114, No 1, 248–254.

Lutzker S, Rothman P, Pollock R, Coffman R, Alt FW (1988): Mitogen- and Il-4-regulated expression of germ-line Ig γ2b transcripts: Evidence for directed heavy chain class switching. Cell, Vol 53, 177–184.

Maggi E, Del Prete GF, Tiri A, Macchia D, Parronchi P, Ricci M, Romagnani S (1987): Role of interleukin-4 in the induction of human IgE synthesis and its suppression by interferon-γ. La Ricerca Clin Lab, Vol 17, No 4, 363–367.

Martens CL, Jardieu P, Trounstine ML, Stuart SG, Ishizaka K, Moore KW (1987): Potentiating and suppressive IgE-binding factors are expressed by a single cloned gene. Proc Natl Acad Sci USA, Vol 84, 809–813.

Mazurek N, Schindler H, Schürholz T, Pecht I (1984): The cromolyn binding protein constitutes the Ca^{2+} channel of basophils opening upon immunological stimulus. Proc Natl Acad Sci USA, Vol 81, 6841–6845.

Nishizuka Y (1984): The role of protein kinase C in cell surface signal transduction and tumour promotion. Nature, Vol 308, 19 April 1984, 693–698.

Norn S, Stahlskov P, Kock C, Andersen P, Pedersen M, Tonnesen P, Pedersen PS, Moller NE, Hertz J, Hoiby N (1982): Intrinsic asthma and bacterial histamine release. Agents and Actions, Vol 12, 1/2, 101–102.

Owen WF, Rothenberg ME, Silberstein DS, Gasson JC, Stevens RL, Austen FK, Soberman RJ (1987): Regulation of human eosinophil viability, density, and function by granulocyte/macrophage colony-stimulating factor in the presence of 3T3 fibroblasts. J Exp Med, Vol 166, 129–141.

Pardoll DM, Kruisbeek AM, Fowlkes BJ, Coligan JE, Schwartz RH (1987): The unfolding story of T-cell receptor gamma. FASEBJ, Vol 1, 103–109.

Pelikan Z (1982): The effects of disodium chromoglycate and beclomethasone dipropionate on the late nasal mucosa response to allergen challenge. Annals of Allergy, Vol 49 (4), 200–212.

Pène J, Rousset F, Brière F, Chrétien I, Bonnefoy J-Y, Spits H, Yokota T, Arai N, Arai K-I, Banchereau J (1988): IgE production by normal human lymphocytes is induced by interleukin 4 and suppressed by interferons γ and α and prostaglandin E_2. Proc Natl Acad Sci USA, Immunology, Vol 85, 6880–6884.

Pincus SH, Whitcomb EA, Dinarello CA (1986): Interaction of Il-1 and TPA in modulation of eosinophil function. The Journal of Immunology, Vol 137, 3509–3514.

Piper PJ (1983): Pharmacology of leukotrienes. British Medical Bulletin, Vol 39, No 3, 255–259.

Ray A, Hemady Z, Rocklin RE (1987): Glucocorticoid-induced enhancement of IgE synthesis. New England and Regional Allergy Proceedings, Vol 8, No 2, 81–84.

Resta O, Barbaro MPF, Carnimeo N (1982): A comparison of sodium chromo-glycate nasal solution and powder in the treatment of allergic rhinitis. The British Journal of Clinical Practice, Vol 36, No 3, 94–98.

Riccardi VM (1987): Mast-cell stabilization to decrease neurofibroma growth. Arch Dermatol, Vol 123, 1011–1016.

Rocklin RE (1983): Clinical and immunologic aspects of allergen-specific immunotherapy in patients with seasonal allergic rhinitis and/or allergic asthma. J Allergy Clin Immunol, Vol 72, No 4, October 1983.

Rocklin RE, Beer DJ (1983): Histamine and immune modulation. Advances in Internal Medicine, Vol 28, 225–251. In: 1983, Year Book Medical Publishers, Inc.

Romagnani S, Del Prete G, Maggi E, Ricci M (1987): Activation through CD3 molecule leads a number of human T cell clones to induce IgE synthesis in vitro by B cells from allergic and nonallergic individuals. The Journal of Immunology, Vol 138, No 6, 1744–1749.

Rothman P, Lutzker S, Cook W, Coffman R, Alt FW (1988): Mitogen plus interleukin 4 induction of Cε transcripts in B lymphoid cells. J Exp Med, Vol 168, 2385–2389.

Sagi-Eisenberg R, Lieman H, Pecht I (1985): Protein kinase C regulation of the receptor-coupled calcium signal in histamine-secreting rat basophilic leukaemia cells. Nature, Vol 313, 59–60.

Sampson HA (1983): Prospects for control of the IgE antibody response. Pediatric Clinics of North America, Vol 30, No 5, 773–785.

Schild HO (1981): The multiple tacets of histamine research. Agents and Actions, Vol 11, 1/2, 12–19.

Schnitzler S, Eckert R, Volk D, Grunow R (1982): Histamin und Immunreaktionen. Allergie u Immunol, Vol 28, 219–235.

Schwartz LB, Bradford TR, Irani AA, Deblois G, Craig SS (1987): The major enzymes of human mast cell secretory granules. Am Rev Respir Dis, Vol 135, 1186–1189.

Snapper CM, Finkelman FD, Paul WE (1988): Differential regulation of IgG1 and IgE synthesis by interleukin 4. J Exp Med, Vol 167, 183–196.

Snapper CM, Paul WE (1988): The role of lymphokines in the immunoglobulin class switch. Lymphocyte Activation and Differentiation, Walter de Gruyter & Co., Berlin, New York, 83–95.

Sullivan KE, Calman AF, Nakanishi M, Tsang SY, Wang Y, Peterlin BM (1987): A model for the transcriptional regulation of MHC class II genes. Immunology Today, Vol 8, No 10, 289–293.

Tasaka K, Mio M, Okamoto M (1986): Intracellular calcium release induced by histamine releasers and its inhibition by some antiallergic drugs. Annals of Allergy, Vol 56, 464–469.

Todd III RF, Liu DY (1986): Mononuclear phagocyte activation: Activation-associated antigens. Federation Proc, Vol 45, 2829–2836.

Tomilets VA (1982); Role of cyclic nucleotides in the immunomodulating action of histamine in mice. Bullet Experim Biol and Medicine, Vol 93, No 6, 79–80.

Uede T, Huff TF, Ishizaka K (1984): Suppression of IgE synthesis in mouse plasma cells and B cells by rat IgE-suppressive factor. The Journal of Immunology, Vol 133, No 2, 803–808.

Uede T, Ishizaka K (1984): IgE-binding factors from mouse T lymphocytes. II. Strain differences in the nature of IgE-binding factor. The Journal of Immunology, Vol 133, No 1, 359–367.

Unanue ER, Allen PM (1987): The basis for the immunoregulatory role of macrophages and other accessory cells. Science, Vol 236, 551–557.

Vercelli D, Jabara HH, Arai K-I, Geha RS (1989): Induction of human IgE synthesis requires interleukin 4 and T/B cell interactions involving the T cell receptor/CD3 complex and MHC class II antigens. J Exp Med, Vol 169, 1295–1307.

Volpi M, Yassin R, Naccache PH, Sha'afi RI (1983): Chemotactic factor causes rapid decreases in phosphatidylinositol, 4,5-bisphosphate and phosphatidylinositol 4-monophosphate in rabbit neutrophils. Biochemical and Biophysical Research Communications, Vol 112, No 3, 957–964.

Wasmoen TL, Bernischke K, Gleich GJ (1987): Demonstration of immunoreactive eosinophil granulae major basic protein in the plasma and placentae of non-human primates. Placenta, Vol 8, 283–292.

Yanagihara Y, Kajiwara K, Kiniwa M, Kamisaki T, Yui Y, Shida T, Delespesse G (1987): Modulation of IgE synthesis by IgE-binding factors released by T cells of asthmatic patients with elevated serum IgE. Microbiol Immunol, Vol 31, 261–274.

Yokota A, Kikutani H, Tanaka T, Sato R, Barsumian EL, Suemura M, Kishimoto T (1988): Two species of human Fcε receptor II (Fcε RII/CD23): Tissue-specific and IL-4-specific regulation of gene expression. Cell, Vol 55, 611–618.

Chapter 6

Abeles JH (1982): Inosiplex in recurrent herpes simplex infection. Lancet, 926.

Andrus L, Granelli-Piperno A, Reich E (1984): Cytotoxic T cells both produce and respond to interleukin 2. J Exp Med, Vol 59, 647–652.

Arvin AM, Kushner JH, Feldman S, Baehner RL, Hammond D, Merigan TC (1982): Human leukocyte interferon for the treatment of varicella in children with cancer. New Engl J Med, Vol 306, No 13, 761–765.

Ashorn RG, Vandenbark AA, Acott KM, Krohn KJ (1986): Dialysable leukocyte extracts (transfer factor) augment nonspecifically keyhole limpet haemocyanin and horseshoe crab haemocyanin skin reactivity in unimmunized human recipients. Scand J Immunol, Vol 23, 161–167.

Attallah AM, Petricciani JC, Galasso GJ, Rabson AS (1980): Report of a workshop on standards for human interferon in clinical trials. J Infect Dis, Vol 142, No 2, 300–301.

Avella J, Binder HJ, Madsen JE, Askenase PW (1978): Effect of histamine H_2-receptor antagonists on delayed hypersensitivity. Lancet, 624–626.

Bach JF, Bach MA, Blanot D et al (1978): Thymic serum factor. Bull Inst Pasteur, Vol 76, 325–330.

Ballet JJ, Morin A, Schmitt C, Agrapart M (1982): Effect of isoprinosine on in vitro proliferative responses of human lymphocytes stimulated by antigen. Int J Immunopharm, Vol 4, No 3, 151–157.

Barret DJ, Wara DW, Ammann AJ et al (1980): Thymosin therapy in Di George-Syndrome. The Journal of Pediatrics, Vol 97, 66–71.

Begley CG, Metcalf D, Nicola NA (1986): Primary human myeloid leukemia cells: comparative responsiveness to proliferative stimulation by GM-CSF or G-CSF and membrane expression of CSF receptors. Leukemia, Vol 1, 1–8.

Bennett J, Zloty P, McKneally M (1982): Cimetidine blocks the development of tumor-induced suppressor T-cell activity. J Int Immunopharmacol, Vol 4, 280.

Bergstrand H, Hegardt B, Lowhagen O, Strannegard O, Svedmyr N (1985): Effects of long-term treatment with low dose cimetidine on allergen-induced airway responses and selected immunological parameters in atopic asthmatics. Allergy, Vol 40, 187–197.

Berkman N, Legoix H, Moubri M, de Saxe E (1979): Action favorable de l'isoprinosine au cours des affections oculaires virales et inflammatoires. La Nouvelle Presse Médicale, Vol 8, No 46, 3829–3830.

Beutler B, Cerami A (1988): The common mediator of shock, cachexia, and tumor necrosis. Advances in Immunology, Vol 42, 213–231.

Bicker U, Ziegler AE, Hebold G (1979): Investigations in mice on the potentiation of resistance to infections by a new immunostimulant compound. J Infect Dis, Vol 139, 389–395.

Blomgren H, Edsmayr F, von Stedingk L-V, Wasserman J (1986): Bestatin treatment enhances the recovery of radiation induced impairments of the immunological reactivity of the blood lymphocyte population in bladder cancer patients. Biomedicine & Pharmacotherapy, Vol 40, 50–54.

Bocci V (1981): Pharmacokinetic studies of interferons. Pharmac Ther, Vol 13, 421–440.

Borden EC (1979): Interferons: Rationale for clinical trials in neoplastic disease. Ann Intern Med, Vol 91, 472–479.

Borden EC, Holland JF, Dao TL, Gutterman JU, Wiener L, Chang Y-Ch, Patel J (1982): Leucocyte-derived interferon (alpha) in human breast carcinoma. Ann Intern Med, Vol 97, 1–6.

Bornemann LD, Spiegel HE, Dziewanowska ZE, Krown S, Colburn WA (1985): Intravenous and intramuscular pharmacokinetics of recombinant leukocyte A interferon. Eur J Clin Pharmacol, Vol 28, No 4, 469–471.

Boylston AW, Vose BM (1983): Potential use of purified interleukin 2 as a therapeutic agent. Clin Immunol Allergy, Vol 3/2, 229–234.

Brandt SJ, Peters WP, Atwater SK, Kurtzberg J, Borowitz MJ, Jones RB, Shpall EJ, Bast RC, Gilbert CJ, Oette DH (1988): Effect of recombinant human granulocyte-macrophage colony-stimulating factor on hematopoietic reconstitution after high-dose chemotherapy and autologous bone marrow transplantation. New Engl J Med, Vol 318, 869–876.

Bricaire F (1981): L'interferon. La Nouvelle Presse Médicale, Vol 10, No 7, 458–461.

Brockmeyer NH, Kreuzfelder E, Mertins L, Chalabi N, Kirch W, Scheiermann N, Goos M, Ohnhaus EE (1988): Immunomodulatory properties of cimetidine in ARC patients. Clin Immunol Immunopathol, Vol 48, 50–60.

Bronchud MH, Scarffe JH, Thatcher N, Crowther D, Souza LM, Alton NK, Testa NG, Dexter TM (1987): Phase I/II study of recombinant human granulocyte colony-stimulating factor in patients receiving intensive chemotherapy for small cell lung cancer. Brit J Cancer, Vol 56, 809–813.

Brown GL, Kellerman JS, Lamont P, Sciutto M, Berbos EA, Polk HC Jr (1985): Muramyl dipeptide and polymorphonuclear leukocyte chemotaxis in vitro. J Surg Res, Vol 39, 128–132.

Burger CJ, Elgert KD, Farrar WL (1984): Interleukin 2 (IL-2) activity during tumor growth: IL-2 production, kinetics, absorption of and responses to exogenous IL-2. Cellular Immunology, Vol 84, 228–239.

Cabrera EJ, Sergio SL (1986): Differential effect of isoprinosine on lymphocyte proliferation: Comparison of two tissue culture media. Int J Immunopharm, Vol 8, 893–896.

Cantrell DA, Smith KA (1984): The interleukin-2 T-cell system: A new cell growth model. Science (USA), Vol 224/4655, 1312–1316.

Carey JT, Lederman MM, Toossi Z, Edmonds K, Hodder S, Calabrese LH, Proffitt MR, Johnson CE, Ellner JJ (1987): Augmentation of skin test reactivity and lymphocyte blastogenesis in patients with AIDS treated with transfer factor. JAMA, Vol 257, 651–655.

Carter WA, O'Malley J, Beeson M, Cunnington P, Kelvin A, Vere-Hodge A, Alderfer JL, Ts'o PO (1976): An integrated and comparative study of the antiviral effects and other biological properties of the polyinosinic-polycytidylic acid duplex and its mismatched analogues. Molecular Pharmacology, Vol 12, 400–453.

Cesario ThC (1983): The clinical implications of human interferon. Med Clin North America, Vol 67, No 5, 1147–1162.

Chalmers ThC, Smith H Jr (1982): Inosiplex for SSPE. Lancet, 1475.

Charieras J-L, Plassart H (1982): Etude en double-insu de 59 cas de rougeole sévère traités par isoprinosine. Médecine tropicale, Vol 42, No 3, 316–318.

Chedid LA, Parant MA, Audibert FM, Riveau GJ, Parant FJ, Lederer E, Choay JP, Lefrancier PL (1982): Biological activity of a new synthetic muramyl peptide adjuvant devoid of pyrogenicity. Infection and Immunity, Vol 35, No 2, 417–424.

Cheers C, Haigh AM, Kelso A, Metcalf D, Stanley ER, Young AM (1988): Production of colony-stimulating factors (CSFs) during infection: Separate determinations of macrophage-, granulocyte-, granulocyte-macrophage-, and multi CSFs. Infection and Immunity, Vol 56, 247–251.

Cheever MA, Greenberg PhD, Fefer A, Gillis St (1982): Augmentation of the antitumor therapeutic efficacy of long-term cultured T lymphocytes by in vivo administration of purified interleukin 2. J Exp Med, Vol 155, 968–980.

Chun M, Hoffmann MK (1982): Modulation of interferon-induced NK cells by interleukin 2 and cAMP. Lymphokine Research, Vol 1, No 4, 91–98.

Cohen MH, Chretien PB, Inde DC et al (1979): Thymosin fraction 5 and intensive combination chemotherapy. Prolonging the survival of patients with small cell lung cancer. JAMA, Vol 241, 1813–1815.

Cohn ZA (1978): The activation of mononuclear phagocytes: Fact, fancy, and future. The Journal of Immunology, Vol 121, No 3, 813–816.

Converse PJ, Mshana RM, Bjune GJ (1987): Cimetidine inhibits suppressor factor production in Ethiopian lepromatous leprosy patients. Int J Lepr Other Mycobact Dis, Vol 55, 548–553.

Creagh-Kirk T, Doi P, Andrews E, Nusinoff-Lehrman S, Tilson H, Hoth D, Barry DW (1988): Survival experience among patients with AIDS receiving zidovudine. JAMA, Vol 260, 3009–3015.

Cryz SJ, Fürer E, Germanier R (1984): Protection against fatal pseudomonas aeruginosa burn wound sepsis by immunization with lipopolysaccharide and high-molecular-weight polysaccharide. Infection and Immunity, Vol 43, No 3, 795–799.

Csaba G, Laszlo V, Kovacs P (1986): Effect of tuftsin on the phagocytotic activity of the unicellular Tetrahymena. Does primary interaction develop imprinting? Z Naturforsch, Vol 41, 805–806.

Cummings NP, Pabst MJ, Johnston RB (1980): Activation of macrophages for enhanced release of superoxide anion and greater killing of candida albicans by injection of muramyl dipeptide. J Exp Med, Vol 152, 1659–1669.

Currie GA (1978): Activated macrophages kill tumour cells by releasing arginase. Nature, Vol 273, 758–759.

Damais C, Riveau G, Parant M, Gerota J, Chedid L (1982): Production of lymphocyte activating factor in the absence of endogenous pyrogen by rabbit or human leukocytes stimulated by a muramyl dipeptide derivate. Int J Immunopharmac, Vol 4, No 5, 451–462.

De Simone C, Meli D, Sbricoli M, Rebuzzi E, Koverech A (1982): In vitro effect of inosiplex on T-lymphocytes. J Immunopharmacol, Vol 4, 139–152.

Delafuente JC, Panush RS (1988): Pharmacologic immunoenhancement in the elderly: In vitro effects of isoprinosine. Clin Immunol Immunopathol, Vol 47, 363–367.

Di Luzio NR, Williams DL, Mc Namee RB, Edwards BF, Kitahama A (1979): Comparative tumor-inhibitory and anti-bacterial activity of soluble and particulate glucan. Int J Cancer, Vol 24, 773–779.

Donahue RE, Wang EA, Stone DK, Kamen R, Wong GG, Sehgal PK, Nathan DG, Clark SC (1986): Stimulation of haematopoiesis in primates by continuous infusion of recombinant human GM-CSF. Nature, Vol 321, 872–875.

Dournon E, Rozenbaum W, Michon C, Perrone C, De Truchis P, Bouvet E, Levacher M, Matherson S, Gharakhanian S, Girard PM, Salmon D, Leport C, Dazza MC, Regnier B (1988): Effects of zidovudine in 365 consecutive patients with AIDS or AIDS-related complex. Lancet, December 3, 1297–1302.

Du Rant RH, Dyken PR, Swift AV (1982): The influence of inosiplex treatment of the neurological disability of patients with subacute sclerosing panencephalitis. The Journal of Pediatrics, Vol 101, No 2, 288–293.

Dunnick JK, Galasso GJ (1979): Clinical trials with exogenous interferon: summary of a meeting. J Infect Dis, Vol 139, No 1, 109–123.

Dunnick JK, Galasso GJ (1980): Update on clinical trials with exogenous interferon. J Infect Dis, Vol 142, No 2, 293–299.

Dyken PR, Swift A, Du Rant RH (1981): Long-term follow-up of patients with subacute sclerosing panencephalitis treated with inosiplex. Annals of Neurology, Vol 11, No 4, 359–364.

Editorial (1982): Clinical uses of interferon. Bulletin of the World Health Organization, Vol 60, No 1, 37–38.

Eisenthal A, Monselise J, Zinger R, Adler A (1986): The effect of cimetidine on PBL from healthy donors and melanoma patients: Augmentation of T cell responses to TCGF, mitogens and alloantigens and of TCGF production. Cancer Immunol Immunother, Vol 21, 141–147.

Eschenfeldt WH, Manrow RE, Krug MS, Berger SL (1989): Isolation and partial sequencing of the human prothymosin α gene family. The Journal of Biological Chemistry, Vol 264, No 13, 7546–7555.

Executive Committee of the Danish Breast Cancer Cooperative Group (1980): Increased breast cancer recurrence after adjuvant therapy with levamisole. Lancet II: 824–827.

Feldmann JL, Mery C, Amor B, Kahan A, de Gery A, Delbarre F (1981): Effectiveness of levamisole in rheumatoid arthritis: Immune changes and long-term results. Scand J Rheumatol, Vol 10, 1–8

Ferguson TA, Krieger NJ, Pesce A, Michael JG (1983): Enhancement of antigen-specific suppression by muramyl dipeptide. Infection and Immunity, Vol 39, No 2, 800–806.

Fibbe WE, van Damme J, Billiau A, Goselink HM, Voogt PJ, van Eeden G, Ralph P, Altrock BW, Falkenburg JHF (1988): Interleukin 1 induces human marrow stromal cells in long-term culture to produce granulocyte colony-stimulating factor and macrophage colony-stimulating factor. Blood, Vol 71, 430–435.

Fidler IJ (1986): Optimization and limitations of systemic treatment of murine melanoma metastases with liposomes containing muramyl tripeptide phosphatidylethanolamine. Cancer Immunol Immunother, Vol 21, 169–173.

Fidler IJ, Sone S, Fogler WE, Smith D, Braun DG, Tarcsay L, Gisler RH, Schroit AJ (1982): Efficacy of liposomes containing a lipophilic muramyl dipeptide derivative for activating the tumoricidal properties of alveolar macrophages in vivo. Journal of Biological Response Modifiers, Vol 1, 43–55.

Fischer GW, Podgore JK, Bass JW, Kelley JL, Kobayashi GY (1975): Enhanced host defense mechanisms with levamisole in suckling rats. J Infect Dis, Vol 132, 578–581.

Fischl MA, Richman DD, Grieco MH, Gottlieb MS, Volberding PA, Laskin OL, Leedom JM, Groopman JE, Mildvan D, Schooley RT, Jackson GG, Durack DT, King D (1987): The efficacy of azidothymidine (AZT) in the treatment of patients with AIDS and AIDS-related complex. New Engl J Med, Vol 317, 185–191.

Fleischmann WR Jr (1982): Potentiation of the direct anticellular activity of mouse interferons: Mutual synergism and interferon concentration dependence. Cancer Research, Vol 42, 869–875.

Flodgren P, Hugander A, Sjogren HO (1985): Recombinant leukocyte A interferon as single agent therapy or in combination with cimetidine in patients with advanced colo-rectal carcinoma. A phase II investigation. Acta Radiol (Oncol), Vol 24, 25–34.

Flury F, Wegmann T (1979): Klinische Erfahrungen bei der Therapie mit Interferon. Schweiz Rundschau Med (Praxis), Vol 68, 1401–1405.

Fogler WE, Fidler IJ (1987): Comparative interaction of free and liposome-encapsulated nor-muramyl dipeptide or muramyl tripeptide phosphatidylethanolamine (3H-labelled) with human blood monocytes. Int J Immunopharm, Vol 9, 141–150.

Fogler WE, Wade R, Brundish DE, Fidler IJ (1985): Distribution and fate of free and liposome-encapsulated (^{3}H)nor-muramyl dipeptide and (^{3}H)muramyl tripeptide phosphatidylethanolamine in mice. The Journal of Immunology, Vol 135, No 2, 1372–1377.

Fraser-Smith E, Waters RV, Matthews TR (1982): Correlation between in vivo anti-pseudomonas and anti-candida activities and clearance of carbon by the reticuloendothelial system for various muramyl dipeptide analogs, using normal and immuno-suppressed mice. Infection and Immunity, Vol 35, No 1, 105–110.

Fraser-Smith EB, Eppstein DA, Larsen MA, Matthews TR (1983): Protective effect of a muramyl dipeptide analog encapsulated in or mixed with liposomes against candida albicans infection. Infection and Immunity, Vol 39, No 1, 172–178

Fraser-Smith EB, Matthews TR (1981): Protective effect of a muramyl dipeptide derivate analogs against infections of pseudomonas aeruginosa or candida albicans in mice. Infection and Immunity, Vol 34, No 3, 676–683.

Frith JA, McLeod JG, Basten A, Pollard JD, Hammond SR, Williams DB, Crossie PA (1986): Transfer factor as a therapy for multiple sclerosis: A follow-up study. Clin Exp Neurol, Vol 22, 149–154.

Gabrilove JL, Welte K, Harris P, Platzer E, Lu L, Levi E, Mertelsmann R, Moore MAS (1986): Pluripoietin alpha: A second hematopoietic colony-stimulating factor produced by the human bladder carcinoma cell line 5637. Proc Natl Acad Sci USA, Vol 83, 2478–2482.

Galbraith GM, Thiers BH, Jensen J, Hoehler F (1987): A randomized double-blind study of inosiplex (isoprinosine) therapy in patients with alopecia totalis. J Am Acad Dermatol, Vol 16, 977–983.

Galelli A, Dosne AM, Morin A, Dubor F, Chedid L (1985): Stimulation of human endothelial cells by synthetic muramyl peptides: Production of colony-stimulating activity (CSA). Exp Hematol, Vol 13, 1157–1163.

Galelli A, le Garrec Y, Chedid L, Lefrancier P, Derrein M, Level M (1980): Macrophage stimulation in vivo by an inactive muramyl dipeptide derivative after conjugation to a multi-poly (DL-alanyl)-poly (L-lysine) carrier. Infection and Immunity, Vol 28, No 1, 1–5.

Galli M, Lazzarin A, Moroni M, Zanussi C (1982): Inosiplex in recurrent herpes simplex infections. Lancet, 331–332.

Gemsa D, Seitz M, Deimann W et al. (1981): Mediatoren aus Makrophagen. Allergologie, Vol 4/6, 308–313.

Gifford RRM, Ferguson RM, Voss BV (1981): Cimetidine reduction of tumour formation in mice. Lancet, 638–639.

Gillio AP, Bonilla MA, Potter GK, Gabrilove JL, O'Reilly RJ, Souza LM, Welte K (1987): Effects of recombinant human granulocyte-colony stimulating factor on hematopoietic reconstitution after autologous bone marrow transplantation in primates. Transplant Proceedings, Vol 19, 153–156.

Girot R, Hamet M, Perignon JL, Guesnu M, Fox RM, Cartier P, Durandy A, Griscelli C (1983): Cellular immune deficiency in two siblings with hereditary orotic aciduria. New Engl J Med, Vol 308, 700–704.

Glasky AJ, Gordon JF (1987): Isoprinosine (inosine pranobex BAN, INPX) in the treatment of AIDS and other acquired immunodeficiencies of clinical importance. Cancer Detection and Prevention, Supplement 1, 597–609.

Goetz O (1981): Die Behandlung der subakuten sklerosierenden Panencephalitis mit Isoprinosin. Mschr Kinderheilkd, Vol 129, 655–657.

Goldstein AL, Rossio JL (1978): Thymosin for immunodeficiency diseases and cancer. Compr Ther, Vol 4, 49–57.

Goldstein G (1975): The isolation of thymopoietin (thymin). Ann NY Acad Sci, Vol 249, 177–185.

Goodman MG (1984): Inductive and differentiative signals delivered by C8-substituted guanine ribonucleosides. Immunology Today, Vol 5, No 11, 319–324.

Gordon J, Minks MA (1981): The interferon renaissance: Molecular aspects of induction and action. Microbiological Reviews, Vol 45, No 2, 244–266.

Granstein RD, Tominaga A, Greene MI (1984): Therapeutic use of interleukins: Experimental results. Surv Immunol Res (Switzerland), Vol 3/2–3, 127–134.

Grekas D, Nakos V, Theocharides A, Spanos P, Arvanitakis C, Tourkantonis A (1985): Prophylactic treatment with cimetidine after renal transplantation. Nephron, Vol 40, 213–215.

Guinan P, Crispen R, Rubenstein M (1987): BCG in management of superficial bladder cancer. Urology, Vol 30, No 6, 515–519.

Gutterman JW, Blumenschein GR, Alexanian R, Yap H-Y, Buzdar AU et al. (1980): Leukocyte interferon-induced tumor regression in human metastatic breast cancer, multiple myeloma and malignant lymphoma. Ann Intern Med, Vol 93, 399–406.

Hansbrough JF, Zapata-Sirvent RL, Bender EM (1986): Prevention of alterations in postoperative lymphocyte subpopulations by cimetidine and ibuprofen. Am J Surg, Vol 151, 249–255.

Heinonen E, Gröhn P, Tarkkanen J, Maiche A, Wasenius VM (1981): Transfer factor immunotherapy in Hodgkin's and non-Hodgkin's lymphoma. Cancer Immunol Immunother, Vol 11, 73–79.

Hermanowicz A, Sliwinski Z, Kaczor R (1985): Effect of long-term therapy with sulphasalazine, levamisole, corticosteroids and ascorbic acid and of disease activity on polymorphonuclear leukocyte function in patients with ulcerative colitis. Hepatogastroenterology, Vol 32, 81–86.

Herrmann F, Mertelsmann R (1989): Tumornekrosefaktor. Dtsch med Wschr, Vol 114, 312–316.

Hersey P, Bindon C, Bradley M, Hasic E (1984): Effect of isoprinosine on interleukin 1 and 2 production and on suppressor cell activity in pokeweed mitogen stimulated cultures of B and T cells. Int J Immunopharm, Vol 6, No 4, 321–328.

Hibbs JB Jr, Remington JS, Stewart CC (1980): Modulation of immunity and host resistance by microorganisms. Pharmacol Ther, Vol 8, 37–69.

Hillerdal G, Kiviloog J, Nou E, Steinholtz L (1986): Corynebacterium parvum in malignant pleural effusion. A randomized prospective study. Eur J Respir Dis, Vol 69, 204–206.

Hirai N, Hill NO, Motoo Y, Osther K (1985): Cimetidine enhances interferon induced augmentation of NK cell activity and suppresses interferon production. Acta Pathol Microbiol Immunol Scand (C), Vol 93, 153–159.

Hirschhorn R (1983): Metabolic defects and immunodeficiency disorders. New Engl J Med, Vol 308, 714–716.

Hofschneider PH, Obert H-J (1982): Stand klinischer Interferonstudien in der Bundesrepublik Deutschland. Münch med Wschr, Vol 124, No 42, 911–914.

Hooper JA, McDaniel MC, Thurman GB et al (1975): The purification and properties of bovine thymosin. Ann NY Acad Sci, Vol 249, 145–153.

Horning SJ, Levine JF, Miller RA, Rosenberg SA, Merigan TC (1982): Clinical and immunologic effects of recombinant leukocyte A interferon in eight patients with advanced cancer. JAMA, Vol 247, No 12, 1718–1722.

Huttenlocher PR, Mattson RH (1979): Isoprinosine in subacute sclerosing panencephalitis. Neurology, Vol 29, 763–771.

Ikic D, Trajer D, Cupak K, Petricevic I, Prazic M, Soldo I, Jusic D, Smerdel S, Soos E (1981): The clinical use of human leukocyte interferon in viral infections. Intern J Clin Pharmacol Ther and Toxicol, Vol 19, No 11, 498–505.

Ingimarsson S, Cantell K, Strander H (1979): Side effects of long-term treatment with human leukocyte interferon. J Infect Dis, Vol 140, No 4, 560–563.

Jones CE, Dyken PR, Huttenlocher PR, Jabbour JT, Maxwell KW (1982): Inosiplex therapy in subacute sclerosing panencephalitis. Lancet, 1034–1037.

Jorizzo JL, Sams WM, Jegasothy BV, Olansky AJ (1980): Cimetidine as an immunomodulator: Chronic mucocutaneous candidiasis as a model. Ann Intern Med, Vol 92, Part 1, 192–195.

Jupin C, Parant M, Chedid L, Damais C (1987): Enhanced oxidative burst without interleukin 1 production by normal human polymorphonuclear leukocytes primed with muramyl dipeptides. Inflammation, Vol 11, 153–161.

Karnovsky ML, Lazdins JK (1978): Biochemical criteria for activated macrophages. The Journal of Immunology. Vol 121, No 3, 809–812.

Kasushansky K, O'Hara PJ, Berkner K, Segal GM, Hagen FS, Adamson JW (1986): Genomic cloning, characterization, and multilineage growth-promoting activity of human granulocyte-macrophage colony-stimulating factor. Proc Natl Acad Sci USA, Vol 83, 3101–3105.

Kawasaki ES, Ladner MB, Wang Am, van Arsdell J, Warren KM, Coyne MY, Schweickart VL, Lee MT, Wilson KJ, Boosman A, Stanley ER, Ralph P, Mark DF (1985): Molecular cloning of a complementary DNA encoding human macrophage specific colony-stimulating factor (CSF-1). Science, Vol 230, 291–296.

Kaye J, Janeway CA (1984): Induction of receptors for interleukin 2 requires T cell Ag: Ia receptor crosslinking and interleukin 1. Lymphokine Research, Vol 3, No 4, 175–182.

Kazanowska B, Steuden W, Boguslawska-Jaworska J, Konopinska D (1987): The influence of synthetic tuftsin and its analogs on the function of granulocytes of children with acute lymphoblastic leukemia. Arch Immunol Ther Exp (Warsz), Vol 35, 169–173.

Khakoo RA, Watson GW, Waldman RH, Ganguly R (1981): Effect of inosiplex (Isoprinosine) on induced human influenza A infection. J Antimicrob Chemother, Vol 7, 389–397.

Khanna OP, Son DL, Mazer H, Read J, Nugent D, Cottone R, Heeg M, Rezvan M, Viek N, Uhlman R (1988): Superficial bladder cancer treated with intravesical bacillus Calmette-Guérin or adriamycin: Follow-up report. Urology, Vol 31, 287–293.

Kikuchi Y, Oomori K, Kizawa I, Kato K (1985): Effects of cimetidine on tumor growth and immune function in nude mice bearing human ovarian carcinoma. J Natl Cancer Inst, Vol 74, No 2, 495–498.

Kikuchi Y, Oomori K, Kizawa I, Kato K (1985): The effect of cimetidine on natural killer activity of peripheral blood lymphocytes of patients with ovarian carcinoma. Jap J Clin Oncol, Vol 15, 377–383.

Kikuchi Y, Oomori K, Kizawa I, Kato K (1986): Augmented natural killer activity in ovarian cancer patients treated with cimetidine. Eur J Cancer Clin Oncol, Vol 22, 1037–1043.

Kirkpatrick CH (1988): Transfer factor. J Allergy Clin Immunol, Vol 81, 803–813.

Klefstrom P, Nuortio L, Taskinen E (1986): Postoperative radiation therapy and adjuvant chemoimmunotherapy in breast cancer. Aspects of timing and immune competence. Acta Radiol (Oncol), Vol 25, 161–166.

Kokoshis PL, Williams DL, Cook JA, Di Luzio NR (1978): Increased resistance to staphylococcus aureus infection and enhancement in serum lysozyme activity by glucan. Science, Vol 199, 1340–1342.

Kook Al, Yakir Y, Trainin N (1975): Isolation and partial chemical characterization of THF, a thymus hormone involved in immune maturation of lymphoid cells. Cell Imm, Vol 19, 151–157.

Kurzrock R, Auber M, Mavligit GM (1987): Cimetidine therapy of Herpex Simplex virus infections in immunocompromised patients. Clin Exp Dermatol, Vol 12, 326–331.

Lamm DL, Harris SC, Gittes RF (1977): Bacillus Calmette-Guérin and dinitrochlorobenzene immuno-therapy of chemically induced bladder tumors. Investigative Urology, Vol 14, No 5, 369–372.

Lang RA, Metcalf D, Cuthbertson RA, Lyons I, Stanley E, Kelso A, Kannourakis G, Williamson DJ, Klintworth GK, Gonda TJ, Dunn AR (1987): Transgenic mice expressing a hemopoietic growth factor gene (GM-CSF) develop accumulations of macrophages, blindness, and a fatal syndrome of tissue damage. Cell, Vol 51, 675–686.

Le Beau MM, Epstein ND, O'Brien SJO, Nienhuis AW, Yang YC, Clark SC, Rowley JD (1987): The interleukin 3 gene is located on human chromosome 5 and is deleted in myeloid leukemias with a deletion of 5 q. Proc Natl Acad Sci USA, Vol 84, 5912–5917.

LeBeau MM, Westbrook CA, Diaz MO, Larson RA, Rowley JD, Gasson JC, Golde DW, Sherr CJ (1986): Evidence for the involvement of GM-CSF and FMS in the deletion (5q) in myeloid disorders. Science, Vol 231, 984–987.

Lederer E (1980): Synthetic immunostimulants derived from the bacterial cell wall. J Med Chem, Vol 23, 819–825.

Lederer E (1986): New developments in the field of synthetic muramyl peptides, especially as adjuvants for synthetic vaccines. Drugs Exp Clin Res, Vol 12, 429–440.

Lifson JD, Benike CJ, Mark DF et al (1984): Human recombinant interleukin-2 partly reconstitutes deficient in-vitro immune responses of lymphocytes from patients with AIDS. Lancet 1/8379, 698–702.

Lomnitzer R, Rabson AR (1987): Depressed 3H-thymidine incorporation by measles infected mononuclear cells can be corrected by treatment with isoprinosine or 5-fluoro-2-deoxyuridine. Clin Exp Immunol, Vol 68, 259–265.

Louie E, Borkowsky W, Klesius PH, Haynes TB, Gordon S, Bonk S, Lawrence HS (1987): Treatment of cryptosporidiosis with oral bovine transfer factor. Clin Immunol Immunopathol, Vol 44, 329–334.

Low TL, Thurman GB, McAdoo M et al (1979): The chemistry and biology of thymosin I. Isolation, characterization and biological activities of thymosin a and polypeptide b from calf thymus. J Biol Chem, Vol 254, 981–986.

Low TLK, Goldstein AL (1980): Thymosin and other thymic hormones and their synthetic analogues. In: Chedid L, Miescher PA, Mueller-Eberhard HJ (eds) Immunostimulation. Springer Verlag, Berlin, Heidelberg New York, 129–146.

Mackaness GB (1964): The immunologic basis of acquired cellular resistance. J Exp Med, Vol 120, 105–120.

Mackaness GB (1971): Resistance to intracellular infection. J Infect Dis, Vol 123, 439–445.

Maguire LC, Roszman TL, Lackey S (1985): Failure of cimetidine as an immunomodulator in cancer patients and normal subjects. South Med J, Vol 78, 1078–1080.

Markiewicz K, Malec P, Tchorzewski H (1985): Changes in the interleukin-1 and interleukin-2 generation in duodenal ulcer patients during cimetidine treatment. Immunol Lett, Vol 10, 19–23.

Martinez-Pineiro JA, Muntanola P (1977): Nonspecific immunotherapy with BCG vaccine in bladder tumors. Eur Urol, Vol 3, 11–22.

Massicot JG, Goldstein RA (1982): Transfer factor. Annals of Allergy, Vol 49, 326–329.

Mathé G (1987): Do tuftsin and bestatin constitute a biopharmacological immunoregulatory system? Cancer Detection and Prevention, Supplement 1, 445–455.

Mathé G, Blazsek I, Canon C, Gil-Delgado M, Misset JL (1986): From experimental to clinical attempts in immunorestoration with bestatin and zinc. Comp Immunol Microbiol Infect Dis, Vol 9, 241–252.

Matsumoto K, Ogawa H, Nagase O, Kusama T, Azuma I (1981): Stimulation of nonspecific host resistance to infection induced by muramyldipeptides. Microbiol Immunol, Vol 25 (10), 1047–1058.

Mattsson L, Blomgren H, Holmgren B, Jarstrand C (1983): Bestatin treatment for the correction of granulocyte dysfunction in patients with recurrent furunculosis. Infection, Vol 11, 205–207.

Mavligit GM (1987): Immunologic effects of cimetidine: Potential uses. Pharmacotherapy, Vol 7, 120–124.

Mayer P, Drews J (1980): The effects of protein-bound polysaccharide from Coriolus versicolor on immunological parameters and experimental infections in mice. Infection, Vol 8, 13–21.

Mayer P, Hamberger H, Drews J (1980): Differential effect of ubiquinone Q_7 and ubiquinone analogs on macrophage activation and experimental infections in granulocytopenic mice. Infection, Vol 8, No 6, 256–261.

Mayer P, Lam C, Obenaus H, Liehl E, Besemer J (1987): Recombinant human GM-CSF induces leukocytosis and activates peripheral blood polymorphonuclear neutrophils in nonhuman primates. Blood, Vol 70, 206–213.

McKneally MF, Maver CM, Alley RD, Kausel HW, Older TM, Foster ED, Lininger L (1979): Regional immunotherapy of lung cancer using intrapleural BCG: summary of a four-year randomized study. In: Muggia F, Rosenzweig M (eds) Lung cancer. Raven Press New York.

Mellstedt H, Ahre A, Björkholm M, Holm G, Johansson B, Strander H (1979): Interferon therapy in myelomatosis. Lancet, 245–247.

Merigan TC (1988): Human interferon as a therapeutic agent. New Engl J Med, Vol 318, No 22, 1458–1460.

Merigan TC, Gallagher JG, Pollard RB, Arvin AM (1981): Short-course human leukocyte interferon in treatment of herpes zoster in patients with cancer. Antimicrobial Agents and Chemotherapy, Vol 19, No 1, 193–195.

Merluzzi VJ, Badger AM, Kaiser CW, Cooperband SR (1975): In vitro stimulation of murine lymphoid cell cultures by levamisole. Clin Exp Immun, Vol 32, 486–492.

Merluzzi VJ, Kaiser CW, Moolten FL, Cooperband SR, Levinsky NG (1975): Stimulation of mouse spleen cells in vitro by levamisole. Fed Proc, Vol 34, 1004.

Metcalf D (1985): The granulocyte-macrophage colony-stimulating factors. Science, Vol 229, 16–22.

Metcalf D (1988): Haemopoietic growth factors. Med J Austral, Vol 148, 516–519.

Metcalf D, Begley CG, Johnson GR, Nicola NA, Lopez AF, Williamson DJ (1986): Effects of purified bacterially synthetized murine multi-CSF (IL-3) on hematopoiesis in normal adult mice. Blood, Vol 68, 46–57.

Meyers JD, Mc Guffin RW, Neiman PE, Singer JW, Thomas ED (1980): Toxicity and efficacy of human leukocyte interferon for treatment of cytomegalovirus pneumonia after marrow transplantation. J Infect Dis, Vol 141, No 5, 555–562.

Mihich E (1986): Future perspectives for biological response modifiers: a viewpoint. Seminars in Oncology, Vol 13, 234–254.

Mihich E, Fefer A (1983): The interferon system. National Cancer Institute Monograph, No 63, 67–104.

Mihich E, Fefer A (1983): Thymic factors and hormones. National Cancer Institute Monograph, No 63, 107–137.

Miller LL, Spitler LE, Allen RE, Minor DR (1988): A randomized, double-blind, placebo-controlled trial of transfer factor as adjuvant therapy for malignant melanoma. Cancer, Vol 61, 1543–1549.

Mitsuyasu RT, Golde DW (1988): Potential role of granulocyte-macrophage colony stimulating factor in patients with HIV infection. Behring Inst Mitt 83, 139–144.

Miyasaka N, Nakamura T, Russell IJ, Talal N (1984): Interleukin 2 deficiencies in rheumatoid arthritis and systemic lupus erythematosus. Clin Immunol Immunopathol, Vol 31/1, 109–117.

Morgan DA, Ruscetti FW, Gallo RC (1976): Selective in vitro growth of T-lymphocytes from normal human bone marrows. Science, Vol 193, 1007–1008.

Morstyn G, Souza LM, Keech J, Sheridan W, Campbell L, Alton NK, Green M, Metcalf D (1988): Effect of granulocyte colony stimulating factor of neutropenia induced by cytotoxic chemotherapy. Lancet March 26, 667–672.

Mulé JJ, Shu S, Schwarz SL, Rosenberg SA (1984): Adoptive immunotherapy of established pulmonary metastases with LAK cells and recombinant interleukin-2. Science, Vol 225, 1487–1489.

Mustafa AS, Godal T (1987): BCG induced CD4+ cytotoxic T cells from BCG vaccinated healthy subjects: Relation between cytotoxicity and suppression in vitro. Clin Exp Immunol, Vol 69, 255–262.

Nagata S, Tsuchiya M, Asano S, Kaziro Y, Yamazaki T, Yamamoto O, Hirata Y, Kubota N, Oheda M, Nomura H, Ono M (1986): Molecular cloning and expression of cDNA for human granulocyte colony-stimulating factor. Nature, Vol 319, 415–418.

Nakamura T, Miyasaka N, Pope RM, Talal N, Russel IJ (1983): Immunomodulation by isoprinosine: Effects on in vitro immune functions of lymphocytes from humans with autoimmune diseases. Clin Exp Immunol, Vol 52, 67–74.

Nathan C, Nogueira N, Juangbhanich C, Ellis J, Cohn Z (1979): Activation of macrophages in vivo and in vitro. Correlation between hydrogen peroxide release and killing of trypanosoma cruzi. J Exp Med, Vol 149, 1056–1068.

Nathan CF, Silverstein SC, Brukner LH, Cohn ZA (1979): Extracellular cytolysis by activated macrophages and granulocytes. J Exp Med, Vol 149, 100–113.

Nicola NA (1987): Why do hemopoietic growth factor receptors interact with each other? Immunology Today, Vol 8 (5), 134–140.

Nienhuis AW, Donahue RE, Karlsson J, Clark SC, Agricola B, Antinoff N, Pierce JE, Turner P, Anderson WF, Nathan DG (1987): Recombinant human granulocyte-macrophage colony-stimulating factor (GM-CSF) shortens the period of neutropenia after autologous bone marrow transplantation in a primate model. J Clin Invest, Vol 80, 573–577.

Nikaido T, Shimizu A, Ishida N, Sabe H, Teshigawara K, Maedam M, Uchiyama T, Yodoi J, Honjo T (1984): Molecular cloning of cDNA encoding human interleukin-2 receptor. Nature, Vol 311, 631–635.

Nimer SD, Champlin RE, Golde DW (1988): Serum cholesterol-lowering activity of granulocyte-macrophage colony-stimulating factor. JAMA, Vol 260, 3297–3300.

North RJ (1978): The concept of the activated macrophage. The Journal of Immunology, Vol 121, No 3, 806–808.

Nyka W (1956): Enhancement of resistance to tuberculosis in mice experimentally infected with Brucella abortus. Am Rev Tuberc, Vol 73, 251.

Ogmundsdottir HM, Weir DM (1980): Mechanisms of macrophage activation. Clin Exp Immunol, Vol 40/2, 223–234.

Osada Y, Ohtani T, Une T, Ogawa H, Nomoto K (1982): Enhancement of non-specific resistance to pseudomonas pneumoniae by a synthetic derivative of muramyl dipeptide in immuno-suppressed guinea pigs. J gener Microbiology, Vol 128, 2361–2370.

Osband ME, Shen YJ, Shlesinger M, Brown A, Hamilton D, Cohen E, Lavin P, McCaffrey R (1981): Successful tumour immunotherapy with cimetidine in mice. Lancet, 636–638.

Pasino M, Bellone M, Cornaglia P, Tonini GP, Massimo L (1982): Methisoprinol effect on enriched B and T-lymphocyte populations stimulated with phytohemagglutinin. J Immunopharmacol, Vol 4, 101–108.

Patrone F, Dallegri F, Pistoia V, Ghio R, Sacchetti C (1985): Restoration of defective EAG-rosetting capacity of cancer patient neutrophils by levamisole. Cancer, Vol 55, 1668–1672.

Pestka S (1983): The human interferons – from protein purification and sequence to cloning and expression in bacteria: Before, between and beyond. Arch Biochem Biophys, Vol 221, No 1, 1–37.

Pettenati MJ, Le Beau MM, Lemons RS, Shima EA, Kawasaki ES, Larson RA, Sherr CJ, Diaz MO, Rowley JD (1987): Assignment of CSF-1 to 5q33.1: Evidence for clustering of genes regulating hematopoiesis and for their involvement in the deletion of the long arm of chromosome 5 in myeloid disorders. Proc Natl Acad Sci USA, Vol 84, 2970–2974.

Pinsky CM, Hirshaut Y, Wanebo HJ, Fortner JG, Mike V, Schottenfeld D, Oettgen HF (1976): Randomized trial of bacillus Calmette-Guérin (percutaneous administration) as surgical adjuvant immunotherapy for patients with stage-II melanoma. Ann New York Acad Sci, Vol 277, 187–194.

Pollard RB (1982): Interferons and interferon inducers: Development of clinical usefulness and therapeutic promise. Drugs, Vol 23, 37–55.

Pollard RB, Merigan TC (1978): Experience with clinical applications of interferon and interferon inducers. Pharmac Ther A, Vol 2, 783–811.

Presser SE, Blank H (1981): Cimetidine: Adjunct in treatment of tinea capitis. Lancet, 108–109.

Priestman TJ (1980): Initial evaluation of human lymphoblastoid interferon in patients with advanced malignant disease. Lancet July 19, 113–118.

Priestman TJ (1983): Interferons and cancer therapy. J Pathology, Vol 141, 287–295.

Pullinger EJ (1936): The influence of tuberculosis on the development of Brucella abortus infection. J Hyg Comb 456.

Renoux G (1978): Modulation of immunity by levamisole. Pharmacol Ther A2, 397–423.

Renoux G, Renoux M (1971): Effet immunostimulant d'un imidothiazole dans l'immunisation des souris contre l'infection par Brucella abortus. CR Acad Sci, Vol 272 D, 349–350.

Renoux G, Renoux M (1972): Antigenic competition and non specific immunity after a rickettsial infection in mice: Restoration of antibacterial immunity by phenyl-imidothiazole treatment. The Journal of Immunology, Vol 109, 761–765.

Renoux G, Renoux M (1972): Restauration par le phénylimidothiazole de la réponse immunologique des souris âgées. CR Acad Sci, Vol 274D, 3034–3035.

Renoux G, Renoux M (1979): Immunopotentiation and anabolism induced by sodium diethyldithiocarbamate. J Immunopharmacol, Vol 1(2), 247–267.

Renoux G, Renoux M, Teller MN, McMahon S, Guillaume JM (1976): Potentiation of T-cell mediated immunity by levamisole. Clin Exp Immunol, Vol 25, 288–296.

Renoux G, Touraine J-L, Renoux M (1980): Induction of differentiation of human null cells into T lymphocytes under the influence of serum of mice treated with sodium diethyldithiocarbamate. J Immunopharm, Vol 2 (1), 49–59.

Rey A, Cupissol D, Thierry C, Esteve C, Serrou B (1983): Modulation of human lymphocyte functions by isoprinosine. Int J Immunopharm, Vol 5, No 1, 99–103.

Richtsmeier WJ, Eisele D (1986): In vivo anergy reversal with cimetidine in patients with cancer. Arch Otolaryngol Head Neck Surg, Vol 112, 1074–1077.

Ridgway D, Borzy MS, Bagby GC (1988): Granulocyte macrophage colony-stimulating activity production by cultured human thymic non-lymphoid cells is regulated by endogenous interleukin-1. Blood, Vol 72, 1230–1236.

Robb RJ (1984): Interleukin 2: the molecule and its function. Immunology Today, Vol 5, No 7, 203–209.

Rosenberg SA (1988): Immunotherapy of patients with advanced cancer using interleukin-2 alone or in combination with lymphokine activated killer cells. Important Advances in Oncology, 1988, 217–257.

Rosenberg SA (1988): The development of new immunotherapies for the treatment of cancer using interleukin-2. A review. Annals of Surgery, Vol 208, 121–135.

Rosenberg SA, Grimm EA, McGrogan M, Doyle M et al (1984): Biological activity of recombinant human interleukin-2 produced in Escherichia coli. Science, Vol 223, 1412–1415.

Rosenthal SR (1988): Surgery, recall antigens, immunity, and bacillus Calmette-Guérin vaccination. Am J Surg, Vol 156, 1–3.

Rossi GA, Felletti R, Balbi B, Sacco O, Cosulich E, Risso A, Melioli G, Ravazzoni C (1987): Symptomatic treatment of recurrent malignant pleural effusions with intrapleurally administered corynebacterium parvum. Clinical response is not associated with evidence of enhancement of local cellular-mediated immunity. Am Rev Respir Dis, Vol 135, 885–890.

Rothstein G, Rhondeau SM, Peters CA, Christensen RD, Gillis S (1988): Stimulation of neutrophil production in CSF-1-responsive clones. Blood, Vol 72, 898–902.

Ruch W, Cooper PH, Baggiolini M (1983): Assay of H_2O_2 production by macrophages and neutrophils with homovanillic acid and horseradish peroxidase. J Immunol Methods, Vol 63, 347–357.

Ruco LP, Meltzer MS (1978): Macrophage activation for tumor cytotoxicity: tumoricidal activity by macrophages from C_3H/HeJ mice requires at least two activation stimuli. Cell Immunol, Vol 41, 35–51.

Ruscetti FW (1984): Biology of interleukin-2. Surv Immunol Res (Switzerland), Vol 3/2–3, 122–126.

Ruscetti FW (1988): Interleukin 2 receptor: Two distinct proteins bind interleukin 2. The Year in Immunology, Vol 3, 129–137.

Saiki I, Milas L, Hunter N, Fidler IJ (1986): Treatment of experimental lung metastasis with local thoracic irradiation followed by systemic macrophage activation with liposomes containing muramyl tripeptide. Cancer Research, Vol 46, 4966–4970.

Schumann G (1986): Antiviral and antitumor effects of liposome-entrapped MTP-PE, a lipophilic muramylpeptide. In Seidl PH, Schleifer KH (eds) Biological Properties of Peptidoglycan, Walter de Gruyter, Berlin, New York, 255–260.

Schumann G (1987): Biological activities of a lipophilic muramylpeptide (MTP PE). In Azuma I, Jolles G (eds) Immunostimulants: Now and Tomorrow, Springer, New York, 71–77.

Schumann G, van Hoogevest P, Fankhauser P, Probst A, Peil A, Court M, Schaffner J-C, Fischer M, Skripsky T, Graepel P (1988): Comparison of free and liposomal MTP-PE: Pharmacological, toxicological and pharmacokinetic aspects. UCLA Symposium "Liposomes in the Therapy of Infectious Diseases and Cancer", 1–13.

Scott GM, Phillpotts RJ, Wallace J, Secher DS, Cantell K, Tyrrell DAJ (1982): Purified interferon as protection against rhinovirus infection. Brit Med J, Vol 284, 1822–1825.

Scott GM, Tyrrell DAJ (1980): Interferon: Therapeutic fact or fiction for the '80s? Brit Med J, Vol 280, 1558–1562.

Scullard GH, Pollard RB, Smith JL, Sacks SL, Gregory PB, Robinson WS, Merigan TC (1981): Antiviral treatment of chronic hepatitis B virus infection. I. Changes in viral markers with interferon combined with adenine arabinoside. J Infect Dis, Vol 143, No 6, 772–783.

Shah I, Band J, Rudnick S, Lerner AM (1982): Pharmacokinetics and tolerance of intravenous recombinant alpha2 interferon (a2 IFN) in patients with lympho-proliferative malignancies. Clin Res, Vol 30, No 4, 732 A.

Shalaby MR, Weck PK (1983): Bacteria-derived human leukocyte interferons alter in vitro humoral and cellular immune responses. Cellular Immunology, Vol 82, 269–281.

Sher R, Wadee AA, Joffe M, Kok SH, Imkamp FMJH, Simson IW (1981): The in vivo and in vitro effects of levamisole in patients with lepromatous leprosy. Intern J Leprosy, Vol 49, No 2, 159–166.

Sieff CA (1987): Hematopoietic growth factors. J Clin Invest, Vol 79, No 6, 1549–1557.

Silvennoinen-Kassinen S, Karttunen R, Tiilikainen A, Huttunen K (1987): Isoprinosine enhances PHA responses and has potential effect on natural killer cell (NK) activity of uremic patients in vitro. Nephron, Vol 46, 243–246.

Simmers RN, Weber LM, Shannon F, Garson MO, Wong G, Vadas MA, Sutherland GR (1987): Localization of the G-CSF gene on chromosome 17 proximal to the breakpoint in the t(15;17) in acute promyelocytic leukemia. Blood, Vol 70, 330–332.

Simon MR, Salberg DJ, Silva J, Ganji S, Desai S, Muller BF, Palutke M (1981): Atypical mycobacterium infection treated with dialyzable leukocyte extracts: evidence for antigenic specificity. Clin Immunol Immunopath, Vol 20, 123–128.

Singh MM, Kumar P, Malaviya AN, Kumar R (1981): Levamisole as an adjunct in the treatment of pulmonary tuberculosis. Am Rev Respir Dis, Vol 123/3, 277–279.

Smith KA (1984): Interleukin 2. Ann Rev Immunol, Vol 2, 319–333.

Smith R, Esa A (1982): In vitro effect of murine-derived transfer factor on Salmonella-specific rosette formation. Infection and Immunity, Vol 38, 588–591.

Socinski MA, Elias A, Schnipper L, Cannistra SA, Antman KH, Griffin JD (1988): Granulocyte-macrophage colony stimulating factor expands the circulating haemopoietic progenitor cell compartment in man. Lancet, May 28, 1194–1198.

Solbach W, Rollinghoff M, Wagner H (1983): Die Rolle von Interleukin-2 bei Aktivierung von zytotoxischen T-Lymphozyten. Klin Wschr, Vol 61/2, 67–75.

Soloway MS (1988): Introduction and overview of intravesical therapy for superficial bladder cancer. Urology, Vol 31, 5–16.

Sone S, Lopez-Berestein G, Fidler IJ (1986): Potentiation of direct antitumor cytotoxicity and production of tumor cytolytic factors in human blood monocytes by human recombinant interferon-gamma and muramyl dipeptide derivatives. Cancer Immunol Immunother, Vol 21, 93–99.

Sone S, Tandon P, Utsugi T, Ogawara M, Shimizu E, Nii A, Ogura T (1986): Synergism of recombinant human interferon gamma with liposome-encapsulated muramyl tripeptide in activation of the tumoricidal properties of human monocytes. Int J Cancer, Vol 38, 495–500.

Sone S, Tsubura E (1982): Human alveolar macrophages: Potentiation of their tumoricidal activity by liposome-encapsulated muramyl dipeptide. The Journal of Immunology, Vol 129, No 3, 1313–1317.

Sone S, Utsugi T, Tandon P, Ogawara M (1986): A dried preparation of liposomes containing muramyl tripeptide phosphatidylethanolamine as a potent activator of human blood monocytes to the antitumor state. Cancer Immunol Immunother, Vol 22, 191–196.

Souza LM, Boone TC, Gabrilove J, Lai PH, Zsebo KM, Murdock DC, Chazin VR, Bruszewski J, Lu H, Chen KK, Barendt J, Platzer E, Moore MAS, Mertelsmann R, Welte K (1986): Recombinant human granulocyte colony-stimulating factor: Effects on normal and leukemic myeloid cells. Science, Vol 232, 61–65.

Steele RW, Myers MG, Vincent MM (1980): Transfer factor for the prevention of varicella-zoster infection in childhood leukemia. New Engl J Med, Vol 303, No 7, 355–359.

Suter E (1956): Interaction between phagocytes and pathogenic microorganisms. Bacteriol Rev, Vol 20, 94–132.

Symoens J, Decree Wf, Van Bever M, Janssen PAJ (1979): Levamisole. In: Goldberg M (ed) Pharmacological and biochemical properties of drug substances. Vol 2, American Pharmaceutical Association, Washington, DC, 407–464.

Symoens J, Rosenthal M, De Brabander M, Goldstein A (1980): Immunoregulation with levamisole. In: Chedid L et al. (eds) Immuno-stimulation. Springer, Heidelberg.

Tandon P, Utsugi T, Sone S (1986): Lack of production of interleukin 1 by human blood monocytes activated to the antitumor state by liposome-encapsulated muramyl tripeptide. Cancer Res, Vol 46, 5039–5044.

Taniguchi T, Matsui H, Fujita T, Takaoka C, Kashima N, Yoshimoto R, Hamuro J (1983): Structure and expression of a cloned cDNA for human interleukin-2. Nature, Vol 302, 305–310.

Thatcher N, Mene A, Banerjee SS, Craig P, Gleave N, Orton C (1986): Randomized study of corynebacterium parvum adjuvant therapy following surgery for (stage II) malignant melanoma. Brit J Surg, Vol 73, Nr 2, 111–115.

Thienpont D, Vanparus OFJ, Raymaekers AHM, Vandenberk J, Demoen PJA, Allewun FTN, Marsboom RPH, Niemegeers CJE, Schellekens KHL, Janssen PAJ (1966): Tetramisole (R8299), a new potent broad spectrum anthelminthic. Nature, Vol 209, 1084–1086.

Touraine J-L, Hadden JW, Touraine F (1980): Isoprinosine-induced T-cell differentiation and T-cell suppressor activity in humans. Current Chemotherapy of Infect Dis, Vol 1, 1735–1736.

Toy JL (1983): The interferons. Clin Exp Immunol, Vol 54, 1–13.

Ts'o POP, Alderfer JL, Levy J, Marshall LW, O'Malley J, Horoszewicz JS, Carter WA (1976): An integrated and comparative study of the antiviral effects and other biological properties of the polyinosinic acid-polycytidylic acid and its mismatched analogues. Molecular Pharmacology, Vol 12, 299–312.

Tsang KY, Donnelly RP, Galbraith GM, Fudenberg HH (1986): Isoprinosine effects on interleukin-1 production in acquired immune deficiency syndrome (AIDS). Int J Immunopharm, Vol 8, 437–441.

Tsang KY, Pan JF, Swanger DL, Fudenberg HH (1985): In vitro restoration of immune responses in aging humans by isoprinosine. Int J Immunopharm, Vol 7, 199–206.

Tsang P, Lew F, O'Brien G, Selikoff IJ, Bekesi JG (1985): Immunopotentiation of impaired lymphocyte functions in vitro by isoprinosine in prodromal subjects and AIDS patients. Int J Immunopharm, Vol 7, 511–514.

Tsang PH, Sei Y, Bekesi JG (1987): Isoprinosine-induced modulation of T-helper-cell subsets and antigen-presenting monocytes resulted in improvement of T- and B-lymphocyte functions, in vitro in ARC and AIDS patients. Clin Immunol Immunopath, Vol 45, 166–176.

Umezawa H, Aoyagi T, Suda H, Hamada M, Takeuchi T (1976): Bestatin, an inhibitor of aminopeptidase B produced by actinomycetes. J Antibiot, Vol 29, 97–99.

Vadhan-Raj S, Keating M, LeMaistre A, Hittelman WN, McCredie K, Trujillo JM, Broxmeyer HE, Henney C, Gutterman JU (1987): Effects of recombinant human granulocyte-macrophage colony-stimulating factor in patients with myelodysplastic syndromes. New Engl J Med, Vol 317, 1545–1552.

Vaith P, Maas D, Feigl D, Hauke G, Lang B, Oepke G, Stierle HE, Bross KJ, Andreesen R, Gross G (1985): In vitro and in vivo studies with interleukin 2 (IL-2) and various immunostimulants in a patient with AIDS. Immun Infekt, Vol 13, 51–63.

Van Haver H, Lissoir F, Droissart C, Ketelaer P, Van Hees J, Theys P, Vervliet G, Claeys H, Gautama K, Vermylen C (1986): Transfer factor therapy in multiple sclerosis: A three-year prospective double-blind clinical trial. Neurology, Vol 36, 1399–1402.

Van der Spruy S, Levy DW, Levin W (1980): Cimetidine in the treatment of herpes virus infections. S Afr Med J, Vol 58/3, 112–116.

Van Eygen M, Znamensky PY, Heck E, Raymaekers I (1976): Levamisole in prevention of recurrent upper-respiratory-tract infections in children. Lancet II, 382–385.

Veys EM, Mielants H, Symoens J, Vetter G, Huskisson EC, Scott J, Felix-Davies DD, Wilkinson B, Rosenthal M, Vischer TL, Gerster JC (1978): Multicentre study group report: A multicentre randomized double-blind study comparing two dosages of levamisole in rheumatoid arthritis. J Rheumatol Suppl 4, 5–10.

Veys EM, Mielants H, Verbruggen G, Dhondt E, Goetnais L, Cherouthre L, Buelens H (1981): Levamisole as basic treatment of rheumatoid arthritis: Long-term evaluation. J Rheumatol, Vol 8, 44–56.

Veys EM, Symoens J (1981): Immunopharmacologic therapy of connective tissue diseases. In: Hadden J, Chedid L, Mullen P, Spreafico F (eds): Advances in immuno-pharmacology. Vol 1, Pergamon Press, Oxford, 140–147 .

Wagner G, Knapp W, Gitsch E, Selander S (1987): Transfer factor for adjuvant immunotherapy in cervical cancer. Cancer Detection and Prevention, Supplement 1, 373–376.

Wara DW, Goldstein AL, Doyle N et al (1975): Thymosin activity in patients with cellular immunodeficiency. New Engl J Med, Vol 292, 70–74.

Warren MK, Ralph P (1986): Macrophage growth factor CSF-1 stimulates human monocyte production of interferon, tumor necrosis factor, and colony stimulating activity. The Journal of Immunology, Vol 137, 2281–2285.

Waymack JP, Alexander JW (1986): Immunostimulation by TP-5 in immunocompromised patients and animals – current status of investigation. Comp Immunol Microbiol Infect Dis, Vol 9, 225–232.

Weir DM, Blackwell CC (1983): Interaction of bacteria with the immune system. J Clin Lab Immunol, Vol 10, 1–12.

Weisbart RH, Golde DW, Clark SC, Wong GG, Gasson JC (1985): Human granulocyte-macrophage colony-stimulating factor is a neutrophil activator. Nature, Vol 314, 361–363.

Welte K, Bonilla MA, Gillio AP, Boone TC, Potter GK, Gabrilove JL, Moore MAS, O'Reilly RJ, Souza LM (1987): Recombinant human granulocyte colony-stimulating factor. Effects on hematopoiesis in normal and cyclophosphamide-treated primates. J Exp Med, Vol 165, 941–948.

Welte K, Ciobanu N, Moore MAS, Gulati S, O'Reilly RJ, Mertelsmann R (1984): Defective interleukin 2 production in patients after bone marrow transplantation and in vitro restoration of defective T lymphocyte proliferation by highly purified interleukin 2. Blood, Vol 64, No 2, 380–385.

82nd WHO Expert Committee on biological standardization (1983): Standardization of interferons. World Health Organization. Technical Report Series, No 687, 35–60.

Werb Z, Chin JR (1983): Apoprotein E is synthesized and secreted by resident and thioglycollate-elicited macrophages but not by pyran copolymer – or bacillus Calmette-Guérin – activated macrophages. J Exp Med, Vol 138, 1272–1293.

Wiedermann D, Wiedermannova D, Lokaj J (1987): Immunorestoration in children with recurrent respiratory infections treated with isoprinosine. Int J Immunopharm, Vol 9, 947–949.

Williams DL, Di Luzio NR (1980): Glucan-induced modification of murine viral hepatitis. Science, Vol 208, 67–69.

Wilson GB, Metcalf JF, Fudenberg HH (1982): Treatment of mycobacterium fortuitum pulmonary infection with transfer factor (TF): New methodology for evaluating TF potency and predicting clinical response. Clin Immunol Immunopath, Vol 23, 478–491.

Wing EJ, Gardner ID, Ryning FW, Remington JS (1977): Dissociation of effector functions in populations of activated macrophages. Nature, Vol 268, 642–644.

Wiranowska-Stewart M, Hadden JW (1986): Effects of isoprinosine and NPT 15392 on interleukin-2 (IL-2) production. Int J Immunopharmacol, Vol 8, 63–69.

Wolinsky JS, Dan PC, Buimovici-Klein E, Mednick J, Berg BO, Lang PB, Cooper LZ (1979): Progressive rubella panencephalitis: Immunovirological studies and results of isoprinosine therapy. Clin Exp Immunol, Vol 35, 397–404.

Wong GG, Clark SC (1988): Multiple actions of interleukin 6 within a cytokine network. Immunology Today, Vol 9, No 5, 137–139.

Wong GG, Witek JS, Temple PA, Wilkens KM, Leary AC, Luxenberg DP, Jones SS, Brown EL, Kay RM, Orr EC, Shoemaker C, Golde DW, Kaufmann RJ, Hewick RM, Wang EA, Clark SC (1985): Human GM-CSF: Molecular cloning of the complementary DNA and purification of the natural and recombinant proteins. Science, Vol 228, 810–815.

Woodruff MFA (1986): The cytolytic and regulatory role of natural killer cells in experimental neoplasia. Biochimica et Biophysica Acta, Vol 865, 43–57.

Woods WA, Fliegelmann MJ, Chirigos MA (1975): Effect of levamisole (NSC-177023) on DNA synthesis by lymphocytes from immunosuppressed C57BL mice. Cancer Chemother Rep, Vol 59, 531–536.

Yang YC, Ciarletta AB, Temple PA, Chung MP, Kovacic S, Witek-Giannotti JS, Leary AC, Kriz R, Donahue RE, Wong GG, Clark SC (1986): Human IL-3 (multi-CSF): Identification by expression cloning of a novel hematopoietic growth factor related to murine IL-3. Cell, Vol 47, 3–10.

Zidek Z, Capkova J, Boubelik M, Masek K (1983): Opposite effects of the synthetic immunomodulator, muramyl dipeptide, on rejection of mouse skin allografts. Eur J Immunol, Vol 13, 859–861.

Zsebo KM, Yuschenkoff VN, Schiffer S, Chang D, McCall E, Dinarello CA, Brown MA, Altrock B, Bagby GC (1988): Vascular endothelial cells and granulopoiesis: Interleukin-2 stimulates release of G-CSF and GM-CSF. Blood, Vol 71, 99–103.

Chapter 7

Adorini L, Muller S, Cardinaux F, Lehmann PV, Falcioni F, Nagy ZA (1988): In vivo competition between self peptides and foreign antigens in T-cell activation. Nature, Vol 334, 623–625.

Bocci V (1985): The physiological interferon response. Immunology Today, Vol 6, No 1, 7–9.

Boss MA, Wood CR (1985): Genetically engineered antibodies. Immunology Today, Vol 6, No 1, 12–13.

Bussel JB (1984): The use and mechanism of action of intravenous immunoglobulin in the treatment of immune haematologic disease. Brit J Haematol, Vol 56, 1–7.

Cahill J, Hopper KE (1982): Immunoregulation by macrophages: Differential secretion of prostaglandin E and interleukin-1 during infection with Salmonella enteritidis. Cellular Immunology, Vol 67, 229–240.

Dattwyler RJ (1982): T cell antigens defined by monoclonal antibodies: A review. Plasma Ther Tranfus Technol, Vol 3, 369–374.

Dayer-Métroz M-D, Wollheim CB, Seckinger P, Dayer J-M (1989): A natural interleukin-1 (IL-1) inhibitor counteracts the inhibitory effect of IL-1 on insulin production in cultured rat pancreatic islets. Journal of Autoimmunity, Vol 2, 163–171.

Duff G (1985): Many roles for interleukin-l. Nature, Vol 313, 352–353.

Dwyer JM (1984): Thirty years of supplying the missing link. History of gammaglobulin therapy for immunodeficient states. Amer J Med, March 30, Vol 76, 46–52.

Fischer GW, Weisman LB, Hemming VG, London WT, Hunter KW, Bosworth JM, Sever JL, Wilson SR, Curfman BL (1984): Intravenous immunoglobulin in neonatal group B streptococcal disease. Pharmacokinetic and safety studies in monkeys and humans. Amer J Med, March 30, Vol 76, 117–123.

Fontana A, Hengartner H, de Tribolet N, Weber E (1984): Glioblastoma cells release interleukin 1 and factors inhibiting interleukin 2-mediated effects. The Journal of Immunology, Vol 132, No 4, 1837–1843.

Jesdinsky HJ et al. (1983): Cooperative group of additional immunoglobulin therapy in severe bacterial infections: Multicenter randomized controlled trial on the efficacy of additional immunoglobulin therapy in cases of diffuse fibrino-purulent peritonitis – study design. Klin Wschr, Vol 61, 445–450.

Kasakura Sh (1985): Suppressor cell induction factor: A new mediator released by stimulated human lymphocytes and distinct from previously described lymphokines. Lymphokine Research, Vol 4, No 1, 31–37.

Kingston AE, Kay JE, Ivanyi J (1985): The effects of prostaglandin E and I analogues on lymphocyte stimulation. Int J Immunopharm, Vol 7, No 1, 57–64.

Lachman LB (1985): Summary of the fourth international lymphokine Workshop. Lymphokine Research, Vol 4, No 1, 51–57.

Lehmann H (1980): Immunglobulinprophylaxe der post-transfusionellen Hepatitis. Therapiewoche, Vol 30, 5997–6002.

Männel DN, Farrar JJ, Mergenhagen SE (1980): Separation of serum-derived tumoricidal factor from a helper factor for plaque-forming cells. The Journal of Immunology, Vol 124, No 3, 1106–1110.

Männel DN, Meltzer MS, Mergenhagen SE (1980): Generation and characterization of a lipopolysaccharide-induced and serum-derived cytotoxic factor for tumor cells. Infection and Immunity, Vol 28, No 1, 204–211.

Matthews N (1981): Production of an anti-tumour cytotoxin by human monocytes. Immunology, Vol 44, 135–142.

McIntyre KW, Unowsky J, DeLorenzo W, Benjamin W (1989): Enhancement of antibacterial resistance of neutropenic, bone marrow-suppressed mice by interleukin-1a. Infection and Immunity, Vol 57, 48–54.

McIntyre KW, Unowsky J, DeLorenzo W et al (1989): Stimulation of hematopoiesis and antibacterial resistance by interleukin-1. Biotherapy, Vol 1, 319–325.

Merluzzi VJ, Last-Barney K (1985): Potential use of human interleukin 2 as an adjunct for the therapy of neoplasia, immunodeficiency and infectious disease. Int J Immunopharm, Vol 7, No 1, 31–39.

Metcalf D (1985): Multi-CSF-dependent colony formation by cell murine hemopoietic line: Specificity and action of multi-CSF. Blood, Vol 65, No 2, 357–362.

Moore RN, Pitruzzello FJ, Deana DG, Rouse BT (1985): Endogenous regulation of macrophage proliferation and differentiation by prostaglandins and interferon a/b. Lymphokine Research, Vol 4, No 1, 43–50.

Nydegger UE, Blaser K, Hässig A (1984): Antiidiotypic immunosuppression and its treatment with human immunoglobulin preparations. Vox Sang, Vol 47, 92–95.

Ochs HD, Fischer SH. Wedgwood RJ, Wara MJ, Ammann AJ, Saxon A, Budinger MD, Allred RU, Rousell RH (1984): Comparison of high-dose and low-dose intravenous immunoglobulin therapy in patients with primary immunodeficiency diseases. Amer J Med, March 30, Vol 76, 78–82.

Pasanen VJ (1979): In vitro enhancement of natural cytotoxicity by tumour necrosis serum. Scand J Immunol, Vol 10, No 28, 1284.

Playfair JHL, de Souza JB, Taverne J (1982): Endotoxin induced tumour-necrosis serum kills a subpopulation of normal lymphocytes in vitro. Clin Exp Immunol, Vol 47, 753–755.

Pluznik DH, Cunningham RE, Noguchi PD (1984): Colony-stimulating factor (CSF) controls proliferation of CSF-dependent cells by acting during the G_1 phase of the cell cycle. Proc Natl Acad Sci USA, Vol 81, 7451–7455.

Ring J, Bode U, Kadach U, Stix E, Burg G (1983): Gammaglobuline und Allergie. Münch med Wschr, Vol 125, No 14, 289–292.

Ruff MR, Gifford GE (1981): Rabbit tumor necrosis factor: Mechanism or action. Infection and Immunity, Vol 31, No 1, 380–385.

Ruff MR, Gifford GE (1980): Purification and physio-chemical characterization or rabbit tumor necrosis factor. The Journal of Immunology, Vol 125, No 4, 1671–1677.

Sakiel S, Schiller B, Buchowicz L, Kotkowska-Tomanek E (1983): Anti-pseudomonas immunoglobulin. III. Preliminary clinical evaluation. Arch Immunologiae et Therapiae Experimentalis, Vol 31, 517–521.

Schmidt RE, Deicher H (1983): Indikationen zur Anwendung intravenöser Immunglobuline. Dtsch med Wschr, Vol 108, Nr 6, 227–231.

Schumacher K, Maerker-Alzer G, Kleinau T, Hügel W, Dalichau H, Dienst C, Mitrenga D (1982): Passive Immunprophylaxe der Posttransfusionshepatitis durch Immunglobulin-Präparationen. Dtsch med Wschr, Vol 107, Nr 39, 1459–1464.

Shirai T, Yamaguchi H, Ito H, Todd CW, Wallace RB (1985): Cloning and expression in Escherichia coli of the gene for human tumor necrosis factor. Nature, Vol 313 , 803–806.

Shirani KZ, Vaughan GM, McManus AT, Amy BW, McManus WF, Pruitt BA, Mason AD (1984): Replacement therapy with modified immunoglobulin G in burn patients: preliminary kinetic studies. Amer J Med, March 30, Vol 76, 175–180.

Skvarc A, Bone G, Ladurner G, Ott E, Lechner H (1982): Die Bedeutung der Immunglobuline in der Therapie der eitrigen Meningitis. Nervenarzt, Vol 53, 701–704.

Todd JA, Acha-Orbea H, Bell JI, Chao N, Fronek Z, Jacob CO, McDermott M, Sinha AA, Timmerman L, Steinman L, McDevitt HO (1988): A molecular basis for MHC class II-associated autoimmunity. Science, Vol 240, 1003–1009.

Todd JA, Bell JI, McDevitt HO (1988): A molecular basis for genetic susceptibility to insulin-dependent diabetes mellitus. Trends in Genetics, Vol 4, No 5, 129–134.

Index

MIX
Papier aus verantwortungsvollen Quellen
Paper from responsible sources
FSC® C105338

If you have any concerns about our products,
you can contact us on
ProductSafety@springernature.com

In case Publisher is established outside the EU,
the EU authorized representative is:
Springer Nature Customer Service Center GmbH
Europaplatz 3, 69115 Heidelberg, Germany

Printed by Libri Plureos GmbH
in Hamburg, Germany